# Psychiatry and Medical Practice
## in a General Hospital

# Psychiatry and Medical Practice
# in a General Hospital

*Edited by*

NORMAN E. ZINBERG, M.D.

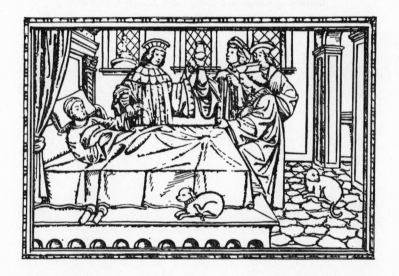

INTERNATIONAL UNIVERSITIES PRESS, INC.

New York

Frontispiece: "The Consultation," Italian School, Seventeenth Century

Manufactured in the United States of America

"I am a sick man . . . I am a spiteful man. I am an unattractive man. I believe my liver is diseased. However, I know nothing at all about my disease, and do not know for certain what ails me. I don't consult a doctor for it, and never have, though I have a respect for medicine and doctors. Besides, I am extremely superstitious, sufficiently so to respect medicine, anyway (I am well educated enough not to be superstitious, but I am superstitious). No, I refuse to consult a doctor from spite. That you probably will not understand. Well, I understand it, though. Of course, I can't explain who it is precisely that I am mortifying in this case be my spite: I am perfectly well aware that I cannot 'pay out' the doctors by not consulting them: I know better than anyone that by all this I am only injuring myself and no one else. But still, if I don't consult a doctor it is from spite. My liver is bad, well—let it get worse!"

FYODOR DOSTOYEVSKY
*Notes from Underground*

# Contributors

HENRY G. ALTMAN, M.D.
   Associate in Psychiatry, Beth Israel Hospital, Boston, Mass.; Assistant in Psychiatry, Harvard Medical School.

EDWARD BIBRING, M.D.
   Deceased. Formerly, Visiting Psychiatrist, Beth Israel Hospital, Boston, Mass.; Associate Professor of Psychology, Boston University; Training Analyst, Boston Psychoanalytic Institute.

GRETE L. BIBRING, M.D.
   Psychiatrist-in-Chief, Beth Israel Hospital, Boston, Mass.; Clinical Professor of Psychiatry, Harvard Medical School; Training Analyst, Boston Psychoanalytic Institute.

LEO BERMAN, M.D.
   Deceased. Formerly, Head, Unit of Psychoanalytic Group Psychology and Visiting Psychiatrist, Beth Israel Hospital, Boston, Mass.; Clinical Associate in Psychiatry, Harvard Medical School; Training Analyst, Boston Psychoanalytic Institute.

RICHARD E. CUTLER, M.D.
   Associate in Psychiatry, Beth Israel Hospital, Boston, Mass.; Instructor in Psychiatry, Harvard Medical School.

EDWARD M. DANIELS, M.D.
   Assistant Visiting Psychiatrist, Beth Israel Hospital, Boston, Mass.; Clinical Associate in Psychiatry, Harvard Medical School; Faculty, Boston Psychoanalytic Institute.

THOMAS F. DWYER, M.D.
   Associate Director, Psychiatric Service and Visiting Psychiatrist, Beth Israel Hospital, Boston, Mass.; Assistant Clinical Professor of Psychiatry, Harvard Medical School; Member, Boston Psychoanalytic Society.

WALTER GRUEN, PH.D.
   Research Psychologist, Canandaigua V. A. Hospital.

RALPH J. KAHANA, M.D.

Associate Visiting Psychiatrist, Beth Israel Hospital, Boston, Mass.; Clinical Associate in Psychiatry, Harvard Medical School; Member, Boston Psychoanalytic Society.

DON R. LIPSITT, M.D.

Head, Integration Clinic and Associate in Psychiatry, Beth Israel Hospital, Boston, Mass.; Assistant in Psychiatry, Harvard Medical School.

CECIL MUSHATT, M.D.

Associate Visiting Psychiatrist, Beth Israel Hospital, Boston, Mass.; Clinical Associate in Psychiatry, Harvard Medical School; Member, Boston Psychoanalytic Society.

EDMUND C. PAYNE, JR.

Associate Visiting Psychiatrist, Beth Israel Hospital, Boston, Mass.; Instructor in Psychiatry, Harvard Medical School; Member, Boston Psychoanalytic Society.

JOHN REICHARD, M.D.

Associate in Psychiatry, Beth Israel Hospital, Boston, Mass.; Assistant in Psychiatry, Harvard Medical School.

DAVID SHAPIRO, PH.D.

Associate Psychologist, Harvard Medical School; Lecturer in Social Relations, Harvard University; Career Investigator, U. S. Public Health Service.

BENSON R. SNYDER, M.D.

Assistant Visiting Psychiatrist, Beth Israel Hospital, Boston, Mass.; Psychiatrist-in-Chief, Massachusetts Institute of Technology; Instructor in Psychiatry, Harvard Medical School; Member, Boston Psychoanalytic Society.

MAX I. WOOL, M.D.

Deceased. Formerly, Associate in Psychiatry, Beth Israel Hospital, Boston, Mass.; Instructor, Harvard Medical School; Member, Boston Psychoanalytic Society.

NORMAN E. ZINBERG, M.D.

Assistant Director, Psychiatric Service and Visiting Psychiatrist, Beth Israel Hospital, Boston, Mass.; Assistant Clinical Professor in Psychiatry, Harvard Medical School; Lecturer on Social Relations, Harvard University; Faculty, Boston Psychoanalytic Institute.

# Contents

## THE PSYCHIATRIC SERVICE AND THE COMMUNITY

# Preface

THIS VOLUME COMPRISES a series of excerpts from the psychiatric-medical workshop of a psychiatric service in a general hospital. It is not intended as a reference book, nor do we claim any finality or total account in reporting on the projects in areas of patient care, teaching of medical students, or research, or on the innumerable informal contacts which developed in the many years of close association between the psychiatric staff and the doctors on the other services.

A great deal of thought has gone into this combined program since its beginning, and a great deal of mutual respect and appreciation has sustained its growth through the years. However, the Beth Israel Hospital in Boston is only one among many others that strive earnestly for the integration of modern medicine and psychoanalytic psychiatry in an effort toward a deeper understanding of the sick person and of his illness. Though this may seem like a relatively limited program whose explicit objective varies from place to place, implicitly it aims toward bridging the gap between the organic and the psychological concomitants in man—an endeavor that deserves infinite determination, patience, and effort. As the different institutions explore this territory, whose boundaries are not drawn clearly and whose pathways are not yet marked carefully, they each develop their individual approach and their specific program according to their own prevailing interest and to the general constellation surrounding their work. It is the intent of this book to present our particular experience in this pursuit, and to point out problem areas which we encountered and the solutions we attempted to reach.

No systematic study has yet been done by us to evaluate objectively the results of this work in our hospital. Impressionistic data suggest that there is a quiet but effective process of mutual assimilation taking place, without dramatic episodes, but with occasional blurring of the sharp line of demarcation between psychiatrists and other doctors in the hospital, a condition which in my opinion holds great promise for progress in medicine of the future.

I want to give thanks to the people who helped in building this project, and find myself at a loss as to where to begin and where to end. There are so many of them, the doctors on my staff as well as on the other services of the hospital, administrators, social workers, dieticians and nurses, as well as other employees, who are carrying their share with us, and sometimes more than just their share. I could not mention the names of all of them without doing injustice one way or the other. Yet there are two persons who stand out in the special effect they had on our work: Dr. Herrman L. Blumgart, our former Physician-in-Chief, whose incisive concern with the future of comprehensive medicine caught my imagination at the outset of my work in 1946, and whose interest and friendship proved of infinite value in times of stress and confusion, and Dr. George Packer Berry, Dean of the Harvard Medical School, without whose wise counsel and genuine understanding of our efforts during all these years I might have lost my way many more times than was the case. I want to express my deepest regard and appreciation for their support.

GRETE L. BIBRING

Cambridge, Massachusetts
March 12, 1964

# Introduction:
# The Development and Operation
# of a Psychiatric Service

NORMAN E. ZINBERG, M.D.

THE SECOND WORLD WAR marked for psychiatry, as it did for many other branches of medicine, the beginning of a new era. Before 1942, psychiatric training centers developed almost exclusively from traditional mental hospitals connected with medical schools, and the psychiatric resident learned about emotional disturbance from patients whose illnesses were so severe that they could not sustain themselves in the usual social or institutional environments. The mental hospital and the general hospital were usually sharply separated, and relatively few psychiatrists worked actively in general hospitals as teachers and therapists. The prevailing attitude in practice, if not in theory, was that an important qualitative difference existed between the emotionally disturbed and the rest of the population, and that, because the patient population in a general hospital was a representative sample of the "normal" population at large, it was not the province of the psychiatrist and certainly not a place for psychiatric training.

Nevertheless, from 1933 until 1942 Dr. M. Ralph Kaufman organized and sustained an active psychiatric department at the Beth Israel Hospital in Boston which not only offered psychoanalytically oriented psychotherapy in an outpatient clinic, but also pioneered in efforts to consult with the physicians about their inpatients and to teach the house officers of the hospital how the knowledge of psychiatric principles might help them to practice medicine more effectively. Before Dr. Kaufman went into the Army in 1942, he had gathered around him a staff which included many of the psychiatrists in the area who cared about broadening psychiatric education and the scope of psychiatric usefulness. Some of these doctors remain as an integral part of the present psychiatric staff. In those war years following Dr. Kaufman's departure, the Beth Israel Hospital fared

1

no better than most of the rest of the medical world. The hospital operated with a minimum staff and innovations were out of the question.

In the armed services, however, diversified use of psychiatrists turned out to be not a luxury but a necessity. The long, painful war required thoughtful attention to the morale of all soldiers, and it was demonstrated once and for all that, while certain mental illnesses were clear-cut and discrete, under overwhelming conditions of stress anyone could develop emotional difficulty, whether caused by physical illness, battle fatigue, or simply situations of tension. The demand for the services of psychiatrists came then not just from the segregated mental-illness sections of the hospitals but from all over. Unquestionably, the government's decision to begin a comprehensive program for the support of psychiatric training, which began after the war and continues, came as a result of the obviously insufficient number of psychiatrists and the equally obvious inadequacy of their training for the tasks assigned to them in the armed services. Nevertheless, the trial-and-error efforts of many brilliant and devoted people accomplished much in treatment and prevention of emotional disturbance in the armed forces. Perhaps time will show that the greatest accomplishment of all was the beginning of the destruction of the wall that separated psychiatry from the other medical specialties.

Following the war, Dr. Kaufman did not return to Boston but accepted the post—newly created as a result of this revolution—of full-time Chief of Psychiatry at the Mt. Sinai Hospital in New York. In the fall of 1946, Dr. Grete L. Bibring accepted the appointment as Head of the Department of Psychiatry at Beth Israel, and in 1955, as Psychiatrist-in-Chief when the Department was officially designated a Service. The choice of Dr. Bibring by the Beth Israel Hospital and the Harvard Medical School implied many things that have become explicit in the intervening seventeen years. That Dr. Bibring, a graduate of a Vienna medical school who trained as a psychoanalyst under Freud and the other members of his circle while still a medical student, was accepted by the medical hierarchy indicated their awareness of the contribution psychoanalysis could make to all of medicine. Dr. Bibring had already indicated in her work the existence in her thinking of a grand design which would show the flexibility and usefulness of psychoanalytic principles when applied in areas other than psychoanalytic practice. She and her husband, Dr. Edward Bibring, had outlined how the basic principles of psychoanalytic theory could aid social work, general medical practice, and general psychiatric practice. Her appointment indicated the beginning of a broad pioneering teaching and training program in these fields.

A recognized and distinguished teacher, Dr. Bibring undertook the task imposed by the new era in psychiatry. This book is intended as a progress report of the Psychiatric Service. It is divided into three sections which describe (1) the underlying tenets of medical psychology; (2) the broad teaching program to physicians other than psychiatrists; and (3) some of the more direct ventures of this psychiatric service, by way of a group approach, into the community. It cannot, of course, include the whole story. It leaves for another occasion many things, principally a report on the training of psychiatric residents as competent therapists and teachers, a program which received equal attention with the one to be described. Its aims were to see that psychotherapy was broadly conceived and carried out as separate from psychoanalysis. At Beth Israel, the competent psychotherapist could and should, when indicated, do anything a good social worker, marriage counselor, educational or vocational counselor, doctor, psychopharmacologist, or (except for psychoanalysis) psychoanalyst could do. Moreover, the psychiatric resident was taught to be a good teacher, in the sense that he was expected to be able to communicate his ideas in reasonably simple language to other doctors, students, nurses, nurses aides, dieticians, and, above all, patients. The success of the program can be measured by the large number of applicants for residency training each year and by the fact that of the 57 residents trained, all but one now spend from 25 to 100 per cent of their time teaching and training. The formation of a residency training program of this scope and depth was part of the grand design of general hospital psychiatry with which Dr. Bibring began her tenure, and complemented the plan to convey the principles of what came to be known as medical psychology into every crevice of all the other services of the hospital.

A special complication of Dr. Bibring's appointment deserves mention. There were then, and still are now, very few women chiefs of service anywhere in medicine. Her appointment was, of course, a tribute to the brilliance of her past work and to her visions of what could come. But more than that, it showed that, in psychiatry, women practitioners were needed as they were in no other medical specialty. In the other medical specialties, particularly gynecology and pediatrics, an occasional patient, usually on emotional grounds, prefers a woman physician, but generally speaking, male practitioners feel they could do approximately as well with almost every patient and bring forth the classic arguments for the preferability of men as doctors: greater stamina, professional dedication without biological diversions, and the traditional image which consoles patients. But in psychiatry, many patients, including adolescent girls, certain homo-

sexuals, some phobics, patients with early complicated relations with one
parent or the other, are treated more successfully by a woman than by a
man. Because they are needed specifically as clinicians, women, almost from
the beginning of the psychoanalytic movement, have been accepted completely as equals. Consequently, women have made proportionately a much
greater contribution to the scientific endeavors of the psychiatric specialty
than they have to any other branch of medicine. Here the implication of
Dr. Bibring's trail-blazing appointment, increasingly borne out each year,
is that for the specialty to be maximally effective in every area, women
practitioners, and more than that, women as chiefs are needed at the
policy level of the academic and hospital hierarchies.

## I. The Derivation of Medical Psychology

The four papers in this section must seem an odd and disparate group
to act as an introduction to a system of thought intended essentially for
physicians. Two were published in a journal of social casework; two, in
psychoanalytic journals. However, all four present facets which, when tak-
en together, make up the underlying tenets and attitudes from which the
system of medical psychology was derived. To understand fully the development of the teaching program based on medical psychology, the
reader needs to comprehend its sources.

One of the psychoanalytic papers deals with countertransference. This
technical word refers to the subjective response of the analyst to the patient. Dr. Leo Berman characterizes countertransference in these sentences:

> Actually most analysts' positive feelings for their patients involve a
> wider range of feeling whose totality we shall describe as *dedication*.
> It is dedication in this wider sense and in the sense of the dedication
> of the good leader and good parent that makes an analyst's attitudes
> of kindly acceptance, patience, and so on, genuine and effective.

Berman's (1949) statement describes the human response that the Psychiatric Service of the Beth Israel Hospital feels underlies the work of
most physicians. It may seem almost a cliché to speak of the dedication
of physicians, yet many contemporary views and studies of medical practice have given short shrift to the traditional acceptance of a physician's
unyielding goodwill.

Dr. Berman does more in this paper for medical psychology than re-
emphasize the dedication of most physicians. He explores many of the interactions between doctor and patient which occur just below the level of

consciousness but which may be crucial to successful rapport. Because the system of medical psychology, as we will show, involves a kind of goal-directed strategy, it is of special importance to make explicit the ordinary human responses of the doctor as well as of the patient. Even though Berman goes into these matters in terms of the psychoanalytic situation, almost all of what he says about the analyst as a person in an intense human relationship is applicable to other physicians with their patients.

The two social work papers of Grete L. Bibring represent the first published expression of the principles which became medical psychology. This is not to suggest that the problems faced by social workers and the problems faced by physicians are so similar that they can be handled by identical techniques. In certain respects, however, the physician's approach is more closely related to that of the counselor or social worker than to that of the psychiatrist.

The physician's medical training admirably prepares him to use two of the principles outlined by Dr. Bibring in her discussion of casework. (1) The social worker must discover the pertinent social and psychological facts of a case through organized interviews, and by paying careful attention to what the client says and to what can be gleaned from what he does not say or omits purposely. Since the well-trained physician similarly relies on an organized history and on inspection for an understanding of the patient's organic condition he can recognize the applicability of the same methods for an understanding of the patient's psychology. (2) Dr. Bibring (1947) states: "The true dynamic nature of the technical procedure is not so much determined by what we actually do but essentially by the effect it has on the patient." A favorite medical joke—but from the opposite point of view—"The operation was a success but the patient died," says the same thing. However, in treating emotional conflicts, it is extremely difficult to evaluate various therapeutic efforts; this fact annoys everyone in the field but causes special restlessness in many medical doctors used to the concreteness and specificity of the clinical laboratory. But even while distressed by the difficulty of evaluating therapeutic efficacy, they will try a therapeutic measure that seems logical. The difficulty in interesting the general physician in psychoanalytic principles, therefore, seems to lie in the absence of a clearly worked out method of application of psychoanalytic principles to medical practice.

For a long time, caseworkers, because of their infatuation with psychoanalysis, attempted to use psychoanalytic techniques in a modified form, often replacing traditional social work functions and skills, as if the patient or client could be helped only with the full-fledged use of all these techniques, including interpretation (Zinberg and Edinburgh, 1964). Dr. Bibring hoped that physicians, as well as social workers, could be taught principles of psychoanalytic theory and some techniques that they could use without attempting to use psychoanalytic methods in their entirety.

Before the principles of psychoanalytic theory could be taught so that they could be applied within the framework of a physician's usual professional practice, it was necessary to have available a thorough delineation of the technical procedures that were derived from the principles. Then it could be determined which techniques should be emphasized for the goals of psychotherapy and which should be emphasized for the goals of casework or medical psychology. "Psychoanalysis and the Dynamic Psychotherapies" supplies a frame of reference for the technical analysis of the interactions between doctor and patient in the individual treatment process. This frame of reference divides the therapeutic interactions into suggestion, abreaction, manipulation, clarification, and interpretation. This division permits an analysis of what interactions are useful in various circumstances, which, in turn, makes possible the delineation of a reasonably definite procedure for their use. Dr. Edward Bibring spelled out what therapeutic measures are and, therefore, made it possible for a physician to puzzle out which of them is most likely to suit his needs. He differentiates therapeutic method from curative process and indicates how each of the divisions of technique seems to work in therapeutic situations. As Dr. Grete Bibring had already shown in the earlier paper, the various forms of manipulation were the procedures most applicable to situations where the person does not primarily seek psychotherapy. Although both Drs. Edward and Grete Bibring carefully state that they define the word "manipulation" as the employment of various emotional systems existing in the patient for the purpose of achieving therapeutic and adjustive change, and illustrate this definition in many ways, people persistently misunderstand, questioning whether manipulation is not the undesirable attempt of the social worker or the physician to force his concepts and plans on the client or patient. Dr. Grete Bibring searched for another word or phrase to describe the same technical process in order to avoid this misunderstanding, and came up with "adaptive intervention." But this term proved to be artificial, and before very long psychiatrists at the Beth Israel Hospital reverted to "manipulation," taking care to define it whenever they used it.

It is worth remembering that, although manipulation is emphasized in the Bibrings' approach to casework and to medical psychology, other forms of interaction are used also. Suggestion as a form of interaction occurs of necessity in every doctor-patient or client-caseworker relationship. For instance, the request of the doctor for full information or for emotional expression promotes the therapeutic or curative aspects of the relationship. While abreaction, the expression or reliving of emotional experiences, does not stand as high in the hierarchy of curative procedure as it did at one time, for the patient and the doctor to understand what a patient is feeling, it is necessary for the patient to express it fully. Clarification—the spelling out of patterns of behavior, the attempt to bring to the patient's attention feelings and attitudes which are vague and obscure—enhances the therapeutic effort and helps the patient to gain perspective on his problems. Only interpretation as a technical procedure remains limited to psychotherapy or psychoanalysis.

Occasionally, when this system of medical psychology, emphasizing manipulation and minimizing interpretation, is presented to professional groups, they express concern that it represents a downgrading of psychiatric knowledge and insight. Their questions about medical psychology raise the perennial problem of defining goals in any form of psychic intervention. To some people, any goal short of thorough insight into unconscious conflicts and the resulting reorganization of the personality is insufficient. Whether or not this proud goal is always achieved even in psychoanalysis is not our concern here. What we do believe is that this system of medical psychology, while shirking such a rigorous task, does not downgrade psychiatric knowledge but rather finds a proper, useful niche for it. The crux of our argument lies in our definition of what the general physician faces with all patients. Every patient who visits a physician is worried about being ill; otherwise he would not be there. It is likely that this worry will institute a psychological regression in the patient, which may vary from mild in the relatively well person to severe in the relatively disturbed person. We view this response to illness as an exceptionally important example of the general human response to external threat or to disharmony with the environment. The physician's ability to understand how the anxiety associated with illness has affected the patient and to use this understanding in medical management may be crucial. The patient may be spared the unnecessary psychic scars that so frequently accompany a period of childish responses or behavior. Here the caseworker's and the doctor's functions differ, as the doctor must deal always with patients who are, or think they are, threatened from outside the psyche, that is, with physical illness. It is not infrequent for a casework client's difficulties to be primarily intrapsychic, even when the client believes that his problems result from external events. Therefore, we believe that, while the caseworker and the doctor must both understand psychoanalytic principles, the difference in their jobs often requires methods as different from each other as both are from those of the psychiatrist or psychoanalyst. All of these professional groups wish to help troubled people; all must find the form and method most appropriate to their professional roles. The four papers in this first section show how the principles of medical psychology were derived initially; in the second section we will show how medical psychology was applied and taught to physicians.

## II.  Teaching Medical Psychology

As teachers, the members of the Psychiatric Service of the Beth Israel Hospital share with an organization as different as the National Association for the Advancement of Colored People an overriding preoccupation with integration. Teaching medical psychology at the Beth Israel Hospital strikingly resembles the uncompromising position that people with differences have something to offer each other without inequities. For the psychiatrists at the Beth Israel Hospital to take the position that certain aspects of their work should be integrated with the other medical specialties is not in itself unique. But the uncompromising way in which this principle dominates the content and method of the teaching program permits the analogy with militant civil rights organizations and separates this psychiatric teaching service from many others. Examples of this principle in action occur in all teaching of medical students, but especially in the second-year course in History-taking and Physical Diagnosis. When several sessions of this course were first designated for Psychiatry, the possibility of using these sessions for a coherent presentation of what psychiatry is and how it works was tempting. Several of the other hospitals at which this course was given taught it that way and taught it well. At the Beth Israel Hospital the decision to renounce individual psychiatric sessions per se came about after long and careful discussions with the medical and surgical instructors. Instead, psychiatry would share the designated sessions with medicine or surgery, continuing the teaching exercise, but insisting that the findings to be discussed at the end of the examination include an estimate of the personality of the patient. Furthermore, during the first and last sessions of the course, when the student was oriented to the procedure or summed up his experience, the instructors' staff at the Beth Israel Hospital included a psychiatrist. The latter presented his specialty not as a study of emotional disturbance but as a specialty of communication, emphasizing that an understanding of the information received in a standard medical history, and even the physical examination, requires evaluation as a many-faceted communication. This form of participation by the psychiatrist put the medical and surgical instructors on their mettle: wishing to offer the maximum to the students, they too tried to puzzle out the levels of interaction between the patient interviewed and the doctor-student interviewer, even in those sessions when a psychiatrist was not present. The psychiatrist, in turn, learned a great deal of medicine in these sessions, which he needed in order to be able to evaluate correctly what was medically relevant in the history of the patient being discussed. This teaching exercise is typical of what is meant at the Beth Israel Hospital's Psychiatric Service by integrated teaching. In fact, this exchange of learning is deemed so important that an applicant for psychiatric residency is asked if he retains an interest in clinical medicine. Without such an interest this kind of joint teaching wearies without edifying the resident, and he had best stick to a psychiatric service in a mental hospital.

Two questions arise at this point: (1) how much does the general physician need to know about psychiatry to make an adequate personality diagnosis? and (2) does it take too much time? The latter question is discussed more fully by Reichard (pp. 169-204), but let it be said here that the use of Grete Bibring's medical psychological approach promises to be time-saving rather than time-consuming. To identify a problem early and head it off by proper medical management is demonstrably less demanding of time than trying to work with the same problem after a faulty start. For example, if a patient is properly diagnosed as a dependent, demanding person who claims large quantities of time then the appropriate treatment may well be to parcel out time in specific quantities, often small, and with definite limits. This treatment, imposed early, can save much annoyance later.

The other question remains more difficult and certainly continues to be a source of anxiety for many physicians. Repeatedly, in our teaching programs, physicians say that they had felt they had learned their job pretty well, but now they see nuances and complexities which they expect themselves to understand. All of the discussions of teaching are concerned with this problem and try to delineate certain broad limits of what is possible and useful. All too often the enormous complexity of trying to learn something about a branch of medicine where each case is different stirs up feelings of insecurity and helplessness which prevent the practitioner from even starting a systematic study of medical psychology. It is for this reason that Dr. Bibring and Dr. Kahana (pp. 108-123) attempt to show that, while each person is different, there is a finite number of personality types that can be outlined generally. The system of medical psychology aims at supplying the physician with something concrete and possible, requiring flexibility in his functioning rather than change. Here it should be emphasized that any attempt to memorize by rote a few characteristics of each personality type, and apply the appropriate management as if it were an exercise in cryptography, misses the point, The number of specific personality types is limited, but the variations and combinations of them are not.

This classification of types, therefore, gives a medical practitioner a good place to begin, but if he thinks that this is all there is to it, his surprise at an unexpected amalgamation or modification may frighten him away altogether. The task of classification, in the long run, abides with the student. Primers prepare the way and perhaps more than anything else demonstrate how useful the understanding of the principles of medical psychology can be in the practice of any medical specialty. But the student of medical psychology must persevere alone.

The foundations of any psychiatric teaching program in a general hospital must include a consultation program to the other hospital services, a direct teaching program to the physicians of those services and the outpatient department clinics and, if it is a teaching hospital, partnership with other physicians in the medical student teaching program. The papers in this section are examples of how these programs were brought about at the Beth Israel Hospital and of concrete applications of the principles of medical psychology. The physical surroundings, personnel, and goals of the various programs where these principles were applied resulted in specific modifications in the teaching methods and objectives. Some of the programs which are described were experimental when begun, and required thoughtfulness and co-operation from the chiefs of the other hospital services and the heads of the clinics where psychiatrists worked and taught.

Many of the factors which we have mentioned probably influenced department heads to request the integration of psychiatric services with their own. The result of so many psychiatric teaching efforts throughout the hospital was that they reinforced one another and made the climate of opinion in the hospital receptive to still more psychiatric programs. This book, of necessity, can report only a small part of all this activity. Two of the largest and most ambitious projects attempted by the Psychiatric Service are presented in part in other publications: the programs on the Pediatric Service and in the Well-Baby Clinic were presented and discussed in Worcester during the Freud Half-Century Anniversary Symposium (G. L. Bibring, 1960; Wermer, 1960). The presentation of the work on Obstetrics was more indirect, as the papers in *The Psychoanalytic Study of the Child* were more concerned with the ambitious research project on pregnancy than with the teaching and service aspects of the psychiatrists' collaboration with obstetricians (G. L. Bibring, 1959; G. L. Bibring, Dwyer, Huntington, and Valenstein, 1961). Others, such as the postgraduate courses for practicing physicians, the fertility clinic study, and the physical rehabilitation project, are not reported.

With all of this going on, the obvious next step is to ascertain in a systematic way what has been and can be learned from all this teaching. Dr. Reichard (pp. 169-204) makes a beginning in his paper. His fascinating and highly ambiguous findings raise, as well as answer, many questions which prepare the way for our next volume, to be devoted entirely to the question, "Can psychiatry be taught?"

One last point, touched on earlier, remained paramount throughout these integrated programs and, while probably a truism, should be reiterated. That is, the psychiatrists try to provide the best possible service for the patient and then, if possible, combine with it a teaching obligation. The comfort and well-being of the patient, the prevention or cure of his difficulty, come first, but then the psychiatrist asks the other physicians to think about how what was learned from this patient might be carried over to the next. To some this teaching zeal appears excessive. But the psychiatrist knows that there is no official place on the medical chart for psychological data and that, consequently, the only indelible recording of the complex process of making a personality diagnosis and deciding on the proper medical management will be made when a case is shared and discussed with other physicians. The basic concept in all of medicine which gives prevention priority over cure, whenever possible, requires this constant preparation for the next case, and the next, and so on.

### III. The Psychiatric Service and the Community

The papers in this section cover one facet of the Psychiatric Service's many community activities, the group program initiated by Dr. Leo Berman. This program has an applied psychoanalytic orientation which is essentially the same as that of the other programs of the Psychiatric Service. The group work Dr. Berman envisaged is delicately balanced between the educational and the therapeutic. The main purpose is not to effect psychotherapeutic results, but to increase the participants' understanding of themselves and others. A second purpose is to use the thoughts, feelings, and acts of a group member's personal life to enhance his professional purpose; a third is the productive discussion of both individual and group process.

The group approach devised by Dr. Berman clearly demands leaders with a wealth of training. All of the group leaders who report in this section are psychoanalysts with an unusually wide working experience in mental and general hospitals, private practice, schools, and clinics; all of them have had extensive group experience and training with Dr. Berman; and all share similar psychoanalytic assumptions about individual and group psychology.

The members of the groups described participated in order to learn something about themselves and others that would help them to be more effective teachers, nurses, doctors, pupils, or parents. Arrangements for the groups varied slightly with the different situations, but certain factors were the same throughout and are considered essential to the Berman group approach. Participation was voluntary (although within school systems teachers inevitably coerced each other directly or indirectly). The number and length of sessions was limited and decided in advance. But the groups were inevitably "groups" and not ordinary "classes" as a result of the subject matter and task undertaken: although the groups were educational, the aim was the understanding of unconscious processes and motivations and some aspects of their workings in human behavior—an aim which cannot be achieved by ordinary didactic teaching methods. Moreover, the leaders were committed to the view that learning depends on the relationship established between teacher and student, an assumption not shared by those educators and psychologists who stress the specific mechanisms of the learning process without due regard to its interpersonal, motivational underpinnings. On the one hand, each member was told that he could participate as much or as little as he chose, but that, if each spoke no more fully about personal matters than he would in an ordinary bull session, there was little point to the formal group with a highly trained leader. On the other hand, since the groups were not therapy groups, members also were allowed to set their own limits on how freely they were willing to talk, a certain privacy being respected.

It is a unique characteristic of the Berman group approach that the leader tries to balance work with individuals and work with the group. Various facets of this approach are illustrated in the papers in Section III. Leo Berman (pp. 253-270), Norman Zinberg, and David Shapiro (pp. 271-282) present the group activity by singling out one group member and showing chiefly those interactions relating to him. Benson Snyder and Leo Berman try to depict the history of a group by describing the high spots and chief themes (pp. 308-321). Edward Daniels (pp. 301-307), Norman Zinberg, David Shapiro, and Walter Gruen (pp. 283-289), show how much can be learned about an involved situation through such groups. Norman Zinberg (pp. 322-336) illustrates problems of leadership technique by showing typical situations calling for intervention by the leader. But the papers do more than offer different, detailed illustrations of group work: they offer a rationale for the use of dynamic groups as an important tool of preventive psychiatry. All of the writers believe, as did Freud, that by reaching those professional people who influence many others, particularly students, they will accomplish more for the mental health of the community at large than they will probably ever achieve in their lifetime as therapists treating individual patients.

However, these papers raise many basic questions which they do not answer. The most complex theoretical issue remains the same as when Fritz Redl mentioned it in 1940. He called attention to the lack of a true psychoanalytic group psychology, deploring the practice of, on the one hand, attempting to apply the language and concepts of individual psychology to groups, and, on the other, using broad sociological concepts derived from studies of entire populations to explain small-group dynamics. In this group of papers are the rudiments of an assault on the problem stated by Redl (1942). Group dynamics are not the sum of individual dynamic responses in a group. Groups follow behavioral laws which, while overlapping the laws governing behavior of individuals, are not identical with them. Once such group laws are delineated and classified, the way will be paved for the formation of a series of hypotheses concerning group psychology that can be tested for reliability.

Another unanswered question concerns the developmental sequence of groups. It is often assumed that group reactions are intricate, disguised repetitions of early responses to family situations—that is, that the genetic forebearer of the group behavior is the family. It is true that early family relationships must lay down the pattern for group development. But we contend that all future groups—the first tentative play groups, the latency gangs, the adolescent crowds or cliques, and others—are more than varied repetitions or distortions of early family responses. The concept of group genesis requires the same careful delineation as do the rules of group dynamics.

Finally, the question of group structures needs classification and organization. If a group arrogates to itself something as complex as a value, we must ask how this process occurs. If it occurs by way of the individual ego structures of each member only (Freud, 1922), how is the consensus arrived at? This question assumes particular importance if a value which is genuinely espoused in the group is at variance with a member's values when he is not in the group. Such an occurrence can be explained in terms of individual ego structure and its operation, but to explain the simultaneous observance of an idea by many people at once requires a concept of group psychic structures.

The papers in Section III do not answer such questions. Nevertheless, they have the virtue of presenting an attempt to relate group content and process to important external content and process so that problems on the job are not seen as distinct from personal problems, or individual experiences from group experiences and, to some extent, therapy from education. This group approach is, of course, very difficult for both leader and members, partly because of multiple points of view—which, however, may also account for its effectiveness. This approach exemplifies, as does all of this book, the flexible use of basic psychoanalytic principles in the service of prophylaxis by way of the deeper understanding of self and others.

# The Derivation of Medical Psychology

# Countertransferences and Attitudes of the Analyst in the Therapeutic Process

LEO BERMAN, M.D.

IT HAS HAPPENED FREQUENTLY in the history of science that what at first was considered to be a troublesome and interfering phenomenon during a given investigation later proved to be an important aspect of the very problem under study. The history of psychoanalysis offers a good example of this in the way the phenomenon of transference was discovered and fruitfully investigated. The leading thought of this paper is that further consideration of the problem of the analyst's emotional reactions to his patient will prove to be similarly rewarding.

Many analysts have come to the conclusion that the various emotional reactions of the analyst to his patient are of importance in the therapeutic process, and of importance not only in the negative sense that the analyst's emotional responses may intrude upon and "blur the transference picture (Fenichel, 1941)." Besides this, they feel that the reality of the analyst's total personality, and its functioning in the analytic situation, probably makes its own positive contribution to the therapeutic process. In this paper, "countertransference" means the analyst's reactions to the patient as though the patient were an important figure in the analyst's past life. By "attitudes" I mean the emotional reactions of the analyst as a person during the treatment hour, including his reasonable and appropriate emotional responses and his characteristic defenses. It is assumed that the totality of the analyst's emotional reactions, as in all interpersonal relationships, represents a blending, to a varying de-

Reprinted from *Psychiatry*, 12:159-166, 1949.

gree, of appropriate, defensive, and transference responses to the patient, but that the appropriate ones largely predominate.

In order to avoid possible misunderstanding I would like to state what this paper will and will not deal with. As was indicated in the title, I am concerned here with the analyst's emotional processes which are present in relation to the patient and which may have a bearing on the therapeutic process. In other words, this paper is not primarily concerned with the full problem of the psychology of the analyst. Furthermore, the psychoanalytic data and considerations mentioned here are mostly drawn from sources sometimes referred to as "orthodox Freudian." Thus, this paper does not deal with a consideration of the analytic situation as it obtains in certain forms of "active" psychoanalysis. Finally, I should like to state that this paper deals with the analytic situation as it usually develops with a competent analyst and does not concern itself with instances of obviously faulty psychoanalytic practice.

### Definition of the Analyst's Emotional Responses to His Patient

Much of the literature on the analytic attitude in the analytic situation, beginning with Freud, has been characterized by two contrasting points of view frequently expressed by the same authors. The first is more familiar and has received fuller attention. It is characterized by statements recommending a "coldness in feeling" and comparisons with a surgeon "who puts aside all his own feelings, including that of human sympathy, and concentrates his mind on one single purpose, that of performing the operation as skillfully as possible." Also, " . . . the analyst must not offer his patients any transference satisfactions" (Freud, 1915).

The other point of view is also familiar to psychiatrists and used in their daily work. But it is infrequently and too briefly referred to. Thus, Freud (1915) stated: "A certain amount of transference gratification must of course be permitted to him, more or less according to the nature of the case and the patient's individuality. But it is not good to let it become too much. . . . I do not think I have exhausted the range of useful activity on the part of the physician with the statement that a condition of privation is to be kept up during the treatment."

Fenichel (1941, p. 74) after noting how the fear of the countertransference may lead an analyst to the suppression of all human freedom in his reactions to patients, continues: "I have often been surprised at the frequency with which I hear from patients who had previously been in analysis with another analyst that they were astonished at my 'freedom' and 'naturalness' in the analysis. They had believed that an analyst is a special creation and is not permitted to be human! Just the opposite impression should prevail. The patient should always be able to rely on the 'humanness' of the analyst. The analyst is no more to be permitted to isolate analysis from life than is a patient who misuses lying on an analytic couch for that same purpose of isolation." A ready answer comes to mind to explain the problem of these two quite contrasting points of view. The answer could simply be that the analyst is always both the cool detached surgeon-like operator on the patient's psychic tissues, and the warm, human, friendly, helpful physician. I think that such an answer is essentially correct.

However, the core of the problem would be missed by thus disposing of it. This problem, as I see it, is how to integrate into the body of psychoanalytic knowledge, theory, and technique, the awareness, clinically, that the analytic situation is, in a sense, a personal one for the analyst, and most if not all patients either dimly sense this fact or have occasion to observe it quite directly. It seems to be disturbing to realize and face fully how cathected, and sometimes highly cathected, the patient and his analysis may be for the analyst.

To return to the two contrasting points of view of Freud and Fenichel, which appear to me to be typical of much of the literature, I am impressed with the following two points. (1) The quality of the emphasis in the first point of view. Although ordinarily an analyst tells himself that he strives for sound attitudes through self-analysis, the language of this point of view has the ring of a call for an unduly strong control of affect. (2) The sketchiness of the second point of view. What is "a certain amount" of transference gratification which is to be "permitted" to the patient, and when is it "too much"? What does "humanness" consist of, and how does one give expression to it? What is a "normal residue" of countertransference? (Stern, 1924).

In a series of papers Freud indicates more clearly his awareness of how real the patient's transference is—in the sense of its relationship to the analyst's real personality and attitudes as defined above—and the relationship of transference and countertransference. In regard to Freud's remarks on the strain imposed on the analyst in the handling of the countertransference, it is of interest to note his statement that ". . . every praiseworthy and valuable quality is based on compensation and overcompensation which, as was only to be expected, have not been absolutely and completely successful" (Freud, 1937).[1]

---

[1] See also Fenichel's (1941, p. 75) discussion of countertransference in which reference is made to the considerable "damming up of libido" which occurs in the analyst.

## The Analyst as Human Being

Technical expressions such as the aim-inhibited libidinal impulses of the analyst, or the normal residue of countertransference, although pertinent, are not sufficiently inclusive. Actually most analysts' positive feelings for their patients involve a wider range of feeling whose totality we shall describe as *dedication*. It is dedication in this wider sense and in the sense of the dedication of the good leader and good parent that makes an analyst's attitudes of kindly acceptance, patience, and so on, genuine and effective.

A few years ago an outstanding analyst remarked that he no longer noticed in himself the zeal and vital interest in regard to his patients that he had felt in his earlier years of psychoanalytic practice. As a result of this change he suspected that he was functioning less effectively as an analyst and that this probably reflected itself in the therapeutic results he was achieving. In this past year in the course of a discussion at a scientific meeting, another well known analyst told of the unusually good results he had obtained with a very difficult case in his first years of analytic work. Half-humorously, he referred to his relative ignorance in those years and expressed some doubts as to whether he could duplicate such achievement at the present time. I would be inclined to explain these two observations on these analysts' early therapeutic experiences in terms of their genuine dedication to the patient's welfare, which the patient sensed. This is apparently the optimal emotional climate for the specific work of the analysis.

I used to take the analytic situation for granted as being a part of my work until various patients repeatedly asked how it was possible for one to sit all day listening to such troubles, taking so much abuse, and so on. I usually analysed such comments as part of the transference, but I have come to realize that perhaps the chief meaning of such remarks, following the viewpoint presented in this paper, frequently derives from the patient's perception of the analyst's real dedication to him and that this is his way of expressing his appreciation and gratitude to the analyst. I became better aware of how much an analyst "gives" and "puts out" for the patient when I noted what a strain it was to focus on the patient and his material on days when, for various external or internal reasons, I was not "all there."[2]

---

[2] It is important to differentiate between an analyst's attitude of realistic and appropriate dedication and the qualitatively different and inappropriate attitude of masochistic submission.

Analysts have probably not sufficiently appreciated the meaningfulness of that reality of the analytic situation which consists of one human being freely consenting to meet with a "stranger" regularly and under difficult and sometimes painful conditions over a long period of time. Low (1935) probably had something like this in mind when she spoke of the "fused living of the patient and the analyst." Child analysts seem to be more aware of their feelings of dedication to their patients.

In brief, the extent to which the psychoneurotic patient is intuitively and sometimes directly aware of the reality of the analyst's feelings toward him requires more careful consideration. Not only, as frequently described, do children, psychotics, and psychopaths possess a high degree of intuitive understanding, but also the psychoneurotic patient is capable of this kind of intuition, especially when his childhood was characterized by particularly cold, harsh, or indifferent parental attitudes.

In the case of the analytic situation with a nonpsychotic adult, it appears that the other side of the analyst's feeling of dedication toward the patient may find expression more often than is generally described. I refer not only to those obvious instances in an analysis when an analyst is, as it were, appropriately firm with the patient, and he knows that the edge of impatience or irritation he feels, for example, at the patient's temporizing, is only "natural" or "human." I have in mind also less obvious instances of "leaks" through temporary crevices of the analyst's ego structure as it is shaken by the patient's subtle or roaring barrage. The analyst's suppressed and repressed aggression may, for example, produce in him minor changes in voice quality, quality and timing of interpretations, and so on. To put it in a more general form: when subjected to a strong stimulus by the patient, the *qualitative* response in the analyst will tend to be about the same as occurs in most people, but the *quantitative* response will be less and its *duration* shorter. The shorter duration is achieved by the working through of the response by self-analysis. According to this formulation, the essence of the analyst's humanness lies in the fact that qualitatively he responds like most human beings. To be more precise, it should be noted that the *range* of his qualitative responses is less restricted and compulsive than in most people because he has learned to function with less repression. To some degree, he has a greater variety of adaptations to different personalities than his patients.

Most of these comments on the role of the analyst's aggressive feelings are applicable to his libidinal feelings. He may for instance, develop feelings of attraction to certain patients and then either mobilize defenses against such feelings or yield to them by becoming too much interested in the corresponding material before his feelings are worked through satisfactorily by self-analysis. Here, too, the problem arises, from the viewpoint of this paper, as to the degree of the patient's awareness of either of these transitory reactions of the analyst and the role that this awareness plays in the therapeutic process.

## Technique and the Therapeutic Process

Waelder (1937), in referring to the dialectical structure of psychoanalysis, described various poles of its dialectic, and then added that analysts try to steer a middle course between such poles. Waelder noted, among others, the poles of transference and real relationships. One may call attention in addition to these, to the related polarities of countertransference and the actual feelings of the analyst—acting out and just plain living—and the unique elements of the analytic situation and its commonplaceness. Although most of the emphasis in the analytic literature has been on the uniqueness of the analytic situation, about two years before his death Freud (1937, p. 381) wrote: "Let us be quite clear that what analysis achieves for neurotics is just what normal people accomplish for themselves without its help." It may be said, I think, that the analytic situation represents a unique way of arranging for the commonplace—the commonplace of experimentation and learning through human intercourse. To an important degree such functioning has been lost to patients largely as a result of earlier unfavorable interpersonal experiences.

Of particular importance is the reaction of the analyst to the fully developed childish elements in the transference neurosis, and it should be emphasized that, as a result of the analyst's emotional reactivity to his patient, the child in the patient not only tries to achieve various childhood goals in regard to the analyst, but *actually does* achieve these goals in a limited and transitory way. If this point is correct, one can indeed say that the analytic situation is also one of experimentation and learning through human relationships. The analyst is then to be seen not only as the detached observer who helps the patient gain insight through discussion, but, to a certain degree, the analyst is an active participant *in* the analytic situation. The analyst is not only the parental figure to the patient, but he actually functions emotionally as such, within limits. The analyst is like a parent in his attitude toward the patient, and the mature parent is the protoype of the analyst at work. The patient has the experience in the analysis of learning to function in a realistic and integrated way through the living demonstration afforded him of such relatively successful functioning occurring in the analyst as the analyst betimes contends with his conflicting feelings toward the patient. It may be that Freud had something like this in mind when he wrote in 1915 that the patient has to learn from the analyst how to overcome the pleasure principle (Freud, 1915 p. 390).

This viewpoint should clarify certain difficulties which commonly arise during the course of analysis. First, it is my impression that some analyses which are abruptly terminated by the patient, and those which are terminated by mutual consent after a dull and frustrating period of analysis, result from the patient's correctly sensing that the analyst is for some reason unable genuinely to warm up to him and feel the dedication of a parent. In the initial exploratory and getting acquainted stage of any relationship between two persons, a multidimensional human experience is not to be expected. However, after this initial period in analysis, the patient will react vigorously if the proper and formally correct analyst does not gradually become a parent in terms of his genuine dedication.

A second type of difficulty arises with certain very sensitive and intuitive patients who know that the analyst is really reacting emotionally and are aware of his tendency toward defensiveness and oversecretiveness. Such a situation may result in two different patterns in the patient, depending on the patient's character structure. In some instances the patient behaves like the analyst and the analysis develops the artifact of a pseudo tranquil atmosphere because important areas remain unanalyzed. In patients of a different character structure, the analyst's attempted denial of certain of his feelings toward the patient results in an excessive storminess of the analysis. The patient is then driven to act out both inside and outside of the analysis to a greater degree than he otherwise would, usually with the unconscious intent of provoking the analyst into even more obvious and unmistakable expressions of his emotional interest in him. He tries to achieve with others outside what he felt he was unfairly deprived of by the analyst, and at the same time seeks to provoke an outburst of jealousy in the analyst.

Frequently the patient gives ample warning before he swings into one of the patterns just noted. There may be a marked increase in material centering around jealousy of the analyst's other patients, and dreams in which the analyst is nice and friendly with others but ignores the patient. The patient may increasingly complain how one-sided the analysis is, why should he talk so much about himself and the analyst doesn't talk about himself. The patient may repeat that he would rather have the analyst angry and upset at him than suffer the analyst's indifference. If adequately dealt with, these points lead to important genetic material centering around the patient's early childhood feelings about his weakness and helplessness, together with his ideas of sexual irresistibility and general power and control in regard to the parents.

A third type of difficulty arises in an analysis when the analyst, impelled by his excessive feelings in regard to the patient, falls into the trap set by the patient. Soon after the success of such a maneuver the patient comes to regard the analyst scornfully and enjoys a brief bitter feeling of triumph over him. In such a setting it does not really matter to the patient whether he has provoked an exaggeratedly aggressive or oversolicitous response in the analyst. All such responses by the analyst are regarded by the patient as incidents in a raging battle which can only have one or two possible outcomes: either the patient or the analyst will win out with the utter castration and annihilation of the other.

There is still another element active in such situations which adds to the patient's bitterness. It is not just that he knows that he has scored a hollow triumph by having uncovered a weak spot in the analyst. It is that the patient had hoped to see in the analyst, at that point when the situation was obviously difficult for both the analyst and himself, a demonstration of wisdom and strength which would lead him out of the maze in which he had been wandering unhappily since childhood, and he now feels that the analyst has failed him. It is at such crucial points in an analysis when the analyst is under considerable stress and *showing some tendencies to react the way the patient's parents reacted in the patient's childhood* that a demonstration by the analyst of genuine dedication and reasonableness is most helpful. It is then that the patient is in the best position to learn to discriminate between past and present, between childhood figures and persons in the present. One might draw a military analogy: behind the lines, an officer does not require maximal ability, nor can he then acquire much standing in the eyes of his outfit; it is only when all are equally under fire and exposed to the same dangers that good leadership by the officer is most helpful to his men and at the same time most effective in establishing him as worthy of his rank. The same elements come into play in regard to the parent and his child when the child's struggle with its inner impulses becomes acute.

In brief, I think it is in the patient's experience of the *process* through which the analyst under stress achieves realistic and well-integrated functioning that an important therapeutic factor is to be found. The sound functioning the analyst had achieved prior to his work with a given patient may not ring very true to this patient until he had, to refer again to the military analogy, exposed the analyst to a fresh baptism of fire.

Recognition of these elements in the therapeutic process demands consideration of what technical means are available for providing this experience for those patients who need it. One aspect of this problem is the circumstances under which the analyst should more overtly express his positive feelings for the patient. The more severely neurotic or more "borderline" a patient is, the more important does the analyst's task of quantitatively regulating the more tangible proofs of his dedication to the patient become. It is obvious that both too much and too little of such proof will result in unfavorable repercussions in the patient.

The "analytic attitude" varies considerably as regards how much warmth and subtle "giving" is blended with the simultaneous remaining "outside" of the patient and his problems. Probably, analysts intuitively try to hit the appropriate dosage of genuine "giving" and of proofs of their friendliness and dedication with each patient according to the point each has reached in the analysis. There are many indirect ways in which this is effectively done. The analyst may vary the amount of friendly discussion of some real life problem or interest—for example, the patient's work. There may be more or less laxity in allowing a session to run beyond its official end. There may be a greater or lesser deviation from a previously agreed upon statement as to when the patient would be charged for a missed session, and so on. However, it seems it is not really possible for the analyst to be consistently so keenly attuned to the patient as to achieve an accurate dosage of what the patient needs all the time. This "failing," if it does not become too marked, probably also plays a part in the therapeutic process. The patient has occasion to experience the reality of a person who dedicates himself to the task of helping him to grow up and who comes through reasonably well in spite of obvious difficulties.

The "giving" by the analyst is of interest in another connection. All patients show impairments in their libidinal and ego development, the latter having reference also to the body ego. Although disturbances of the body ego have received relatively little systematic attention, its importance is evident in Freud's (1923, p. 31) statement that "the ego is first and foremost a body ego." There is some reason to believe that one indispensable step in the building of a mature body ego consists of an oral incorporation of parental body parts. If pronounced ambivalence is present in the child, this process takes on a strong sadistic coloring and may lead to various body ego disturbances (Berman, 1948). In this regard, the appropriate and genuine "giving" by the analyst also represents unconsciously to the patient a friendly offer to share his body psychologically with the patient and to help him, as it were, grow up physically as well as emotionally.

In regard to the technical question of how open and truthful the analyst should be about his various feelings toward the patient in order to provide the emotional experience the patient requires, it seems that the verbal expression of such feelings is needed only infrequently and to a limited extent. In some cases the analysis of the transference leads to the question of the patient's ideas as to what the analyst really feels toward him. The patient may then find an easy way out through a kind of official answer to the effect that the analyst feels the way any doctor feels toward his patient, that to the analyst he is just one of the many patients who come to the analyst for treatment, and so on. Such an answer may also suit the defenses of the analyst, and valuable material may thus be lost. In order to deal effectively with such a defense it may sometimes be necessary for the analyst to express himself verbally as to his feelings toward the patient.

In conclusion, a few remarks about the psychology of the analyst may be appropriate in view of the stress placed in this paper on the personal nature of the analytic process as it pertains to the analyst. These remarks are limited to some notes on the art of healing and the sublimation of sadistic impulses. Freud (1937, pp. 400-401) and others have correctly referred to the practice of psychoanalysis as an art. According to various studies of artistic creativity (Fenichel, 1937; Klein, 1929), the artist's unconscious sense of guilt in connection with his sadism, and his need to make reparation, seem to be important components in such activity. In the case of an analysis in which the patient shows little or no improvement over a long period of time, the analyst may begin to feel a certain concern about it beyond what would appear to be appropriate. Pronounced situations of this kind are frequently a result of unconscious needs in the analyst to think of himself as a powerful healer. The narcissistic hurt he suffers when he finds that he is not so effective may then activate various of his repressed conflicts, for example, his unresolved sadism. However, the instance now under consideration can be considered as approximately "normal" and is, in part, to be understood as follows: the improved patient is, in a sense, the product of the analyst's successful artistic creativity and the tangible proof of his adequately sublimated sadism. Thus a patient who does not get well temporarily impairs the smooth working of the analyst's libidinal economy since there is an interference with one of his channels of sublimation. When analysts note that a strong motivating force in the patient's getting well is to please the analyst, one may add that in getting well the patient pleases the doctor in more ways than one. Some patients are more or less aware of this point and unless adequately analyzed, it may become the center of a stubborn area of resistance.[3] From the point of view of the analyst's mental hygiene, these considerations lend emphasis to the recommendation that the analyst should as a rule have more than two or three patients in treatment at any one time.

[3] The subject of the patient's role in helping to further the analyst's self-analysis and professional maturity, and the place of this role in the therapeutic process, are essentially unexplored. Experiences in group psychotherapy make it evident that the conscious therapeutic activity of the patient is an important part of the therapeutic process.

# Psychiatry and Social Work

GRETE L. BIBRING, M.D.

THIS DISCUSSION IS AN ATTEMPT to formulate the relationship between psychoanalysis and social work, the sphere of influence that should be kept open for psychiatric thinking, and the interplay between psychiatry and social work in general.

I should like first to tell when and how my interest in this general problem began. In one of my earliest consultations I discussed with a social worker at length the psychological structure and difficulties of his client as the basis of his problems, until we felt sure that we understood each other completely. Toward the end of the consultation, when we had just started to discuss the application of our findings to the case, the worker asked me, "And what of all that should I interpret to the client?" This question was what started me off on my thoughts about psychiatry and social work, and it is this question that I shall try to discuss in some detail.

When I talk about psychiatry I have, essentially, dynamic or psychoanalytic psychiatry in mind.

We know that social work has not always been as systematic and as well disciplined as it is nowadays; that it started on a more or less amateur basis of good will and warm-heartedness or feeling of obligation; that social, religious, and ethical motives created it for the deprived and underprivileged persons. This unsystematic, more individualistic attempt became organized—very much under the strong influence of Mary E. Richmond's *Social Diagnosis* (1917)—which led to an abundant collec-

Reprinted from *Journal of Social Casework*, 28:203-211, 1947.

tion of social data in each case. This type of material was very helpful but not quite adequate for a total grasp of the client's situation. After the first World War, with the return of veterans with war neuroses, and with the increasing need for a better understanding of the personality of the client, social work turned to psychiatry, especially to psychoanalytic information. With this it went to another extreme: the abundant gathering of psychological data and a lessening of interest in the social factors. Yet the great amount of accumulated material was difficult to integrate and to evaluate. It finally represented more of a burden than of a real help. What took place then was another shift, a kind of reductive movement perhaps best represented by Virginia P. Robinson's *A Changing Psychology in Social Case Work* (1930), which represents an attempt to integrate the findings of medical psychology and social work.

To return to our initial question, the relationship between dynamic psychiatry and social casework, there is no doubt that a deeper psychological knowledge is essential in a field that deals with individuals in their needs and failures, in their maladjustments or conflicts. There are obviously many cases where, beyond the social problems involved, the social worker in his planning faces complications and difficulties not related to outer circumstances but presented by the personality of the client. There the social diagnosis has necessarily to be combined with the personality diagnosis.

It would not be correct to say that good casework has existed only since social workers began to study more psychiatry. Many workers did and still do good work with what we call intuition. This term refers to a kind of psychological empathy that eludes the logical, analytic thinking, to an immediate perceptiveness for apparently insignificant but actually very informative details in the client. But intuition alone—however brilliant its results sometimes may be—is not sufficient because it is dependent on our changing state of mind, on our momentary disposition, and is easily upset or colored by our own emotional conditions. On the other hand, with knowledge alone, understanding remains intellectual and exposed to the errors of a rational approach. Intuition therefore has to be supplemented by systematic psychological knowledge, and —especially in practice—this knowledge by intuition.

What or how much systematic knowledge does the social worker need, how should he apply it, what are his specific needs, how do they differ from the psychiatrist's application? Is his use of this information similar to the psychoanalyst's or the psychotherapist's and, if not, where are the boundaries? Or, more specifically, what do both psychiatrists and social workers have to know in general? What in each particular case? How do the psychiatrist and the social worker gain the necessary knowledge in the particular case? Finally, how does the psychiatrist or the social worker use this knowledge for his particular purpose?

## General Knowledge

What have we to know in general? Both psychiatrist and social worker should be as completely informed as possible about everything that promotes the understanding of human nature. Experienced social workers are sometimes puzzled by the fact that young workers frequently like to express themselves in psychoanalytic terminology (a phenomenon that can be observed just as well in the newly trained psychiatrist). This is only too human and a sign that these individuals have not reached the necessary distance from their theoretical knowledge. This "children's disease" has to be overcome, but it should not lead to withholding theoretical knowledge from the student. Intensive theoretical knowledge is the basis for understanding. The knowledge has to be sound and alive, however, so that we do not use the concepts as a lingo but are guided by their real meaning. To that end, extensive training in the practical application of these concepts has to follow so that they become part of our work and not only part of our studies.

What and how much must we know in each particular field? Here we come to the crossroads where the psychoanalyst parts from the social worker. With the hope of indicating some of the differences, I should like to compare the process of psychoanalytic therapy with the process of social casework.

## Psychoanalytic Goals and Methods

The goal of psychoanalysis is to change the patient's neurotic personality in the sense of removing the basis of his neurosis through insight. It is a proud goal and not always achieved, but it stands foremost in our minds. Everything we do is determined by it. To reach this goal we have not only to understand the actual dynamics of our patients' disturbances, but also to trace them back through all their vicissitudes to their infantile origin.

To gather the necessary extensive and very detailed information, we use a special method, that of free association. This technique of unrestricted expression of nondirected, spontaneously produced thoughts, fantasies, feelings, impulses, and so on, provides the most intimate material, which is used as a basis for our further procedure. The technical handling of this material can be described mainly under two headings: interpretation and manipulation. Interpretation in the psychoanalytic sense refers to the unconscious meaning of, and the unconscious connections between, the patient's thoughts, attitudes, dreams, symptoms, and tendencies in the present and in the past. Interpretation, therefore, plays a leading role in analysis since the cure is based on the patient's comprehension of the unconscious roots of his symptoms and consequently on the more adequate disposal of his pathogenic, infantile conflicts.

This insight into—and re-experiencing of—hidden connections, meanings, and motivations is as a rule not easily achieved. It frequently requires a laborious and time-consuming "working through" which consists of mitigating and removing the opposing forces of the ego, on the one hand, and furnishing repeated, detailed, and multiform evidence of the repressed, on the other hand. Frequently, though not always, it leads to a temporary reactivation of the unconscious tendencies and conflicts. The self-experience thus developed confronts the patient with a new situation which he has to settle anew in accordance with his mature attitudes and values. To achieve this, much skill, patience, and watchfulness are needed.

This leads to the second technical treatment means of importance, which consists of the proper handling, the manipulation of the patient's personality and his relationship to the therapist—the so-called transference—throughout the various ever-changing situations in the therapeutic process. Manipulation in the sense used here is not identical with gross interference, guidance, advice, running the patient's life, and so on. Manipulation in the psychoanalytic sense is based on an intimate knowledge of the various aspects of the patient's personality and refers to the therapist's attempts to influence the patient in immediate ways, verbal and nonverbal, by making use of his actual or habitual emotional systems for the purpose of the cure. Manipulation is a direct method of influence as distinct from the indirect method of interpretation and insight. Manipulation may be positive (trying to achieve certain results) or negative (tending to avoid certain complications). The patient may be aware of this manipulation or not, the latter being more frequently the case. Manipulation may be a personal one (within the therapist-patient relationship) or an environmental one (through suggesting change in the patient's external circumstances). Since the concept of manipulation frequently encounters much misapprehension, mainly on rational grounds, I should like to make perfectly clear in which sense I am using it here by quoting some illustrations from a nonpsychoanalytic setup. A patient comes to the therapist under some authoritative influence about which he seems to be resentful. When the therapist points out that he does not want him to think that he has to come, that it is entirely up to him, the patient, to decide whether he would like to discuss his problem, the therapist reaches the patient by removing the reason for his resentment through re-establishing his freedom of choice, Another patient may come to the therapist because he wants to please an authoritative person who suggested the treatment. The therapist may utilize this tendency to please by developing the patient's self-responsibility in making him sense (perhaps subconsciously) that self-direction is expected from him. This is another way of manipulation. In contrast to this immediate utilization of emotional attitudes in the process of management, insight therapy would first confront the patient with his tendency to please by living up to the expectation of his environment. Then the analyst would attempt to uncover the underlying motives such as perhaps fear of tension, or of being rejected, or excluded, and so on, and finally the background of these fears. By increasing the patient's insight into the dynamics and genetics of his tendency to please, the analyst would finally help him to become independent and self-responsible.

The described types of manipulation, except—as a rule at least—the environmental manipulation, find various applications in the course of psychoanalytic treatment. We handle the transference by promoting or inhibiting tendencies or by noninterference. Our friendly neutrality, our understanding without any condemnation, our acceptance of his personality, represent various forms of management. Using the patient's confidence in and attachment to us, we help him give up his defenses, face many a painful fact, live through reactivated conflicts, stand a temporarily unsettled tense situation, and so on. This is manipulation in the sense described before. Since we cannot interpret everything at once, we have temporarily to mitigate certain anxieties and feelings of guilt through reassurance, devaluation, or by other means. Even the process of interpretation is intimately linked up with manipulation. The choice of what to interpret and in which ways, the timing and dosing of interpretation are again forms of manipulation. We interpret usually only one element at a time, to avoid an attack on different layers with resulting confusion and anxiety. We do not break into deeper levels if the more superficial ones have still to be worked through. We do not offer more than the patient can assimilate at the time. Although, in analysis, interpretation and manipulation have to be handled equally well, they are not of the same theoretical and technical significance. Manipulation is subordinate to interpretation in that it prepares the way for efficient interpretation and subsequent "insight."

This is roughly how psychoanalysis deals with the individual case: the analyst has to know as much as possible; he gets his knowledge through the patient's free association and the observation of his conduct; and he uses it for manipulation and interpretation. All that is dictated by the aim of psychoanalysis to remove the basis of the patient's disorder through insight and reorientation. The insight into the resisting forces and methods of defense as well as insight into the repressed and the reorientation in both are the most important curative factors in analysis. Change in both is identical with change in personality.

## Goals and Methods of Psychotherapy

I shall turn now to a brief discussion of methods of psychotherapy in distinction from the methods of psychoanalysis. I do not intend to present psychotherapy fully as an entity of its own, but wish to refer to it as a link that leads to the next problem: the problem of any profession dealing with humans in their needs, conflicts, and struggles. The professions—such as education, applied law, guidance of any kind, and social work—all engage in activities that, to a certain degree, must be considered psychotherapy .

According to our scheme, we shall start with the aim. The goal of psychotherapy is in a sense different from that of psychoanalysis. It does not strive for a causal solution of the patient's conflicts, for a basic reorientation of his ego, but—as a rule—for a limited adjustment of the neurotic patient to his own possibilities and to the necessities of life. This does not mean to say that psychotherapy can achieve only so much and not more.

That the psychotherapist needs, generally speaking, the same basic knowledge as the analyst, goes without saying. The difference appears in regard to the individual case. In this respect he needs much less information than the analyst. Since he usually deals more with the actual dynamics of the patient's disorders than with their genesis, he has to know the main structure of the patient's symptoms and personality, his essential relations to his environment, his basic conflicts, and to have perhaps a general acquaintance with the most important parts of the infantile background. He acquires this knowledge through interview and observation, not by the technique of free association in the strict sense. He does not look for the detailed evidence one tries to reach in analysis nor for the intimate interplay between the different mechanisms and drives, nor does he intend to trace the actual disorders back through their various transformations to their infantile origin. Nor is he interested in analyzing and removing the resisting forces, the various mechanisms of defense, and so on, to the degree that this is done in analysis—not even approximately so. Psychoanalysis is active in the utilization of the material and in handling the various situations, especially of transference and resistance, but more expectant (though by no means rigidly) in relation to the production of the material. Psychotherapy is active in both respects and much more so than psychoanalysis.

How does the psychotherapist use his general and specific information? It is self-evident that what we may briefly term confidence-transference is the basis of any kind of psychotherapy. More specifically, all types of psychotherapy can, I think, easily be reduced to five groups of technical procedures: suggestion, emotional relief, immediate influence (or manipulation as defined above), clarification, interpretation (or insight as defined above). One principal remark is necessary at this point. The true dynamic nature of the technical procedure is not so much determined by what we actually do but essentially by the effect it has on the patient, a viewpoint much neglected by many writings on psychotherapy. Unfortunately, the effects of the various therapeutic measures are readily evaluated and explained according to the therapist's theoretical viewpoint and in terms of his favored explanatory scheme without much investigation into their actual dynamic nature.

Suggestion is not likely to appear in the evaluations of the dynamics of present-day methods of psychotherapy though it indubitably plays an actual role in many of them. Interpretation, for example, though not intended to be "suggestion," as a matter of fact often works in this way. This is especially the case in brief psychotherapy which does not permit much, if any, investigation into the true effects of interpretation, in contrast to analysis where by necessity these effects have to be checked constantly. Be it as it may, in analysis we try as a matter of principle to avoid suggestion, though in certain cases and situations its use may be quite legitimate.

Emotional relief refers to all forms of expression, primarily verbalization, and is of greatest significance in those cases of acute neuroses where pent-up tension is a strong determinant. In subtle ways, emotional relief seems to be a factor in all kinds of psychotherapy. It is not simply identical with abreaction, but represents a more complex process with various gratifications involved.

Clarification refers to the establishment of the right perspective—concretely speaking, to the separation of objective and subjective factors, of actuality and personal meaning, of the mature attitudes of the ego and its neurotic conceptions and patterns. As a matter of principle, it does not (or need not) include unconscious factors. When we convince the patient that his troubles are psychogenic or self-imposed, when he begins to see the people in his environment in an objective sense (their neuroses where he saw bad will, their concern where he saw suppression and attack, and so on), we have clarified his relation to himself and to others. The result of such clarification is the patient's capacity to conceive of himself and others in a less biased way.

Interpretation, as distinguished from clarification, refers to the exposition of unconscious dynamic factors in the patient's actual personality (dynamic interpretation) or in the various periods of his past in reference to his present condition (genetic interpretation). In analysis, as we have seen, dynamic and genetic interpretations are used both extensively and intensively. The role of interpretation in psychotherapy is receiving technical study but has not yet been definitely clarified. Interpretation in psychotherapy is often identical with what we call clarification, establishing detachment and control. It may often be functionally identical with suggestion. Frequently, interpretation in psychotherapy consists in the adequate verbalization of preconscious material which the patient himself has no capacity to verbalize. Such interpretations are—as a rule—very effective. In any case, dynamic interpretation ( as distinguished from genetic interpretation) is strongly predominant. It is difficult to say, however, how much deeper interpretation (of deeply repressed or strongly modified material) leading to true insight is possible in brief psychotherapy, since there is little chance to investigate into how the patient "takes it." This refers even more to genetic interpretations. Be it as it may, true insight is, as a rule, only possible if the opposing forces are removed or at least considerably reduced. This is usually the result of a laborious process, although insight may sometimes take place rather suddenly.

In psychotherapy, as far as we can see, widest application is made of immediate influence on emotional systems (similar to manipulation in psychoanalysis) whether the therapist is aware of it or not. The unawareness is probably due to the fact mentioned before that limited investigation is made into the actual dynamics of the therapeutic procedures, and that they are often explained in terms of a favored conceptual scheme. What enters the description is mainly the achieved result, as manifested in changes of attitudes and in the patient engaging in new activities. This redirection takes place within the personal therapist-patient relationship. It may vary in extensity and intensity, may make use of superficial or "deeper" emotional systems in the patient, and may have temporary or more lasting effects. Well handled, it may, under favorable circumstances, offer to the patient new experiences of himself and of the world which may become the basis of a new orientation toward life.

In general, one may say that psychotherapy makes use of all the technical measures described above. The techniques actually used may vary according to the various constellations in the individual cases but also largely with the personality of the therapist and his approach. All these methods differ in certain basic aspects from the psychoanalytic one.

## Goals and Methods in Casework

If we now turn to casework and the question as to what use it can make of dynamic psychiatry in general and psychoanalysis specifically, I should like to indicate from the start that I do not consider it my task to discuss here the total realm of casework, and its particular problems of classification of types of treatment. What I have in mind is casework that consciously assumes responsibility for the treatment of personality difficulties.

I should like to follow the same scheme by defining first the aim of psychologically oriented casework. The situation of social work is different right from the outset. First of all, the client often comes to the agency for reasons other than the need for psychic help. If psychological problems are involved in his difficulty, he may or may not know of their existence. In the second place, the worker does not deal with the client exclusively, as psychiatry mostly does, but often with his family and with his environment. Finally, because of the specific nature of the client's request, the worker often has to act almost immediately. In general, the aim of casework is not to eliminate the internal causes underlying the client's character disturbances but to help him find the satisfactory form of social adjustment—on the basis of psychological understanding, yet frequently through direct help with the social problem. This is true not only of the rather trivial instances but also of more complicated situations. To make this clear, a brief remark on some of the psychological principles involved may be permitted.

Psychiatric and psychoanalytic literature has recently paid increasing attention to the function of actuality in the onset and the development of psychoneuroses. This applies even to the analytic treatment itself. The traditional assumption, that among the determinants of a neurosis the infantile predisposition has to be considered as the crucial factor, is now considered valid only to a certain extent. The assumption is based on analytic experience that has shown that a thorough resolution of the infantile predispositions removes the ground of a given neurosis. But this is not the whole truth, especially not from the practical point of view. It is a well known fact that change of a real condition of life not only creates neuroses but also makes neuroses disappear. We know of such changes from trivial experiences. Some people are well balanced on vacation, free from tension, fear, and other symptoms, but they develop all their neurotic fears, psychosomatic and other disorders after their return to normal conditions of life. Others are more neurotic than usual during the weekend or while on vacation. The war, too, has taught us a similar lesson. The conditions of war both created and eliminated tension. They made neurotic reactions manifest or more intense, or created new neuroses, or they made neuroses of civilian life disappear. Such changes need not be of a temporary nature. Just as unfavorable conditions may produce a lasting neurosis, so favorable experiences in life may result in a lasting "cure" without any "treatment" of the infantile predisposition. From the theoretical point of view, both disappearance of neurotic reactions and their appearance or reappearance are equally important.

Here one is inclined to make the distinction between a "true cure," consisting of the removal of the infantile predisposition, and a pseudo cure, as it were, characterized by the disappearance of the neurotic symptoms due to favorable circumstances of life. Such a distinction is justified only to a certain extent. As a matter of fact, psychotherapy imitates in a condensed and systematic form the curative conditions of life and achieves similar results in essentially similar ways. This is in certain respects true also of psychoanalysis. We know that the process of the psychoanalytic treatment, as well as its results, is to a varying degree conditioned by actual circumstances. We treat and sometimes cure our patients under practically limited conditions, due to the actual circumstances of the treatment and of life, and for the average conditions of life; that is, conditions favorable to the cure and, later, to the maintenance of the result, if they remain approximately the same after the treatment. A person cured in this way may, when later exposed to traumatic experiences specific to the individual, nevertheless fall back to the former neurosis or develop a new one.

All this permits the conclusion that the onset of an actual conflict—its nature, the course of its development, and its outcome; the disappearance of a neurosis, whether it occurs under favorable conditions of life or under the influence of a treatment; the treatment itself, its contents and course and its final result; the eventual recurrence of a neurosis after a successful treatment—is at least to a considerable extent determined by the intimate interplay of internal and environmental conditions.

In other words, in all these problems we are dealing with a dynamic system or sphere of mutual influence, consisting of both the dynamic structure of the individual and that of his actual environment. At whatever point in this system change takes place, it influences the rest of it. Such changes may occur in the individual first affecting the instinctual setup, and/or the ego, and consequently the relation to the outside world. Or relevant changes may occur in the environment first and then bring about corresponding changes in the individual.

The conclusion to be drawn at this point is not at all new: the treatment of personality disorders can be undertaken either way, from within or from without or by a combination of both approaches. The environmental approach is the genuine contribution of casework. In current practice, it is frequently combined with the "internal" approach. But what we should like to emphasize here is that with the increase of our knowledge of the intimate interplay of the external and internal factors, certain procedures in casework will take on new significance.

From this point of view the question, what the social worker has to know in general, answers itself. His knowledge has to comprise the psychological development of the personality, its main phases and their disturbances, the various outcomes of these disturbances, the different personality types as a result of inner development and outside influence, the main mechanisms of these different types, the basic sources of conflicts, failures, the main possibilities of success and adjustment, the role sublimation plays, and transference; in short, the fundamentals of the psychology and psychopathology of the personality. This is a large program, but the more familiar the caseworker is with these concepts in theory and their application to his work, the easier it will be for him to see and to plan.

The social worker gains his specific knowledge in the individual case not by free association but through interviews and careful observation, paying equal attention to what the client expresses and what he does not say. It is, therefore, one of the essential tasks to organize the first interviews, if possible, in such a way that they touch most of the pertinent social and psychological facts. Here our growing experience, based on the common work of psychiatry and social work, promises to become increasingly helpful.

This leads to the question as to how the worker uses the specific information he has gained in a particular case. In general, the caseworker will not use his impressions for interpretations in the analytic sense. One may say that such interpretations either will not help the client if they are not carefully prepared, unfolded, and controlled as described above with regard to the psychoanalytic setup, or they might even harm the client, cause anxiety, increase his resistance, or drive him away. What we said about interpretation in psychotherapy refers equally to social work. One can effectively interpret the nearly obvious, what almost exists in the client's mind but for which he has no formulation and thus no releasing understanding. One may in the same way explain his environment to him or him to his environment. The latter leads to what I would like to emphasize here—that casework treatment that utilizes both environmental and personal treatment, often in combination, has in it the potentials for effective reorientation of the client. Such treatment—based on psychological understanding of the client's needs and difficulties, and on our awareness that we are capable of influencing him by our attitudes, our activities, and our arrangements (partly in an inhibiting and partly in a promoting way)—offers him the opportunity of achieving a basic readjustment.

To illustrate this, I should like to discuss briefly a rather familiar problem as it was presented, nearly identically by three different clients. The instances have been selected because of their relative simplicity. Three patients in a hospital setup exhibited the same reaction to the suggestion of the physician, namely, refusal to go to a tuberculosis sanitarium. The one patient stressed his illness, always discussing it, turning from one doctor to the other, from one nurse to the next with his complaints, but he did not appear too eager to use the prescribed medication, almost seemed not to want to get better, easily complaining about being neglected, and so on. But he did not take up the suggestion made to him. His childhood history indicated a feeling of being overlooked by his mother, having had a sick brother who secured all her attention. (Or, to mention another possibility, the patient himself may have been a sickly child and therefore always been favored.) The diagnosis of this patient is that of a masochistic (or infantile) dependent type whose need for love and attention makes him choose the way of suffering since nothing else seems gratifying to him. The worker's attitude as a result of this diagnosis would be to show special interest in his other achievements, to offer him full support and sympathy, but to avoid dwelling on his sickness. In other words, the worker will through his conduct demonstrate to the patient that by his getting well and by going to the place where he can get well he will gain more affection and appreciation.

The second patient conspicuously avoids talking about his symptoms, is irritated when reminded of his illness, shows in every way that he looks upon it as a weakness, and that he feels almost hurt by it in his pride. In this case the worker will in various ways express belief in his strength, will in one way or another present his going to the sanitarium as a task for which he is ready to respect him. He will help him to comprehend especially the necessity to fulfill his obligation toward his family or toward his future, and thus offer him compensation for his unconscious fears with regard to his self-esteem.

A third patient shows the same resistance but he does not hide this fact. He does not permit you, like the first one, to overlook this resistance, and you cannot help feeling that there is an element of aggression and an irritating, sadistic attitude in it, some triumph over you or his wife or his mother. In this case one will try to avoid as much as possible functioning as an object of his sadistic tendencies. On the contrary, one would wish to show an almost detached, completely unruffled attitude and give similar advice to his wife or mother, thus removing the source of his unconscious gratification. The relevant point is not only that one can help such a patient accept the idea of a sanitarium much more by impressing him with the fact that it does not mean a thing to you whether he goes or not than by pleading for it. It is more than that. One helps him to learn that his attitude does not pay, that other attitudes pay better. In other words, just as people learn from "life," from experience, we give him an opportunity to learn in similar ways, with the difference that this experience is well directed by an adequate understanding of the patient's or client's internal and external setup and their interplay. It is clear that such learning from organized experience is possible only against the background of a well balanced relationship between worker and client, the development and control of which is again determined by the worker's understanding of the total situation.

Numerous examples could be added of the ways in which we may use our understanding of a client's structure for our planning. The presentation of cases with a more detailed and extended treatment of this type must be reserved for a more thorough discussion of the problems involved. We can certainly expect that with more systematic experience and with growing insight the field of application will broaden successfully.

# Psychiatric Principles in Casework

GRETE L. BIBRING, M.D.

I SHOULD LIKE to concentrate on one question that has held my interest from the beginning of my personal contact with casework. Previously I had encountered the same problem in my work at the Extension School for Teachers of the Vienna Psychoanalytic Institute; lately it has occurred again in my attempts to teach medical students and doctors how to apply dynamic psychiatry to general medicine and to the medical specialties. The question widens the topic of this symposium to a more general one; namely, what can psychoanalysis offer to the professions that deal with human problems and adjustments in one form or another? To what extent and in what way can psychoanalytic principles be assimilated by these professions?

There are two main possibilities. The first is best represented by a trend observable in some of the mentioned professional groups; that is, after contact with psychoanalytic techniques, to take them over in a somewhat modified form and to use them as the predominant or exclusive tool, thus largely replacing the traditional professional functions and skills. This refers not only to some groups in casework but also in clinical psychology, education, and even in the field of general medicine. It may be due to the difficulties that people encounter in their dealings with human problems or to the fascination that comes with the new understanding, that the non-psychiatrist often surrenders to psychiatry so completely. As the specialty that has systematic information on these problems, psychiatry seems to

Reprinted from *Journal of Social Casework*, 30:230-235, 1949.

hold a promise of final solutions—a promise which it does not always keep, not even for the psychiatrist. Often there ensues the wish to convey this knowledge to the client or patient in the form of direct interpretation.

To illustrate the tendency to identify psychotherapy with insight therapy and to see in interpretation the fundamental tool of dealing with personality problems, I should like to quote from a recent article (Ormsby, 1948):

> When the client's achievement of a fair degree of social adjustment is blocked by emotional difficulties, the caseworker must consider the techniques of interpretation as an essential part of psychotherapy. . . . If we can help the client to understand material that is "almost on the tip of his tongue" but is just short of verbalization, the way may be cleared for the client later to bring material from deeper layers of repression to the sub-surface which may then be susceptible to interpretation.

The second possibility consists of a true integration of the principles of psychoanalytic psychiatry and therapy into the aims and skills of the respective professions, that is, in utilizing them in various typical ways in which they can be applied to the different fields. In a recent article (G. Bibring, 1947) I discussed some of the relations between psychoanalysis, psychotherapy, and casework, attempting to show how basic knowledge and basic principles of techniques are employed differently in these three fields, according to their different goals. I tried to demonstrate that casework methods of helping people to adjust to their social tasks comprise more than conveying "insight"; that the principles of abreaction, clarification, and manipulation find a wider application in casework than interpretation proper (in the sense of offering insight into unconscious material).

We all know how important psychiatric knowledge is for the interviewing technique—how much more pertinent information we can gather, how much more meaningful the gained material becomes if we bring to it a profounder understanding of psychological processes. This knowledge is certainly necessary for intelligent clarification, which consists of attempts to bring to the patient's attention feelings and attitudes which are vague and obscure but which still are on a conscious or preconscious level. Clarification helps the patient to gain an adequate perspective of his problems—a step in the direction of understanding himself and, consequently, of handling his problems differently. Furthermore, psychiatric knowledge is important for the understanding and handling of the transference situation and for the careful observation and control of the countertransference. Above all it plays an important role in the skill of "manipulation."

We do not use the term "manipulation," as it sometimes is used in casework, to describe the undesirable attempt of the worker to force his concepts and plans on the client. We use the term in a more positive sense. After listening to and observing the client we may use our understanding of his personality structure, his patterns, his needs and conflicts, and his defenses in order to "manipulate" him in various ways. We may make suggestions as to what steps may or may not help this individual to cope better with his problems; we may plan with him as to his emotional, professional, and recreational activities; we may give appropriate advice to members of his environment; we may modify our attitude and approach to his problems; or we may purposely activate relevant emotional attitudes in the client for the sake of adjustive change. It is in this specific sense that we use the term "manipulation."

Before discussing it further, I should like to present some clinical examples, somewhat simplified, in order to show the application of this concept to various cases. The material is largely—not exclusively—taken from my experience in a general hospital in co-operation with the social service department and other personnel.

### Case 1

Data on Mrs. X., thirty years old, were presented by a social agency for psychiatric consultation about her marital and vocational problems.

Her husband, a writer, had been employed steadily before their marriage, but since then had been working only irregularly, and lately had been out of work for quite a period. Mrs. X., therefore, took a well-paying but rather strenuous job in a war factory in order to provide for herself and her husband. She had recently been feeling tired. One day she fainted at work without any demonstrable reason and was advised to give up this type of work. Her husband then tried to take over the financial responsibility, but Mrs. X. developed symptoms of depression and Mr. X. then stayed home to take care of his wife. A quite similar incident had happened about two years previous when Mrs. X. had become depressed and Mr. X. had to leave his job to stay with her at home. But usually Mrs. X. was the wage earner and Mr. X. took life easier, wrote poetry, and went out with other women. Mrs. X. had turned to the agency in order to get help with a divorce, because of her husband's unfaithfulness, and to get advice about the kind of job that would not exhaust her as her last one had.

The childhood history of Mrs. X., as told to the worker, showed that she came from a nice family, had three younger sisters, and was her father's favorite. She had almost always taken care of her sisters, thus helping an ailing mother. In her teens, she fell in love with a musician. She gave him up because of her family's resistance. They did not want her to marry this man who, because he was an artist, might be an unreliable person. She left home suddenly in order to look after her next younger sister who, unbeknown to her family, was at that time illegitimately pregnant. Mrs. X. looked after her sister until the baby died, which happened shortly after the delivery. At this point, Mrs. X. felt ready to leave her sister and to marry.

Mrs. X. seemed like a nice, responsible, and competent person. Mr. X. gave the impression of being a less strong or competent personality, but he too seemed a likable man of considerable artistic talent. The question the agency raised was whether a divorce was necessary or whether Mrs. X. could be helped to solve her problems in a different way.

My first impression was that this woman lived according to a masochistic pattern. We can see that she had a tendency to sacrifice herself for the people close to her: for her family by taking care of her younger sisters, first in order to help her mother, and second, probably, in order to retain her father's approval. Her choice of the first love object was, according to the tradition of the family in which Mrs. X. grew up, an undesirable one because this type of man would exploit her and not stand by her as a husband. The following important step Mrs. X. made was again an act of mercy—giving up her own interests in order to help her sister carry the burden of her illegitimate pregnancy and motherhood. When this sacrifice became superfluous, Mrs. X. chose as a husband a man who was very similar to her first boy friend. This time she did succeed in marrying him because he seemed more reliable than her former fiancé. But she made it somehow possible for her husband to give up his employment and live on her income; when he decided to go back to work, Mrs. X. interrupted this activity twice by her depression, which forced him to stay at home with her.

On the basis of this material, I doubted strongly that Mrs. X. could come closer to solving her problems by getting a divorce, since one had to expect that she would probably soon get into a similar situation; that is, find another person who would need her help and self-sacrifices and take advantage of her. One fact seemed especially significant in this connection: Mr. X. had been a good worker before his marriage and obviously was deteriorating now under the influence of his wife's masochistic behavior; she apparently provoked tendencies existing in him which he had under better control prior to his marriage.

We suggested that only a little interpretation and clarification be given Mrs. X. at this time. Only her "behavior pattern" was pointed out to her in order to let her gain some perspective and make it possible for her to consider and observe her own unconscious share in her life experiences. Besides, it was suggested to the worker that she talk with Mrs. X. about the possibility that her behavior may have originated in her desire to be accepted by her father as the nicest and most responsible one among his four daughters, thus helping the client not to become confused and bewildered by her own behavior but to understand some of its meaning.

The important thing to decide was what attitude to take toward the patient and how to manipulate the situation in order to be helpful to her, since we could not provide intensive and prolonged treatment to achieve considerable structural changes. Both—attitude and manipulation—were based on our understanding of Mrs. X.'s masochistic personality. We felt that we should be very sympathetic, letting the client know that we appreciated her painful efforts to carry the burden for her husband, that we were aware of her difficulties in living with this type of man and of the amount of sacrifices she had made. (This was in intentional contrast to any attempt to emphasize her strength in the past or to suggest that she take her life easier—an approach which, in my opinion, would be more justified with a person whose problem is, for instance, anxiety or a feeling of loneliness or helplessness. But with any kind of masochistic personality it would only increase the tendency to reach the masochistic goal: being loved for the suffering. She might, under this condition, unconsciously feel that she had not "done enough" for it and try to do more by more self-denial.)

Since we felt that her husband had to get back to normal, we suggested (based on the evaluation of Mrs. X.'s personality) that it was her responsibility, not to earn the living, but to help Mr. X. to fulfill his function as a man in which he had failed by letting her take over the financial care. We tried to explain to her how essential it might be for this man to assert himself instead of becoming dependent and comfortable under her protection. This changed her role of a breadwinner into the position of an understanding wife; from direct masochistic suffering to moral responsibility.

The next step consisted of helping the client to direct her unchanged masochistic pattern into different channels. Instead of work in a factory, we suggested that she should work as a nurse's aide, and, later on, take up some training in nursery school work. Through this, we hoped, if Mrs.

X. was under the compulsion to repeat her behavior to serve others so that she would be loved, it would be done in a more constructive way than up to then, and outside of her family situation.

To summarize: Very little interpretation was given. The patient was made aware of her behavior pattern and its significance for her life, especially her marriage and its failure. Her basic need was redirected into helping her husband to regain his former status; simultaneously, a more sublimated direct gratification was offered in the form of more adequate professional activities. It seemed justified to neglect other obvious tendencies. The main technical principles employed in this case were clarification and redirective manipulation.

### Case 2

A boy of eighteen came to our hospital with a severe physical condition. Psychiatric consultation was requested because he presented a behavior problem. He was, in spite of his severe sickness, rather unruly and difficult. He started fights, insulted the young doctors, threw on the floor food that the dietitian had just brought for him. He refused to do exercises the physiotherapist requested. Because of all this, transfer to a Veterans Hospital was considered. The anamnesis showed that he had been taken off a sinking ship after hours of standing in cold water in the machine room. He had been on this ship on a secret mission, but he did not want to give any further information on it. It seemed obvious, nevertheless, that the patient was keen about letting people know that he was involved in some kind of underground activity: he had asked immediately that his bed be put in a corner so that if he talked in his sleep nobody would hear him.

During the last part of the war, before he went on this trip and while still a rather young boy, he had been in the Marines. Prior to this, he was employed as a war worker in a plant, although he avoided helping in the store owned by his family where he was urgently needed. He had the feeling that by his plan he could serve the "cause" better. He had run away from high school when a teacher doubted his honesty: he had reported that he had a headache and had to go home, but the teacher wondered whether he did not look too well for a sick boy. After this episode, the patient refused to return to school. When he was visiting in his father's shop as a boy of fourteen and businessmen came in to see Mr. M. (his father), the patient would introduce himself as Mr. M. If the customer refused to take him seriously as a partner for business negotiations, the patient angrily demanded that he leave.

He was a sensitive, difficult patient on the ward and the words one heard most frequently from him were: "Who are you to tell me?" Everything pointed here toward a very narcissistic, adolescent attitude, with anxiety, behind this defense. There was material that indicated that this fear referred primarily to his father.

In our treatment—which, first of all, served the purpose of coping with his very disturbing and self-damaging behavior—we strictly avoided, for the whole acute period, touching on his basic conflicts, nor did anybody talk directly about his misbehavior or about his lack of co-operation. We started out on the assumption that for a boy of his structure the acute disease, which interrupted his important adventures, acted as a severe blow to his self-esteem. Thus his underlying insecurity was aroused, which he tried to master, according to his habitual defense pattern, by an exaggerated aggressive performance.

On the basis of this impression we changed our approach completely. No pressure or direct persuasion, no criticism of his acts were used. We referred frequently to his unusual past, how bad he must feel that he could not go on with his buddies for the time being; what it must mean for a young man with his urge to be active and heroic to lie flat on his back in a hospital. In a cautious interview, I wondered whether he sometimes feared that his buddies who went back into another ship thought that he stayed behind because he had lost courage, that he was a deserter. He confessed that this idea made him feel very bitter. It was interesting to find out why he had thrown the food on the floor—not a very appreciative attitude toward the dietitian who tried so hard to prepare the nicest dishes for him. When asked about the food, he complained that "these fancy salads are no food for a man." He wanted no "sissy" trimmings.

The staff was instructed to deal with this patient with special respect in every contact. The therapeutic activities and demands, including the painful exercises conducted by the physiotherapist, were not suggested in a comforting, soothing form but discussed with him as rather difficult tasks which are for the average patient of his age usually hard to accept but which one could perhaps expect a young man of his courage and stamina to carry out faithfully. The dietitian came up and took the boy's "orders" for the day's menu as if he were a general.

The change that took place in the patient's reaction was rather marked and sudden. He turned into a co-operative and easily manageable patient, made friends with the doctors and nurses, accepted diet and physiotherapy, all of which was essential in order to achieve any therapeutic progress in his severe and painful condition. It is beyond doubt that any attempt to meet his initial behavior with firmness and counter-aggression would have only led to more scenes and finally to his removal from the hospital.

Summary: In this case an acute problem of adjustment was dealt with by manipulation in the sense of adjusting the attitudes of the persons around him to the patient's basic needs. Through it his anxiety and insecurity were reduced, his need for self-assertion considerably met, and his aggressive defenses thus rendered unnecessary. One may speak of manipulations through attitude, or, since such "attitude" acts as a new experience on the patient, of manipulation through experience. It remains to be discussed whether such experience may have a more lasting influence.

### Case 3

To give one more instance of a general nature which one might easily encounter in casework or counseling or in medical practice, I should like to cite the case of a mother who reacts to the adolescence of her daughter with signs of psychological strain and severe headache. She may come to an agency to get help in handling her daughter; she may visit her doctor in order to get help for her fatigue or headache. In such a case there are various possibilities open, according to the respective personality type of the mother. If the mother's personality is one closer to hysteria, one may try to show her the importance of the adolescent phase, the promise that lies in the still confused state, the things that are nice about it, and may plead with her to understand, to help, and to enjoy it. In the case of an obsessional mother, one would better turn to the discussion of the problems and difficulties of adolescence, and not so much to the beauty of it. We would not ask such a mother to be happy about the beginning freedom of her daughter (which may just be the unconscious cause for her conflicts and anxiety). We would suggest methods of handling the situations that arise in adolescence. We would try to replace for this mother the system she applied in order to raise a well-behaved child by a new system of responsibility in her behavior and reactions toward the adolescent.

In brief, we utilize in these different types of personality their characteristic emotional structures, their physical potentialities, partly in order to prevent conflicts, tensions, anxieties, and defenses, partly in order to effect adjustive change. One may speak of manipulation in the form of mobilizing certain emotional systems in a given patient and utilizing them for the purpose of adjustment.

I have tried to demonstrate how, with little or no interpretation, with some clarification, but essentially with the aid of manipulation in its various forms, we attempted to solve sometimes quite severe problems of adjustment. One may ask whether this is reliable help, whether these results are comparable to those achieved in psychotherapy. Before answering these questions I would like to quote a case from the literature.

Karl Abraham, one of the pioneers of psychoanalysis, published an interesting article in 1925 (Fliess, 1949). In it he describes his contact as a military psychiatrist with N, a twenty-two-year-old swindler who from the age of 5 on was constantly breaking the law by stealing, forging, pretending social standing, and, later, higher military rank than was his real one, and so on. The basis of N.'s behavior was, according to the author, a severe rejection in childhood by both parents. Dr. Abraham felt rather pessimistic about any therapeutic results and expressed this viewpoint in his report to the military court.

Five years later Abraham met N. again. His career had changed suddenly some years ago. Since his marriage to an older, motherly widow whose sons were already grown up and independent, he had settled down completely and had become a very popular, respected member of the community. Abraham analyzed the constellation carefully: what infantile needs were fulfilled by this marriage, what conflicts avoided, so that it could lead to the obvious success. He wondered how long the change would last and the answer to this problem was offered by the former delinquent: as long as his relationship with his wife—whom he called his "little mother" —remained intact. Abraham called this "cure through love."

This spontaneous cure in life can be applied to the therapeutic situation by saying that a change achieved through manipulation may last as long as the transference lasts, and this we know lasts beyond the actual treatment and may be practically permanent. But more than pure transference cure seems to be involved. Manipulation offers in many ways a new experience to the patient which may have a more or less lasting influence on him in the same way that similar experience in life may result in changed attitudes in a positive, or negative sense. As we know, the onset of a neurosis may be due to an isolated traumatic experience. On the other hand, a change of attitude, as, for instance, represented by religious, political, scientific, and other conversions, also frequently takes place in reaction to one more or less isolated experience. Adjustive change through a specific experience, which probably happens only rarely in life, can be approximated in the therapeutic setup, including casework therapy.

Without being too modest we have to admit that even with intensive psychotherapy we do not always achieve permanent results, especially if outside conditions remain unfavorable. Besides, such adjustive changes seem worthwhile, since many persons who could never be reached by the psychiatrist and many who do not need direct psychiatric treatment can be helped through this method.

I think, therefore, that casework should remain flexible and not take over one or the other of the existing *methods* of psychotherapy, but that it can and should assimilate—within its own framework—certain fundamental *principles* of psychotherapy and apply them according to its own goal and to the structure of the individual case.

# Psychoanalysis and the Dynamic Psychotherapies

EDWARD BIBRING, M.D.

A COMPARATIVE STUDY as defined by the title . . . can be approached in different ways. In the following paragraphs an attempt is made to approach the task from a technical point of view by applying to it a conceptual scheme consisting of certain basic concepts of psychotherapy, which are called therapeutic principles and procedures, and which are considered to be applicable to all methods of psychotherapy independent of their respective ideologies or theoretical systems.

## I

To start with the terminology: 1. We make a distinction between "technical" and "curative" application of the principles, notwithstanding the fact that they are frequently overlapping, the former referring to the techniques employed in the various psychotherapies, the latter to the factors or agents which are responsible for the adjustive changes by originating or constituting them. The term "therapeutic'" comprises both the technical as well as the curative aspect of the treatment process.

2. The term "techniques" refers to any purposive, more or less typified, verbal or nonverbal behavior on part of the therapist which intends to affect the patient in the direction of the (intermediary or final) goals of the treatment. One can roughly distinguish between five groups of basic techniques: (a) suggestive; (b) abreactive; (c) manipulative;[1] (d) clarifying; and (e) interpretive techniques (G. Bibring, 1947, 1949).

---

Reprinted from *Journal of the American Psychoanalytic Association*, 2:745-770, 1954.

[1] Some objection has been raised against the terms "manipulation" and "manipulate." To my mind there are no more suitable terms available. They are used here in a completely neutral sense.

3. The term "curative agents" relates to those psychic forces in the patient which are brought about by the corresponding techniques and which in turn constitute or originate those changes which we call curative effects. Thus, suggestive techniques result in suggestion (in the sense of induced irrational beliefs); abreactive techniques bring about relief from acute tension through emotional discharge; manipulative measures correspond to a number of curative agents which may be outlined under the general heading "learning from experience"; and finally the techniques of clarification and interpretation which produce the corresponding types of insight, which we propose to call insight through clarification and insight through interpretation.

4. The principles are supplemented by the processes and procedures which constitute the total course of a treatment process and represent more complex concepts. Though they are most intimately interwoven, it seems possible to separate four major types of therapeutic operations, namely: (a) the production of material; (b) the utilization of the produced material, (mainly) by the therapist and/or by the patient; (c) the assimilation by the patient of the results of such utilization; and (d) the processes of reorientation and readjustment. I shall refer to these partial activities as basic therapeutic procedures (as far as the technical operations of the therapist are concerned) or therapeutic processes (with reference to the activities going on in the patient).

We believe that these basic therapeutic (technical and curative) principles and basic therapeutic procedures and processes furnish a suitable framework of references for the technical analysis of the concrete individual treatment processes as well as for the comparative study such as the one suggested by the title of this panel, for we shall see later on that the dynamic psychotherapies (by which term we understand methods derived from psychoanalysis proper) are characterized by particular selections and combinations of the basic principles with their inherent goals, and by certain modifications of the procedures.

II

I shall discuss briefly the therapeutic principles first.

1. To begin with *suggestion*. The psychiatric meaning of the term refers to the induction of ideas, impulses, emotions, actions, etc., in brief, various mental processes by the therapist (an individual in authoritative position) in the patient (an individual in dependent position) independent of, or to the exclusion of, the latter's rational or critical (realistic) thinking.

In psychotherapy, suggestion—frequently combined with hypnosis—is purposefully employed in a technical as well as in a curative sense. The technical employment of suggestion aims at the promotion of the treatment process in its various aspects. Technical suggestion may be predominantly formal (for example, to induce the patient generally to fantasy or to dream, whatever fantasy or dream it may be) or predominantly content suggestion (for example, to dream about specific topics or to remember specific events). Curative suggestion aims at that direct change which is characteristic of induction of beliefs, be it a negative belief (denial: making symptoms or attitudes "disappear"), or a positive one (inducing desirable attitudes, etc.). In modern psychotherapy therapeutic suggestion, in the stricter sense, seems less frequently applied, as compared with the employment of technical suggestion. Suggestion is frequently used in the service of other therapeutic agents. On the basis of a more or less intimate knowledge of the personality, suggestion is purposefully employed, with or without hypnosis, in numerous ways such as to facilitate emotional expression, to help the patient face reality, to overcome or to circumvent resistance, to produce recollections, fantasies and dreams or imaginary or symbolic conflicts, to tolerate anxiety or depression, to encourage the finding of new solutions, even to gain "insight," etc. Many problems are implied in these applications of suggestion which to discuss is beyond the scope of this paper.

2. *Abreaction* or emotional discharge played an important role in the cathartic method as employed by Breuer and the early Freud, the underlying theory being that dammed-up tensions which have found abnormal discharge, such as in symptoms, must be revived in memory and the normal expression re-established mainly in the form of emotionally charged verbalization.

At present, however, the therapeutic significance of abreaction represents a controversial issue. Some therapists emphasize its value in the belief that plain abreaction, as such, cures in a kind of automatic or mechanical way as a one-act treatment; others dispute its curative values regarding the common neuroses or deny it completely. A brief historical survey may help to clarify the question.

The concept of abreaction has suffered from certain ambiguities due to the fact, first, that the three different etiological conceptions were originally presented together: the conceptions of hypnoid hysteria (Breuer-Freud), of retention hysteria (Freud), and that of defense hysteria (Freud); and second, that the concept of "abreaction" underwent a change of function with the development of psychoanalysis proper.

Abreaction as a one-act therapy referred only to the "pure" retention hysteria which was etiologically the simplest type of hysteria, in that for social and similar reasons the "reaction" (emotional discharge) did not occur, but without causing any dissociation of the mind (Freud, 1893, p. 60).

It was different with the two other forms of hysteria, hypnoid and particularly defense hysteria, where splitting did occur: in the former passively and prior to the traumatic events, in the latter actively and as the result of the warding off of upsetting impressions or ideas. In both cases the therapy was assumed to consist of two steps. The first consisted in a complete abreaction of the affects, in form of verbalization, simultaneously with the reminiscence of the events. The request that the traumatic impression should be remembered in all clarity, details, completeness, and intensity, obviously served the purpose of finding all emotional "pockets," of achieving full abreaction. In other words, not the slightest quantum of emotional tension should be left dissociated as a source of symptom formation.

The second step referred to the necessity that the pathogenic "idea" also had to be dealt with. To quote Freud:

> By providing an opportunity for the pent-up affect to discharge itself in words the therapy deprives of its effective power the idea which was not originally abreacted; by conducting it into normal consciousness (in light hypnosis) it brings it into associative readjustment or else dispels it by means of the physician's suggestion, as happens in cases of somnambulism combined with amnesia [Freud, 1893, pp. 40-41].

According to this view, the healing process consisted of several different activities: (1) the recollection of split-off experiences which makes them accessible to the influence by the conscious personality; (2) the transformation of an emotionally strong idea into a weak one through abreaction, i.e., through the discharge in normal ways of displaced emotional tensions, thus make the "idea" manageable; (3) the adjustment of the idea which had been deprived of its intensity, by way of normal working-off mechanisms or by countersuggestion. The term abreaction refers only to the first two aspects of the total process, strictly speaking only to the second one. Thus abreaction, being a part of a therapeutic process cannot be conceived of as one-act therapy "automatically" resulting in cure.

The change in the concept of the function of abreaction was a logical consequence of the further development of psychoanalytic theories and techniques, primarily of the development of the concepts of defense and resistance with the subsequent abandonment of the trauma theory of the neuroses, of hypnosis and with the introduction of the method of free association. Abreaction, now in the sense of "emotional reliving," came to be thought of as offering evidence and establishing conviction in the patient as to the actuality of his repressed impulses, etc. Abreaction, originally considered a curative agent, thus came to be employed as a technical tool in the process of acquiring "insight" through interpretation with all its implications and consequences. This difference in function between abreaction as curative principle and abreaction as technical principle in the process of insight is illustrated, among others, by the fact that the first function required maximum intensity, whereas the second function requires optimal intensity, not too little, and not too much.

Abreaction as a curative principle is to a certain degree maintained in acute emotional conditions. It is a generally recognized fact that acute or chronically retained emotions cause uneasiness, and that finding a normal outlet for them offers sometimes considerable, though only temporary, relief. It is well known that cathartic therapy plays an important role in the treatment of the acute traumatic neuroses including the traumatic neuroses of war, particularly those combined with amnesia or similar conditions due to acute repression of overwhelmingly upsetting impressions. An additional factor of its therapeutic significance in such cases is the preventive function of abreaction, in that early abreaction of acute traumatic impressions frequently prevents the development of a "chronic neurosis."

What then is the curative mechanism of abreaction? Various therapeutic principles other than "abreaction" (i.e., discharge of emotional tension) are involved in the process of emotional expression. In verbalizing feelings, thoughts, reactions, impulses, conflicts, etc., one learns to see them more clearly, in a more objective perspective. Emotional expression of painful tendencies, when met with sympathy, results in the gratifying feeling of being "accepted" and "understood," of sharing responsibility and thus offers reassurance. The active part played by the ego in such expression may gratify certain narcissistic needs, etc.

In brief, the curative value of emotional expression in the treatment of psychoneuroses is not due to abreaction itself, but to a combination with other principles such as manipulation and clarification which will be discussed in the following paragraphs.

3. The concept of *manipulation* covers a wide field of therapeutic measures. Crude forms of manipulation such as advice, guidance, and similar ways of running a patient's life, may be excluded from this dis-

cussion because they do not represent proper curative principles. Manipulation, in the sense used here, can be defined as the employment of various
emotional systems existing in the patient for the purpose of achieving
therapeutic change either in the technical sense of promoting the treatment, or in the curative sense, for manipulative measures too can be employed in a technical as well as a curative way (Hart, 1929, pp. 141f.).

Technical manipulation can be employed in a positive or a negative
form: either to produce favorable attitudes toward the treatment situation or to remove obstructive trends. To give a simple instance for the
latter: a patient comes to the therapist under some authoritative influences
which he seems to resent. When in reaction to this, the therapist makes the
patient understand that it is entirely left to his own free decision whether
or not to discuss his problems and that his decision, whatever it might
be, will be met with acceptance, the therapist re-establishes the patient's
freedom of choice and thus removes the motive for his resentment and fear
regarding the treatment.

This is technical manipulation in so far as it primarily serves to promote
the treatment (in this case, to keep the patient in it). It is also technical
manipulation when we assure a patient who is afraid of being influenced
"against his will and his better knowledge" that he should never accept
any explanation unless he is fully convinced of its validity and of the
evidence offered. It is manipulation in the sense of *neutralizing* certain
emotional forces which represent obstacles to the treatment. It is manipulation of the opposite, the *mobilizing* type when we try to promote the
treatment by persuading a phobic patient to expose himself to his fears
or by activating in other ways a patient's anxieties, feelings of guilt, etc.

More important are the therapeutic types of manipulation which intend to produce adjustive change, though it may be difficult at times to
separate the two functions clearly because one and the same measures may
serve both purposes. To cite again a simple instance: a patient comes to
the therapist for help, not because of a genuine desire to be helped, but
because he wants to please an authority who suggested the treatment.
When the therapist, aware of the situation, makes the patient feel that
he is expected to act on his own responsibility, the patient's desire to please
will influence him in the direction of assuming responsibility. This cannot
be considered as a case of technical manipulation only, particularly since
the patient has no objection to the treatment; it may appear rather as
a first step toward a new adjustment, even though it is initiated by utilizing the patient's desire to please. In such instances one may speak of
manipulation in the sense of *redirecting* emotional systems existent in a

patient toward "adjustive" change (from submissiveness toward independence).

There is another aspect of therapeutic manipulation, however, which is not covered by the types of manipulation discussed thus far. It may be called *experiential* manipulation. One may expose a patient to a "new" experience, new in the sense of not having been experienced before (or since childhood) either because the opportunity did not arise or because—more likely—the opportunity was not recognized due to inhibition or distorted conceptions. To examine the instances quoted above from this angle: the fact that in one case the therapist offered freedom of choice where the patient perhaps resentfully expected to be forced, and that in the other case the therapist did not simply accept the patient's submissiveness but encouraged and even expected him to assume self-responsibility, may be a first experience of this kind in the patient's relations to an authority. (His former experience or distorted conception may have been that authorities demand submission.)

There seems more to it: when the patient actually takes responsibility he may have another "new" experience. He learns—perhaps again for the first time—that he can take responsibility, and do so succesfully. Repeated experiences of this kind may increase his self-confidence and thus his capacity for self-responsibility. In other words, the patient has not only a novel experience in relation to an object (authoritative person) but also in relation to himself.

The common denominator of these therapeutic measures seems to be "influence through experience." Such experience may neutralize or correct existent attitudes based on opposite (actual or imaginary) experiences in the infantile past or reinforce latent tendencies or perhaps even establish "new" emotional systems in the patient, which would act toward adjustive change. One may refer to it also as "learning from experience." Such impressions, if frequently repeated, may be equivalent to what has been called *emotional training* (Alexander & French, 1946).

To summarize: through our words or attitudes we may neutralize certain emotional systems in the patient, mobilize others and utilize them for technical purposes or curative aims; one can redirect existent emotional attitudes from neurotic toward adjustive goals, or one can intensify latent emotional systems favorable to readjustment which represent the patient's readjustive reserve; or one can, perhaps, establish "new" attitudes. To put it briefly, one can speak of two basic types of manipulation: a utilizing type and a formative type.

The boundary line between technical and therapeutic manipulation or between utilizing and creative therapeutic manipulation may frequently be difficult to draw, especially since one and the same manipulative activity may serve more than one purpose, as has been pointed out above.

The theoretical implications of therapeutic manipulation vary according to the type. The mobilizing and redirecting type do not present any serious problem. The "corrective" as well as the "formative" types of (manipulative) experience require further clinical and theoretical investigation. What are the dynamics of the effects of an "experience" in individual cases and in general? When have such impressions only a temporary effect, and when a lasting one? When are they more profound, when more superficial, i.e., of steadily growing, or of very limited effect? Under what conditions is a single experience effective (if this occurs at all), or a prolonged or repetitive experience required? What role does the type of neurosis and the type of the patient's personality play in this respect? Are some patients more accessible to "new experience," others more refractory? How much are certain constellations in the therapeutic interrelationship responsible for it, etc.? Finally the crucial question: what effects do such new experiences have on unconscious trends? The psychology of conversion could be helpful. Perhaps the conception of a "positive" adjustment promoting experience could be formed in analogy to the pathogenic trauma theory (Abraham, 1925a; Alexander, 1953).

4. Suggestion, emotional relief and manipulation per se do not furnish any self-understanding on the part of the patient. This is fundamentally different with the next two therapeutic principles, clarification and interpretation. They constitute the basic principles of what is called *insight therapy*, in the sense that the curative factor consists essentially in the extended self-understanding of the patient. As stated earlier, it is necessary to distinguish between two types of insight which differ not only dynamically but also in regard to the techniques employed to achieve them and to the type of material they are dealing with. I proposed to call the two types of insight—with reference to the techniques—insight through clarification, and insight through interpretation.

The term *clarification* was, to my knowledge, introduced into the vocabulary of psychotherapy by Carl Rogers. Clarification means to help the patient to "see much more clearly" (Rogers, 1942, p. 41), to achieve "clearer differentiation of the meanings of things to him" (Combs, 1948, p. 684), to "assist him to differentiate his personal organization more clearly" or to "gain a clearer and more accurate differentiation of his self-organization and its relationship to the world in which he moves" (Combs, 1948, p. 880). The therapist aids the client or patient to clarify his feelings, including the nature of his fears, object relationships, attitudes, the different choice of actions, etc. (Rogers, 1942, p. 381).

The technique of clarification—as characteristic of Rogers' (1942, p. 38) nondirective method—consists mainly in restating in more precise form the feelings which accompany the main train of thought by "verbalizing them in somewhat clearer form than he [the client] has put them," "by recognizing and stating their meanings clearly and sharply" (Combs, 1948, p. 884). This restating or reflecting has to be entirely based on the "statements" made by the client-patient; that means it must not transcend the phenomenological or descriptive level. It is evident that his "nondirective" technique is not the only one to achieve clarification.

The process of "clarification" is frequently contrasted by Rogers and his collaborators with the process of "interpretation" which is defined as the "attempt to change the individual attitude by means of explanation" of the "factors which underlie behavior" and of "the causes of specific behavior patterns" (Rogers, 1942, p. 25) or "to *inform* the client as to his patterns, to *interpret* his actions and his personality to him" (Combs, 1948, p. 195).[2] However, the difference between interpretation and clarification is not always clear as, for instance, in the following sentences: "Under certain conditions, it is possible to *interpret* to the client some of the material which he has been revealing. When the interpretation is based entirely upon statements which the client has made, and when the *interpretation is merely a clarification* of what the client has already perceived for himself, this type of approach can be successful" (Rogers, 1942, p. 196).[3]

Clarification, in the sense used here, does—*ex definitione*—not refer to unconscious (repressed or otherwise warded off) material but to conscious and/or preconscious processes, of which the patient is not sufficiently aware, which escape his attention but which he recognizes more or less readily when they are clearly presented to him. Many, if not all, patients are often rather vague about certain feelings, attitudes, thoughts, impulses, behavior or reaction patterns, perceptions, etc. They cannot recognize or differentiate adequately what troubles them, they relate matters which are unrelated, or fail to relate what belongs together, or they do not perceive of or evaluate reality properly but in a distorted fashion under the influence of their emotions or neurotic patterns. In brief, there is a lack of awareness (recognition) where awareness is possible. Clarification in therapy aims at those vague and obscure factors (frequently below

[2] Italics mine.
[3] Italics mine.

the level of verbalization) which are relevant from the viewpoint of treatment; it refers to those techniques and therapeutic processes which assist the patient to reach a higher degree of self-awareness, clarity and differentiation of self-observation which makes adequate verbalization possible.

We clarify the patient's feelings, e.g., when we show him that what he describes as fatigue or feeling of being tired is actually an expression of depression. It is clarification when we elaborate his patterns of conduct, demonstrating to him that he reacts in typical ways to typical situations; or that certain of his attitudes which appear to him unrelated are in fact related to each other, representing various manifestations of the same attitude or that certain reaction patterns form a characteristic sequence, etc. We clarify when we demonstrate to a patient that her enthusiasm about "analytic" minds which are readily aware of and skillfully elaborate differences of thought, feelings, etc., and her idea of two worlds which have to be kept apart (the clean and the dirty, the fine one and the low one, school and home, father and mother, etc.) and also her heightened interest in the conception of a class society and class struggle, etc., are various expressions of the same attitude. (Consequently, she was less appreciative of "synthetic" thinkers who were prone to discover more readily the common denominator between seemingly disparate things.) We clarify when we point out to a patient that his strong, nearly compulsive need to put books on a shelf side by side when they were "separated" by space; that his somewhat contented compulsive laughing when he witnessed people discussing in a friendly manner divergent conceptions of how to tackle a certain problem, or his passion to be the middleman between disputing parties, or his interest in telling people every friendly remark they made about each other, that all this represented related attitudes. (What Rogers [1942, p. 195] describes as "informing the client as to his patterns" is here subsumed under clarification.)

We clarify a patient's reality situation, for instance, when we separate the objective reality from his subjective distorted conception of it, when we make him understand the actual, perhaps neurotic motivations of his love objects' attitudes toward him, whereas he may have misinterpreted them as rejection or condemnation or attempts to dominate him, etc.

In all these therapeutic measures we are—by definition and in fact in so far as we exclude any references to unconscious warded-off material— dealing with vague, not adequately perceived or differentiated (conscious and/or preconscious) factors on a phenomenological descriptive level. Consequently clarification as a rule does not encounter resistance, at least not in the proper sense as originating from unconscious defenses against the material being made conscious, as it appears in reaction to interpretation. If resistance does occur, it is of a conscious nature or stems from heterogeneous generalized sources, "habitual" resistance (e.g., the fear of being influenced or criticized or rejected or misunderstood) or from a negative relationship with the therapist, etc., or when the therapist did not succeed in properly elaborating the patient's patterns or formulating them adequately. The latter form of resistance, e.g., has nothing to do with defenses but more with feelings of disappointment or fear or increased insecurity or confusion. As a rule patients react to (successful) clarification with surprise and intellectual satisfaction. The insight resulting from it provides—so to speak—a bird's-eye view for the patient with regard to his attitudes, feelings and impulses, character traits, and modes of conduct, in relation to himself as well as to the environment, his love objects, etc. By seeing his difficulties more clearly and in a more objective realistic perspective he is no longer overwhelmed or frightened by them; he is less "identified" with them; no longer takes them for granted, nor does he consider them as constitutional parts of his personality; in brief, he is less involved. In terms of energy, one may say that the charge of (neutral) ego energy which was added to the neurotic formations by a yielding ego thus reinforcing them ("co-cathexis") is withdrawn now and shifted onto the observing and discerning, differentiating, reality-testing functions of the ego which can now gain control over its difficulties. In general, the neurotic problems are not resolved in the process of clarification but are seen in a different light by a "detached ego." It seems justified, therefore, to consider insight through clarification as a curative agent, though of limited value. It is to a varying extent employed in nearly all forms of psychotherapy.

5. The insight gained through interpretation is dynamically different from that obtained through clarification. Interpretation in the sense as used here refers exclusively to unconscious material: to the unconscious defensive operations (motives and mechanisms of defense), to the unconscious, warded-off instinctual tendencies, to the hidden meanings of the patient's behavior patterns, to their unconscious interconnections, etc. In other words, in contrast to clarification, interpretation by its very nature transgresses the clinical data, the phenomenological-descriptive level. On the basis of their derivatives, the analyst tries to "guess" and to communicate (to explain) to the patient in form of (hypothetical) constructions and reconstructions those unconscious processes which are assumed to determine his manifest behavior. In general, interpretation consists

not in a single act but in a prolonged process. A period of "preparation" (e.g., in form of clarification) precedes it. Every interpretation, whether accepted by the patient or not, is considered at first as a working hypothesis which requires verification. This is done in the process of "working through," which thus has two functions. It serves as an empirical test in that it consists in the repeated application of the hypothetical interpretation to old and new material by the therapist as well as by the patient, inside and outside of the analytic session. By the same token it enables the patient (if the interpretation is correct) to assimilate it and thus to acquire full insight.

The fact that interpretations are explanatory concepts carries with it the danger of intellectualization. This term covers different meanings. It refers, on the one hand, to the defense mechanism of "intellectualization" (A. Freud, 1946) which consists in the transformation of unconscious conflicts into intellectual problems; e.g., when the patient is emotionally preoccupied with the problem of "free will" on a philosophical or meta-physical level but is actually trying in this way to deal with his unconscious problems of guilt and punishment in connection with death wishes against his parents and siblings. On the other hand, it refers to a form of resistance in that the patient "accepts" interpretations on the basis of their plausibility, their ability to make sense (i.e., to explain certain clinical data) but without "feeling" that it is so; or when the patient adopts the analytic language and readily produces all kinds of interpretations with great ease but without any emotion, etc.

Insight through interpretation is dynamically different from insight obtained through clarification. Whereas clarification results in the detachment of the ego (with the implication discussed above), interpretation causes the ego at first to become more involved, since it leads to the re-activation of painful tendencies, memories and conflicts. The effects of insight through clarification consist in "strengthening" the ego through greater objectivity, whereas insight through interpretation initiates a process of reorientation and learning which results in more adequate solutions of the pathogenic infantile conflicts. In practice the processes of interpretation are closely knitted together with the processes of clarification.

The technical and curative agents discussed so far are assumed to represent basic principles of psychotherapy. They proved to be helpful in studying the course of (recorded) therapeutic interviews from the point of view of what is actually going on in a given treatment process from a technical angle; more specifically, the study was concerned with the question of which of the principles (and under what conditions) was actually (and spontaneously) employed by the therapist at a given phase of the therapeutic process, i.e., within the constant interplay between him and the patient, etc. Such investigation is apt to furnish in return the basis for the establishment of a system of indications as to when and where and how to employ planfully in psychotherapy one or the other of the principles singly or in various combinations.[4] Finally it provides what we believe to be a suitable, though limited, frame of reference for a comparative study of the various methods of psychotherapy from a technical point of view. This formal technical approach has to be supplemented by the basic theoretical concepts of the respective psychological and psychopathological systems.

## III

It cannot be denied that there is some overlapping theoretically as well as practically between some of the principles. Suggestion, for instance, could just as well be discussed under the heading of manipulation, in the sense of using emotional systems existing in a given patient for the sake of promoting treatment and achieving cure. There is a difference, however, between suggestion and manipulation which can be defined in the following way: suggestion takes place exclusively within the transference situation, that is, suggestive techniques use emotional systems which constitute a primitive type of positive transference relationship, whereas manipulation proper aims at utilizing emotional forces outside and independent of the transference systems (for instance, when we evoke the patient's moral feelings or mobilize his latent anxieties or feelings of guilt or his narcissism, his pride, etc.) in order to achieve certain therapeutic aims (Hart, 1929, p. 141).

The various types of manipulation are in practice frequently closely interrelated. Letting a patient know that he need not accept any interpretation unless he is convinced neutralizes his fear of being forced into submission or influenced. Simultaneously, his need to form his own independent judgment may be stimulated. Finally, by the same statement the impression may be conveyed that his need for independence is accepted, and so on.

There exists—as mentioned above—a close relationship between abreaction on the one hand, and clarification and manipulation on the other.

---

[4] Such a study of the actual treatment process has been conducted at the Department of Psychiatry, Beth Israel Hospital, Boston, during the years 1948-1950.

Finally, the close relationship between clarification and interpretation has been pointed out.

Each of the curative principles implies a specific goal. Therapeutic suggestion proper aims at a symptomatic change (transference cure), at a "parasitic" change, so to speak, even where it seems to attack some of the causal determinants of the disorder. The goal of abreaction, in the strict sense of the term, is relief from tension and secondarily, in cases of acute traumatic neurosis, also prevention of chronic pathological formations. The various types of manipulation intend to produce changes by rearranging the dynamic field through "experience," either by neutralizing or activating or instituting certain emotional forces, and in this way promoting the establishment of a dynamic equilibrium. The principle of clarification aims at the detachment of the ego through more differentiated self-awareness and subsequently at a better control through a more realistic "knowledge" of himself and the environment. Finally, interpretation aims at those changes of the ego, and indirectly of the other functional systems of the personality, that permit to lift the unconscious conflicts to the level of consciousness with the result that the causal determinants of the various disorders are modified or removed.

## IV

The therapeutic principles are supplemented by the four therapeutic processes and procedures mentioned at the beginning, namely: first, the production of material; second, the utilization of material mainly by the therapist; third, the assimilation of the results of this utilization by the patient; and finally, the processes of reorientation and readjustment. Though they represent highly complex activities, and are in practice strongly overlapping, the usefulness of these concepts for a (comparative) study of the psychotherapies will justify their differentiation.

The process of *production of material* refers to the way in which it is produced: free association as in analysis; free communication, as in "nondirective" counseling; active interviews as in "directive" therapies, etc. The important point which cannot be discussed here is that the particular method of material production largely determines the scope and the quality of the produced material.

The material thus produced may be *utilized* in various ways, either only for understanding, or for guidance, advice, suggestion, relief, for manipulation, clarification, interpretation, etc.—exclusively, or in any combination. Here, too, one has to emphasize that the ways by which the material is utilized largely determine the type of material produced in return.

The process of *assimilation* refers to the patient's positive reaction to the activities of the therapist by which he makes use of the material, to their absorption by the ego and to those changes which we named "curative agents." The processes of assimilation are basic for the evaluation of any method of dynamic psychotherapy, since they represent the decisive links between the utilizing activities and the actual effects on the patient, the resulting curative changes. The true evaluation of the results of a given treatment method depends largely on whether it is possible to recognize the assimilative processes in their true dynamic function.

The processes of *reorientation and readjustment* are intimately linked up with the function of certain curative agents, such as the two forms of insight. They may require an additional, sometimes prolonged and repetitive process of testing out and learning. It is beyond the scope of this paper to discuss them here in detail.

## V

To turn now to psychoanalysis and the dynamic psychotherapies. I shall confine myself to the discussion of a few points to illustrate rather than to apply fully the approach tentatively outlined in the preceding pages. Before doing so, however, I would like to survey briefly the function of the therapeutic principles in the psychoanalytic treatment process.

In psychoanalysis proper, all therapeutic principles are employed to a varying degree, in a technical, as well as in a curative sense, but they form a hierarchical structure in that insight through interpretation is the principal agent and all others are—theoretically and practically—subordinate to it.

*Suggestion,* in the technical sense, is at work right from the beginning. When the patient has confidence in the analyst from the start, when he expects to be cured or markedly improved, though one does not guarantee anything and promises very little, this is due to suggestion. When later in the treatment he is encouraged to face painful experiences or the distress of frustration, this again is achieved with the help of the suggestion that this is a necessary step in the process of treatment and cure. (We have no actual proof for this to offer since we usually cannot demonstrate to the patient those who were treated successfully.) When we point out that better solutions exist to his old problems and that he will achieve mature pleasures instead of the neurotic gratifications and secondary gains, he usually believes us and follows our suggestive influence, though he sometimes has to give up what he actually has here and now in favor of something which he hopes to get in some, perhaps not too near, future, etc.

*Abreaction* as such plays a rather insignificant curative role in psychoanalysis. The patient may get relief from acute emotional tensions as they become reactivated in the therapeutic situation, but as curative agent abreaction has no place. It serves an important purpose, however, in offering evidence for the correctness of the interpretations and constructions and in providing conviction through emotional reliving of the past conflicts.

*Technical manipulation* has a wide range of application in analysis. It refers in the first place to the handling of the transference. The transference relationship of confidence is constantly interfered with by the reactivation of strong positive and negative neurotic tendencies. Adequate handling of the transference requires keeping an equilibrium between too little and too much reactivation. Besides this, all types of technical manipulation are employed in psychoanalysis; however, it is used less frequently the more the treatment progresses, i.e., interpretation replaces manipulation. We have, e.g., temporarily to neutralize what cannot be interpreted at the time, etc.

Therapeutic manipulation has a definite, though perhaps not sufficiently appreciated, function in analysis. The analyst's accepting attitude, his friendly neutrality and objectivity, his readiness to understand and not to judge, etc., represent not only technical tools which help the patient to release his self-expressions, but offer him also the "new" experience in relation to parental and other images as well as in relation to his own self, in a multitude of respects.

The most characteristic principles in analysis, however, are *clarification* and interpretation. *Interpretation* is the supreme agent in the hierarchy of therapeutic principles characteristic of analysis, in that all other principles are subordinate to it; that is, they are employed with the constant aim of making interpretation possible and effective. Particularly since the introduction of the ego-psychological approach which requires the broadest phenomenological exploration of behavior, clarification became a very important part of the psychoanalytic technique, not only in establishing the so-called therapeutic dissociation of the ego, but also, and more so, in carefully elaborating the patient's present and past pattern of behavior as a basis for interpretation (Kris, 1951; Waelder, 1939, 1945). The two techniques are intimately interwoven: interpretation follows clarification and vice versa. To quote (Kris, 1951): It starts with "singling out a patient's present patterns of behavior and arriving, by way of a large number of intermediate patterns, at the original infantile pattern. The present pattern embodies the instinctual impulses and anxieties now operative, as well as the ego's present methods of elaboration (some of which are stereotyped responses to impulses and anxieties which have ceased to exist). Only by means of the most careful phenomenology and by taking into consideration the ego mechanisms now operative can the present pattern of behavior be properly isolated out." Frequently the reason why the patient does not accept an interpretation is to be found in the fact that the clarification (elaboration) of the patterns of behavior did not proceed distinctly enough to make the patient accessible to their interpretation.

The basic therapeutic processes and procedures as discussed above have been mainly abstracted from the psychoanalytic process of treatment which makes full use of them in characteristic ways. Though they have to serve as a frame of reference for this comparative study, not more than a brief outline can be given here.

The analytic material consists, as a matter of principle, of the total verbal and nonverbal behavior of the patient. It is obtained in analysis mainly by the method of free association on the part of the patient and by careful observation of his behavior by the analyst. The goal of dynamic and genetic insight determines the scope and quality of the material and consequently the procedures. The essential point is to get the intimate and minute data which are of so much significance for analysis, for the understanding of the unconscious defensive and instinctual processes, and the reconstruction of the development looked for in analysis.

Utilization of the material takes place with the help of *all* principles, mainly in form of manipulation, clarification and interpretation, according to the requirements of the varying situations and the intermediary and final goals. The utilization is carried out more systematically, more exactly and more completely in modern classic analysis than before the introduction of the structural approach which comprises the total personality by taking detailed account of the ego and id aspect of present and past behavior patterns. To quote (Waelder, 1945): We are "inching downward and backward from a broad base of character study with a view to arriving at more exact reconstructions of unconscious fantasies and of the whole process of the neurotic career. . . . The ultimate technical ideal (of the approach) . . . . is actually to transform the neurosis into its earlier stages, and finally into the precipitating conflicts—to roll the process of neurosis back along the path of its development" (pp. 87-88).

The relative passivity of the analyst intends not to interfere too much with the spontaneity of the patient. The usual "rituals" mean not to inhibit the spontaneity of the patient and of the analyst. That they can be "misused" by the patient for purposes of resistance is well known and requires interpretive or manipulative measures. Situations of resistance or unproductive and nonresponsive cases require more activity on the part of the therapist, productive cases with good response less. The principle of passivity has been exaggerated by some analysts, but perhaps more so by its critics.

The process of assimilation takes place as a result of "working through," which includes the reactivation of the pathogenic infantile conflicts. It is this process of reliving which completes the process of assimilation by producing the final insight. This process of gaining insight through reactivation of the original conflict in the transference situation is particularly characteristic of psychoanalysis (Gill, 1954).

Confronting the ego with the "repressed" or otherwise warded off means to confront it with the task of reorientation and readjustment of finding new solutions to the partly reactivated infantile and later conflicts, on a mature level. The outcome of this process of "working out" depends on the learning capacities of the ego, its adjustive reserve, on the degree of its distortion, on the "strength" of the drives, and on the conditions of environment, etc. (Freud, 1938a). The result may consist in successful repression, in the abandonment of infantile positions, in their acceptance in modified form, in their absorption into the ego, etc.

The relationship between psychoanalysis and the various types of dynamic psychotherapies derived from it are characterized (1) by different selections and combinations of the therapeutic agents which imply a corresponding difference in goal; (2) by a modification of one or more of the four groups of therapeutic procedures; as a matter of fact any modification of one of the basic therapeutic procedures sooner or later carries with it corresponding changes in the other ones, either in their technical aspect or in their theoretical evaluation; (3) there seems to develop a general trend to shift the emphasis from insight through interpretation toward "experiential" manipulation, that is, learning from experience seems to become the supreme agent rather than insight through interpretation. One could add the minor tendency to consider the therapist as a catalyst and to leave to the patient most of the "working through" and "working out" of his problems. Some therapists go even farther by relying heavily on the patient's unconscious understanding.

Regarding point one, the main goal of analysis is, generally speaking, the type of change which results from the reactivation on the conscious level of the pathogenic conflicts. It is achieved mainly through interpretation. It consists—to put it briefly—in changes of the ego (undoing its fixations to pathogenic defense mechanisms, establishing the ego's freedom of choice which is further made feasible through the analysis of the motives of defense) and concomitantly through the ego in a change of the id (establishing the mobility and flexibility of the drives) and of the superego (mitigation and eventual extinction of the rigidity and severity of its archaic formations).

A different selection and combination of the basic therapeutic principles implies a correspondingly characteristic combination of the inherent goals, or in reverse, the goals characteristic of a given method of psychotherapy can be defined with reference to the goals inherent in the curative agents *actually at work* and their combinations. Rogers' "nondirective counseling" (client-centered therapy) may serve as illustration. It lends itself readily for such a purpose because of the relative transparency of its system. The nondirective therapy consists mainly in experiential manipulation (in the sense of offering the "new" experience of being accepted, of successfully assuming self-responsibility, etc., thus gaining in self-reliance and independence) and in clarification. Both seem to work on an equal level. Some authors, however, assume predominance of one over the other, one group being inclined to subordinate the principle of clarification to that of manipulation, whereas another group tends to assign the main role to the insight through clarification and to consider the manipulation toward independence as subordinate to it. Be that as it may, the inherent goal can be defined as the establishment of a realistic, objective perspective to oneself and to the environment, in an ego which is at the same time strongly manipulated toward independence and self-reliance. It is characteristic that even the production of material in client-centered therapy serves simultaneously as a manipulative measure, taking place in "independence" and self-responsibility with a minimum of help from the therapist. In brief, the strengthened ego will exert better control over the clarified reaction patterns, etc., which are seen now in an objective light.

Regarding point two, the various dynamic psychotherapies are characterized by the modification of one or more of the partial therapeutic processes and procedures of psychoanalysis, e.g., when various techniques are employed with the aim to accelerate any one of these operations. Accordingly, one can distinguish between psychotherapies whose technical modifications aim *predominantly* at the acceleration of the process of material production; or those which favor active and quick utilization;

those which tend to facilitate the process of assimilation, and finally those which focus on the acceleration of the processes of reorientation and readjustment.

It is evident that the techniques which aim at the production and utilization of the material can be more easily adjusted to the purpose of active psychotherapy than the processes of assimilation, particularly the achievement of insight through interpretation, and the process of readjustment.

Since production of material is the easiest process to speed up, many devices as to how to achieve this have been recommended and employed. It is common to all material-accelerating methods that they are confronted with the problems of assimilation. It seems relatively easy to obtain material through short-cuts (though the problem is that the short-cut method is bound to affect the type of material produced by it). It seems also easy to utilize it in one way or another, and least easy to influence the process of assimilation and readjustment.

Usually two ways of solving these problems are employed. One is of a predominantly theoretical nature, by adopting the classical abreaction theory or a modification of it (such as Ferenczi's "neocatharsis"). The production of material and the process of cure are assumed to be identical or coincidental, taking place in one act. Such theoretical reinterpretation seems apt to circumvent the problem instead of solving it. The second, technical, way out of the dilemma consists, e.g., in employing a two-act treatment, trying first to "expose" the unconscious material "directly," and then to aid the patient actively in the process of assimilation and readjustment, e.g., in manipulating him in various ways (e.g., by "emotional training").

This leads us to the third point, namely, to the shift in emphasis from insight through interpretation to experiential manipulation. It seems to have become a common trend in various methods of dynamic psychotherapies. Alexander and French's (1946) statements may serve as illustration of this shift: "Insight is frequently the result of emotional adjustment and not the cause of it." And: "The role of insight is overrated."

In child analysis (particularly with unusual children) and in psychotherapy of delinquents and psychotics this shift of emphasis represents a legitimate adaptation of the method of psychoanalysis to special conditions. Now this shift is applied to the original method (Gill, 1954). This shows not only in the technique, but also, to some extent, in the attempt to adjust the theory of neurosis to the manipulative technique, as for instance in form of a revival of the original trauma theory or in adapting the theory that neurosis originates from failure in interpersonal relationship in infancy and childhood (Waelder, 1945).

Be this as it may, the increasing tendency among certain groups of psychotherapists to rely on manipulative principles in combination with or in place of insight makes a theory of experiential manipulation for its proponents a very urgent task.

# Teaching Medical Psychology

# Psychiatry and Medical Practice in a General Hospital

GRETE L. BIBRING, M.D.

VARIOUS INTERESTING facets of the complex problem pertaining to the integration of psychiatry and medicine have been presented of late by a great number of psychiatrists and internists. The purpose of this paper is not to discuss "psychosomatic medicine" or psychiatry as a medical specialty concerned mainly with neuroses and psychoses, but rather to delineate certain important aspects of the role of psychologic thought in medical practice. When referring to psychologic thought, I have in mind psychoanalytically oriented psychology, or what is frequently called dynamic or depth psychology. This psychologic system maintains that there is more to a person's emotional processes than appears on the surface and that his behavior patterns and attitudes are the result of conflicts between his deep strivings and his defensive methods against these strivings developed in a slow adaptive process under the impact of environmental pressures and demands. However fixed these habitual behavior patterns may seem, one may recognize and diagnose the original underlying conflict. These conflicts are revived and intensified in times of stress. Illness always has to be understood as a stress situation, potentially traumatic and threatening to the psychologic equilibrium.

In this context the psychiatric—or, better, the medicopsychologic and medicopsychotherapeutic—approach is a most helpful tool, providing insight into the patient and into oneself, and increasing the doctor's skill within his own specialty by blending his medical knowledge with the

Reprinted from the *New England Journal of Medicine*, 254:366-372 (February 23), 1956 understanding of the patient's personality and psychological needs. There are three main areas in which this knowledge proves to be especially helpful.

### The Diagnostic Area

Differential diagnosis between organic and psychogenic conditions is of utmost significance. The diagnosis of psychogenic origin cannot be made simply by exclusion—for example, the fact that no organic basis can be found for a patient's symptoms is certainly not sufficient grounds for a diagnosis of hypochondriasis. Hypochondriasis is a specific entity, characterized by a pathologic, anxious preoccupation with one's body, by the tendency to describe the subjective symptoms in an irrational, unrealistic form and by the tenacity of the complaints and an over-all suspicious attitude toward the doctor's reactions and comments. Another diagnosis that is frequently ventured on this general basis is that of hysteria. Hysteria is also a specific neurosis, in which the body's functions or dysfunctions are used to express certain meaningful emotional experiences or fantasies. It is characterized by phobic or conversion symptoms, or both, by a dramatic onset and by other signs of the hysterical personality. In brief, the diagnosis of a psychiatric condition must be made, like any medical diagnosis, only on the basis of positive clinical findings.

The differential diagnosis can be further complicated if there are anxiety reactions to organic disease or neurotic symptoms whose onset precedes and that are not directly related to the existing organic conditions. The difficulties of correct diagnosis under such circumstances are admittedly great, even for the psychiatric specialist, but there is reason to believe that they will diminish as medical schools and postgraduate training centers become increasingly aware of the importance of psychiatric knowledge and incorporate it into their teaching programs.

### The Therapeutic Area

#### Psychotherapeutic Medicine

Not every psychiatric diagnosis requires intervention by the psychiatrist. The case may remain in the hands of the medical specialist for reasons of medical management as long as the diagnosis does not refer to a gross emotional disturbance. To decide such questions a psychiatric consultation may be necessary.

Beyond these special cases there is a broad, general area in medicine in which psychologic knowledge is basic and indispensable. I believe that this insight is necessary for the doctor to judge, first of all, what to tell a patient about his disease and how to inform him without traumatization but also without arousing his distrust that essential information is withheld. There is a great difference between the type of patient who "must not know" ("it is his doctor's responsibility") and the other who "*has* to know" and "does not want to be deceived."

A second problem is how to mobilize in the patient the greatest readiness to co-operate and accept the medical procedures and thus to share the responsibility with his doctor—whether by keeping the recommended bed rest or the dietary restrictions or by carrying out exercises in physiotherapy and so forth.

Third, the physician should know how to consult with the family, so that he may add to his medical efforts the support of essential figures in the patient's environment if this proves necessary.

Finally, one should learn how to plan convalescent care or rehabilitation most effectively.

To illustrate the helpfulness of correct appreciation of psychologic factors, one may cite the case of a patient with myocardinal infarction who also suffers from claustrophobia. When taking his bed rest alone in his room, this patient is thrown into panic. Since it is equally undesirable to expose a patient to physical or emotional exertion, he is permitted to take his "bed rest" in a deck chair on the front lawn.

More subtle and requiring deeper understanding is the question of what should be done with a forty-five-year-old man with myocardial infarction who has been accustomed to leave his bed every morning by way of a somersault. He is not an acrobat, which might make his behavior seem less noteworthy, but a "master electrician," as he constantly called himself—not just an electrician. This man, called "the Tiger" by the medical service because of his roaring irritability, came to the attention of the Psychiatric Department because, in spite of strict bed rest and prohibition even to shave, he fought with his sisters and slapped two of them at different visiting hours. He became highly excited and upset; the medical service considered restraining him in his bed. If one could understand what causes a man to leave his bed with a somersault in the morning in spite of being forty-five years of age and not a professional acrobat and why he calls himself, without any provocation, not an electrician but a master electrician, one might also learn to understand how to proceed in his medical management so that he could be kept in bed more quietly.

Before attempting this, one may consider more carefully the psycho-

logic aspects of four patients lying in bed next to each other—all with
the diagnosis of tuberculosis and all refusing to go to a tuberculosis sanatorium.

### The Overconcerned, Worrying Patient

This type of patient appears anxious, is often phobic toward medical
procedures such as hypodermics, talks to many people about "T.B.," tries
to find out from nurses and visitors about his condition, asks his doctors
over and over again how dangerously sick he is, observes with apprehension and obvious involvement the sickest people on the ward and, quite
flustered, refuses to go to the sanatorium.

### The Self-willed, Independent Patient

He seems somewhat aloof, keeps to himself or runs the ward, knows
everything a little better than anyone else, including the professional staff.
He does not like to talk about his sickness and is inclined to make light
of it. He is sure he can manage on his own and adamantly refuses to go
to a sanatorium.

### The Dependent, Demanding Patient

He is always in the doctor's way, resents it deeply if one spends less
time with him on rounds than with a dying neighbor, and turns to the
physician with every question that he could probably solve on his own
(whether he should chew or swallow his pills, take them with water or
juice, whether he can lie on his back at night, and so forth). He is dis-
inclined to let anybody distract him from his illness or, as he puts it, "make
light" of his condition. In spite of this, one gains the impression that he
does not take his medication regularly when nobody is around to pay
attention to him. In general, he seems to mind being sick less than not
being taken care of with the most devoted and intense attention. He plead-
ingly refuses to leave the hospital and go to the sanatorium.

### The Hostile, Querulous Patient

He likes to start arguments with everyone. Nothing is right—neither
the food, nor the care, nor the thinking of the doctors or nurses. Nobody
can fool *him*. Nobody can take it easy with *him* and shove him off to a
sanatorium and thus get rid of the responsibility for him.

## Anxiety Based on Disease

Observing the difficult behavior of these four patients, one can classify them as four different types. It does not seem too far-fetched to assume that all of them suffer from anxieties connected with the diagnosis of tuberculosis. They cannot deny the threat of this illness, though they may try very hard to do so. The idea of an institution, with all its implications, and the ensuing reality problems seem to increase their anxiety and tension. But each of them reacts to this anxiety with his characteristic habitual methods and attitudes. These behavior patterns have to be understood as part of the patient's personality. They represent his leading reactions to stress and are the result of a long history of adjustment. In brief, as he grows up with his constitutional endowment and environmental experiences, he learns to find ways and compromises between his needs and wishes on the one hand and the prohibitions against fulfilling them at any price and at every moment on the other. If these inner conflicts between impulses and defenses arrive at a certain equilibrium in the adjustment process, the results of it appear as personality traits. In times of increased conflicts, as under the pressure of anxieties, these personality characteristics increase in intensity in the attempt to maintain the inner balance. They therefore become more marked and less manageable than under average life conditions. This is the reason why the four patients behaved as described. It can easily be understood that none of them in their mounting anxiety could be expected to act differently, even though this would make it easier for him and for his doctor. One must therefore ask at this point not so much what one can request from the patient, but what one can do to help him overcome his emotional resistance so that he can accept his doctor's recommendations.

In the *overconcerned, worrying patient* every potentially threatening situation will be linked with and increased by a variety of old anxieties, mainly stemming from childhood; sometimes, they are of quite irrational character, like the early nightmares. The patient's main problem lies in the helplessness of his childlike state and in the fact that these imagined dangers are almost always far more threatening than the reality may be. Thus, for the doctor in charge, two main avenues of approach are indicated, the first being to give the child in the patient the feeling of being protected by a strong, knowing, helpful doctor. It is the overly anxious patient with whom the doctor can take the position of the omnipotent, omniscient parental figure of the early years of childhood—a role that incidentally would create quite a problem with the next type, the "self-willed, independent" patient. Furthermore, in recognition of the fact that this overconcerned patient's imagination usually exceeds by far the actual danger of his illness, it is advisable to discuss with him the facts of his disease and the rationale of the treatment and of the expected cure. This will have to be done in a simple, appropriate, comprehensible form, with avoidance of any frightening or vague formulations. Never must one forget that what seems for the experienced doctor an ordinary phrase or everyday professional term may have a most alarming connotation for the worried lay person.

*The self-willed, independent patient* is accustomed to handling his apprehensions by being strong and by acting decisively, not letting any feeling of anxiety or insecurity develop. He is the patient who must not be patted on the head and told soothingly that everything will be all right. He must not be told that everything will be taken care of by his doctor or family or friends. This for him merely emphasizes the fact that he is sick and helpless and therefore, which he can tolerate least, weak. In contrast to this, one should let him know that one appreciates the difficulty in which he, as a man of his responsibilities, finds himself suddenly through his illness. But it also has to be emphasized at the same time that one does believe in his strength. "A man like you can do the seemingly impossible and accept the reality of the disease," represents the most helpful and acceptable approach. In brief, to maintain his equilibrium, the patient has to be helped to shift his self-respect, from being healthy and physically intact, to accepting the challenge of his illness and to manage it intelligently in spite of its threatening implications.

If one realizes that for *the dependent, demanding patient* the satisfaction derived from attention and care is more important even than his health and independence, some way has to be found by which he can obtain this essential gratification in a form that leads to cure. Therefore, he cannot be requested to be stronger and more mature and to accept his doctor's recommendations on the basis of this strength. He will have to be supported in this difficult decision and shown how much it means to his doctor to have him get well. Furthermore, one must emphasize how important it is for the patient's well-being to have all the special care that a sanatorium is designed to give for his condition. One must ask him not to forget to keep the doctor or the social worker regularly informed of his situation. When his fears of being abandoned and deserted are thus allayed, he will no longer resist but will accept the recommendation because the idea of a sanatorium promises even more attention and consideration than he would receive in general practice or in a general hospital.

*The hostile, querulous patient* may well be the most difficult problem for the busy and harassed doctor. Occasionally, at least, his doctors lose patience with him and suddenly react with anger and counterattacks to his critical and aggressive behavior. With this type of patient, to lose one's temper is especially contraindicated. This is exactly what he is looking for: to get into an argument—the more, the better. Then he does not have to pay attention to his own fears any longer and can blame his doctor for mismanaging the situation. If he refuses with anger to accept the doctor's advice, insists that insufficient attention has been paid to his condition, and that the doctors therefore are probably mistaken in their diagnoses, though they think they know all the answers, there seems to be only one constructive way of dealing with the situation. The doctor simply has to say, without taunting the patient, without getting tense and without having to control any anger, that he is sorry but would prefer not to answer all this. He has to state firmly and kindly that all he can do is to give advice as he sees it to the best of his conviction; that it is truly up to the patient to take this advice or to leave it; that the doctor sincerely would like to help, but that he cannot be expected to battle this out; and that it is the patient's health that is at stake and that he, therefore, has the final decision about his choice of physician and course of action. The doctor can only offer his opinion as a responsible advisor—the rest has to be up to the patient. By doing this the physician removes himself as a partner of this hostile scene and hands back to the patient the problem that he must decide, instead of letting him avoid the true issue by attacking his doctor and thus discharging his tension.

The same principles apply to other areas of medical planning such as dietary restrictions and rehabilitation. Whatever measures have to be instituted, the gain from understanding the patient's structure and his dominant central needs is considerable, permitting the doctor to deal with the patient's problems in a more appropriate and positive form.

The patient called the "Tiger" (the man who left his bed in the morning with a somersault) revealed his main problem in a few psychiatric interviews. Coming from an immigrant family, with a disappointingly weak father, he was the youngest child and the only son among three aggressive, domineering older sisters. Having always been his mother's favorite and main emotional support, he acquired his place in the family by ruling them sternly but justly; from an early age providing for all of them financially, he in turn insisted on being consulted and listened to in all family matters. Nevertheless, it seemed that in spite of his constant effort to hold this key position, his self-confidence had never been genuine. The somersaults and his insistence on being called a master electrician can be regarded as signs of his need to prove his strength and manly leadership. Characteristic for this inner insecurity was also one symptom in his marital relationship: he complained about disturbance of potency with his very quiet and meek young wife. The conclusion at which the service arrived was that the illness and the expected invalidism presented a threat to this man that might well increase the existing reality problems. It was clear that he could not go back to his job as a "master" electrician, and his aggressive and unreasonable outbursts against his visitors were expressions of his anxiety and sensitivity at being seen there in his weakness; they served the purpose of demonstrating that he was not down and out yet.

The medical management, therefore, carefully included whatever could be summoned up to re-establish the patient's hopes and self-esteem. In the whole approach, everything was emphasized that helped express tactfully how much the staff believed in him and in his ability to handle trying situations such as irritating relatives and their "condescending" concern. (This was, according to the patient, the attitude of his sisters to which he had reacted by attacking them physically.) Furthermore, as the central area of his anxieties was recognized, the therapeutic efforts concentrated already at this early stage on rehabilitation plans—to provide a program that was appropriate to his future physical condition, that was in keeping with his aptitude and skills as a technician in the field of electricity and, of greatest psychologic importance, that trained him for an activity to fulfill his need of being a "master something" instead of leading merely to a menial occupation providing for his basic financial needs. It was suggested that he switch to radio repair "because it requires expert understanding of technical problems." The patient was found, after a very short time, surrounded by books on radio, studying them with great interest. And, finally, he was promised—and this promise was kept— that he would receive therapy for his impotence later, on an outpatient basis. As could be expected, the "Tiger" became one of the well-adjusted and co-operative patients on the medical ward.

To summarize the aspects of rehabilitation as they developed in this case, it is not sufficient to consider the patient's physical condition, nor is it enough to test and evaluate his aptitude in the vocational field. Rather, one must add to these important factors the third essential one, the psychologic: What kind of activity holds a promise for the patient of fulfilling his emotional needs so that he will want to get well, and to get at it as soon as possible? This does not always require training for a job that has prestige attached to it, as in the case just discussed, but it may be equally necessary with other patients to put the emphasis in the opposite direction. For the dependent personality, for instance, it will be frightening to have to become a foreman or to have to take special responsibility on his future job. Training for a job in a work group or in an organized institution can fulfill far better such a patient's basic emotional needs. Experience with this type of patient has shown that jobs in hospitals, as elevator men or maintenance workers or librarians, offer ideal solutions. Or, when rehabilitation of a young girl with a hysterical personality with all the colorful affective, artistic and seductive qualities and needs that are part of it is evaluated, one must realize that even though she may be a good mathematician, she probably would be a misfit emotionally in an accountant's office; whereas a young compulsive woman, with her characteristic exacting attention to details, and her reserved, controlled and reliable, systematic ways of living, would be equally misplaced as a beautician or milliner.

These considerations enter into numerous problems of medical management, including the prescription of diets. To take only the last two patients as illustrations, if a diet is prescribed for the compulsive type of patient, one will do well to ask him to balance his calories on his own as skillfully and completely as he balances his checkbook. By doing this he is permitted to replace the frustrations of dieting by substitute gratifications in other areas of his personality needs. However, when one is dealing with a hysterical patient, it will be better to avoid adding to the burden of his diet the strain of being systematic about it. Instead, he will need as compensation for these restrictions his doctor's unfailing interest as well as frequent contact with his physician, who represents an emotionally important figure. Similar considerations are possible for the childlike, dependent type, whose diet should be set up around the foods that are most desirable and tempting for him, whereas the anxious patient may do best when the emphasis is put on the healthiest aspects of his diet.

A question frequently raised is, why is this called psychotherapy, and why does it look like simple common sense and not at all like what is mostly expected as the result of complicated psychiatric thinking? What is called medical psychotherapy here differs in certain aspects from psychiatric therapy proper, which is concerned with neuroses, psychoses and severe emotional disturbances and has its special technics and special goals. However, psychiatric psychotherapy involves, in addition to many more complicated technical principles, the same aspects and technics that I have outlined here (E. Bibring, 1954 & G. L. Bibring, 1947). As far as the similarity to simple common sense is concerned, it may be said that any good psychiatric procedure comprises common sense. The complications of the psychiatric approach lie in the evaluation of the clinical data and in the elaboration of the theoretical system by means of which one arrives at one's conclusions. Once the main structure and probable etiology of the presenting symptom, in this case the leading personality trait, have been understood the therapeutic intervention follows logically and simply as in any clinical science.

## The Area of Self-Awareness

There is a third area of significance to which psychologic insight may be applied constructively. Though it refers in the first place to the doctor and his self-awareness and to his understanding of himself and of his own emotional needs and conflicts, it is reflected in a variety of ways as it affects the treatment of his patients.

First and foremost, the doctor's intuitive functioning, his diagnostic ability, is at its best when unhampered by inhibitions, resistances, apprehensions and prejudices.

If with some patients a good and effective relation cannot be established, this is not always because the doctor does not understand the patient, but rather because he does not understand his own reaction to the patient or to the situation. Most doctors try to deal with this difficulty by relying on their habitual bedside manners: "the good, warm, understanding," the "strong, reserved all powerful," "the jovial, slightly teasing," "the charming, captivating" type of doctor. This armor seems usually to be acquired during medical school between the second and fourth years and is then often carried for good, regardless of whether it fits the situation or not, and whether it fits the patient or not (Romano, 1950). It generally serves the purpose of a defensive system behind which the doctors hide whenever they are troubled or concerned over a patient or do not understand him or feel insecure.

It has become the interest of this service to study and discuss these attitudes with the professional personnel, especially with the house officers of the hospital. They are encouraged to observe how they relate themselves to their patients and how the patients in turn react to them. They are asked whether they can discover certain types of patients or certain situations that repeatedly lead to unsatisfactory interpersonal relations or specially smooth and good relations. Furthermore, they compare the results of their self-study with the experiences of their colleagues.

On this basis they are enabled to determine whether there are differences in the skill with which they handle complaining, demanding, stubborn, clinging, independent, overanxious or unconcerned patients. After this has been established, the doctors, contrary to their usual tendency of maintaining that these patients simply are more difficult to handle than others, attempt now to add some self-investigation to learn why a certain type may seem more irritating or less manageable to them. It is gratifying to see how much can be discovered in this way.

For instance, a woman doctor thoroughly disliked "whining, delicately complaining female patients." She even tried to transfer them, whenever possible, to other doctors. On the other hand, she preferred and took on with real enthusiasm any patients who showed some "fighting spirit," though these patients usually present greater difficulties to most doctors. She requested an interview to find out what lay behind this aversion and almost dysfunction in her role as a physician. There was hardly anything one could contribute beyond what she told spontaneously in one hour. Since her early years, she had disliked the way her mother controlled the household, and especially her father, by headaches and failing health. She suspected her mother of being quite well and of using complaints purposefully and without true justification. She made up her mind always to be a good sport and to stand by her father as a strong, reliable soldier. (This decision greatly influenced her whole behavior— she really acted like a soldier, somewhat tough and rugged.) In going over these points, she understood clearly that she had carried this conflict into her professional relations, fighting innocent strangers as if they were her own mother, who had tried to subdue her by illness and complaints.

It should not be too difficult to understand that such insight helped to decrease the tension and difficulties that this doctor had lived out before with some of her patients.

For all physicians there are situations that are more charged than others in which unknown anxieties, prejudices against certain types of behavior, and personal involvement with patients interfere with one's ability to function freely. Unless these problems are understood and controlled, doctors cannot achieve their best potentialities.

This may be illustrated further by a special discussion pursued with the young medical doctors of this hospital. In a series of conferences, the marked lack of genuine interest in aging patients that the doctors showed was investigated and found to be due to a number of emotional factors, none of which had been recognized by the doctors before the extensive discussion but all of which were clearly perceived in the course of the conference.

It was discovered that it is not true, as many of them thought at first, that "aging patients do not offer the same interesting variety of diagnostic problems." Actually, they do, in addition to the more common general conditions characteristic of the aging organism. Thus, they are not "less interesting medically" than younger patients, but might be even more interesting. However, "they are less promising as far as restitution is concerned." The emotional background of this criticism proved to refer to an adolescent daydream that determines for many young people the choice of medicine as their profession—namely, a rescue fantasy centering around the wish to be the benevolent figure in whose hands the fates of people are put. This daydream of restoring all that goes wrong with human beings, of saving people, of being of supreme service and thus of becoming a beloved leader is certainly severely thwarted in work with the uncomfortable, ailing invalids in the older age group.

There is another, not too small group among the future doctors who are concerned with their own health and who choose a medical career to learn the secrets of how to fight disease and death. For these doctors, the elderly patients and particularly the patients with chronic conditions or cancer represent a threat, pointing up the fragility of the body and its gradual decline—unavoidable in spite of intense medical effort. Thus, they seem to be "less desirable" patients because of the discomfort, uneasiness and anxiety they create in these doctors.

Working with older patients involves another important factor that the doctor must become aware of if he is not to get entangled in it. This is especially true of the younger men and women who at the time of their internship have scarcely consolidated their feeling of independence. Having just broken away from the protective or controlling influence of their elders, they are suddenly, at this early stage of their professional existence, confronted with familiar figures resembling their parents and grandparents, aunts and uncles, who demand that they be taken care of and that the house officers be at their disposal, spend their time with them and listen respectfully to all that the patients find essential to complain about. The doctor easily feels put upon and uncomfortable in his new, faltering authoritative position and thus is inclined to avoid and, somewhat, to neglect these patients. He usually finds some kind of rationalization to justify his attitude. On the other hand, the same similarity between the parents and the older patients might stimulate some of the doctors to devote themselves most lovingly to the aged—and as long as this enhances their work and is not complicated by overwhelming concern, no objection to it is necessary.

## Conclusions

In the doctor's work, psychologic understanding is of profound importance. It enables one to gain the most helpful perspective and awareness of one's own involvement as well as to comprehend the patient's life pattern and his basic reactions to his sickness and all it entails, including his relation to his physician. The doctor's own feeling of freedom and security provides clarity of thinking and the best potential for his intuitive diagnostic functioning. It permits him to observe the patient fully, protects him and the patient from rigid, defensive bedside manners, and secures for the patient a great feeling of safety derived from this medical care. This, in turn, evokes in the patient all his positive strength, his willingness to co-operate, and his constructive wish to get well and to do right by himself and by his doctor. Thus, the optimal psychosomatic condition is established that may make the difference between a patient who wants to live and the apathy and sabotage of the patient who lets himself die.

# Psychiatry for Medical School Instructors

THOMAS F. DWYER, M.D.

NORMAN E. ZINBERG, M.D.

THIS PAPER DESCRIBES a course in psychiatry developed for the surgeons and internists responsible for the clinical teaching to the second year Harvard medical students at this hospital. The aim was to direct the teaching of these instructors toward a greater consideration of personality factors in patients. Increased attention is being given to the need for integration of psychiatry and medical training, and experiments to achieve this have been described (Aldrich, 1953; Appel, 1953; Berry, 1953; Cohen, 1953; Fox, 1951, 1953; Pincoffs, 1954; Steiger, Hansen & Rhoads, 1956; Saslow, 1948; Whitehorn, Hanau & Robinson, 1952; Lidz et al., 1956). Reports on additional psychiatric training for the medical faculty as one solution to the problem have not come to our attention.

Psychiatry, and particularly psychoanalysis, developing primarily outside the main stream of medical progress, has for a number of years been moving into closer alliance with medicine. Especially in general hospitals, psychiatrists have gained experience in learning what part of psychiatric knowledge is useful to medicine generally, and how it may be taught. (Bibring, 1951, 1956; Grinker, 1947; Groen, 1956; Kaufman, 1953; Kligerman, 1952; Levine, 1947; Lindemann, 1946; Romano & Engel, 1947; Silverman, 1956). Since 1946, when the Department of Psychiatry was reorganized at Beth Israel Hospital under Dr. Grete L. Bibring, a special interest and activity of the department has been to study and apply the methods by which basic principles of dynamic psychiatry can be taught to physicians who are not psychiatrists and applied by them in their practice. Experi-

---

Reprinted from *Journal of Medical Education*, 32:331-338, 1957.

ence derived from this study was an essential factor in the initiation and completion of the experiment in teaching herein reported.

### Historical Development

Harvard Medical School uses four Boston hospitals for the clinical teaching in the second-year course in history taking and physical diagnosis. The course comprises forty-eight three-hour periods divided equally between medicine and surgery. Since 1951, six of these periods were made available for psychiatric teaching to the students.

The psychiatric departments of the teaching hospitals were allowed latitude in the manner in which they used the allotted time. This paper deals only with the program at Beth Israel Hospital. During 1951, the psychiatric sessions with the students were conducted as seminars by a psychiatric instructor with medical instructors present at some of the meetings. In 1952, for the purpose of greater integration, the medical and surgical instructors were explicitly invited not only to attend, but also to share some of the teaching in the "psychiatric" sessions. The students who interviewed and examined a patient before the small group were given techniques for eliciting and evaluating physical and psychological data in the same session. In 1953, this procedure was essentially repeated with some further integration of teaching as the instructors had additional experience in working together as a team.

In periodic meetings of all instructors to evaluate the effectiveness of the teaching, the medical and surgical instructors expressed a developing awareness that in their clinical teaching to the students, they paid less attention to the "whole patient" than in their own practice. Their initial explanation of this was that lack of time prevented them from considering personality and social features in more than a cursory manner. Further discussions around this point, however, made it apparent that a different factor was operating; although in their own practice, the instructors intuitively made and used personality evaluation, they were often unable to describe these impressions explicitly because of a lack of systematized knowledge of personality. This aspect of medical practice was thus omitted from their teaching, giving the students a distorted picture of how an experienced physician functions.

The psychiatric teaching had been added to the second year course, partly, to correct such distortions. After the third year of such teaching, however, it seemed evident to the instructors that six isolated psychiatric sessions would not alter significantly the basic approach to patients that the student was learning in his much more frequent and vital contact with the medical and surgical instructors. Even when the psychiatric periods were truly joint affairs shared by the psychiatric and other instructors, the students still tended to separate their "psychiatric" and "medical" approaches to the patient.

Consideration of these factors led to the plan to set up a course that would give the medical and surgical instructors a systematic training in some basic elements of psychiatry that had not been part of their own medical training. The medical and surgical instructors initiated the request for such a course after sharing in the joint teaching experiences, and realizing that there was a body of psychiatric knowledge which could be useful in their medical practice. The expressed aim of this course was to improve their teaching to the students; there was neither expectation of, nor interest in, their teaching psychiatry as such.

## Considerations in Teaching

Two members of the department of psychiatry undertook to work out the details of the course to the medical instructors. These psychiatrists had taught medical students in the joint sessions with the medical and surgical instructors, and also had several years experience in the department's special program of teaching psychiatry to nonpsychiatric physicians. This experience influenced their decision toward a systematic, theoretical presentation illustrated by case material. It was believed that without an outline of the essentials of dynamic psychiatry, clinical material would be of little permanent use no matter how interesting.

To support the conviction that a sufficient theoretical knowledge could be imparted to nonpsychiatric physicians was the several years experience of the department in developing techniques and content of teaching "medical psychotherapy." The latter is a well defined psychotherapeutic approach elaborated specifically for the use of the nonpsychiatric physician, and contrasts with psychotherapy applied by the psychiatrist for definitely neurotic disorders (Bibring, 1956). The method provides the physician with the means of recognizing the leading psychological patterns of his patients and utilizing this knowledge in management toward specific goals, without attempting substantial personality changes.

Much of the material, in any course in psychiatry, involves areas that are emotionally weighted to a degree that may interfere with learning. An additional difficulty requiring consideration in the present teaching was the fact that the "students" were physicians of status who had not been students in a formal sense for many years. These factors, plus the nature of the already existing relationship between the instructors contributed to the decision that the psychiatric instructors would not make use of any "group techniques" for educators, elaborated by Leo Berman and others in recent years (Berman, 1953a). If emotional resistance to the course material impeded learning, it was intended that this be recognized and coped with by altering the method of presentation, the content, or by other methods short of a group discussion of the emotional reactions of the participants. It was decided by agreement of all participants that the meetings would take the form of seminars.

## Description of the Course

There were three medical and seven surgical instructors in the first year of this teaching. To the original group were added two medical and two surgical instructors in the second and third year. The course met evenings for one and a half hours weekly for approximately ten weeks each year.

### Content

A systematic presentation of personality development based on psychoanalytic psychology was made. Normal development was emphasized, but neuroses and psychoses were discussed in sufficient detail to illustrate the contribution of early childhood conflicts to these disturbances as well as to adult character structure in the normal.

The course began with hysterical neurosis and the character formations thought to be primarily based on conflicts of the age period 4-6. Illustrative case material on the hysterical personality was used to form a bridge between the theoretical and practical, the unfamiliar and familiar. All these doctors were acquainted with the picture of the emotionally labile patient in their office. Using the physicians' own observations, it was possible to sketch a more detailed picture of such patients, which included consistent patterns of behavior. The next question—what lay behind such personality features developmentally—led naturally to a discussion of the theoretical.

In subsequent meetings, the earlier periods of development, particularly those having to do with the child's training for sphincter control, and with the vicissitudes of the early feeding relationship with mother, were discussed in terms of their effect on later personality development.

The concepts of ego, superego and id were defined and returned to throughout the course as the instructors attempted to relate the clinical pictures that were being discussed to a theoretical scheme. The defensive functions of the ego were given particular attention (as related directly to adult character formation). The greater prominence of some defense mechanisms in certain personality types was illustrated, for example, projection in paranoid types. Wherever possible case material contributed by the participants was used. There was emphasis on the meaningfulness of the everyday behavior of patients in their contact with physicians. A patient was occasionally interviewed before the group to demonstrate some of the principles being discussed.

Throughout the seminars, the complicated nature of the subject matter was emphasized as was the fact that personality understanding cannot be reduced to any simple standard formula. The teaching re-enforced this point of view by avoiding oversimplification and overgeneralization and by repeatedly emphasizing the still imperfect understanding of personality factors. The fact that this was a joint venture and an experimental one was frequently brought to the attention of the group. The aims were periodically redefined: (1) to provide a framework within which behavior and personality development might be understood in a more systematic way, and (2) to find ways to apply this knowledge in the management of medical patients.

Both psychiatrists were present at all meetings although not always for the entire session. At each meeting, one served as the principal teacher and the other intervened when he felt a point needed clarification, or that anxieties in the listeners had begun to interfere with learning. The experimental nature of the teaching and particularly the probability of emotional reactions to the content contributed to the choice of this method.

### Responses to the Course

Only the more general or prominent reactions to the course are reported. The psychiatric instructors met at least briefly between each session to evaluate trends; and teaching in subsequent sessions was altered according to estimates of the reactions of the participants. There was, however, no systematic recording of the teaching sessions, nor detailed analysis.

The sustained attendance through three years, and the recruitment by first year members of additional candidates for the subsequent years, was observed as one indication of positive interest. On those few occasions where attendance was off (3-4 trainees present), examination of previous trends in the teaching often suggested a probable reason. The factor most frequently held responsible by the psychiatrists was an excessive presentation of theoretical and therefore unfamiliar material, and adjustment was made with a temporary greater emphasis on clinical cases.

There were, periodically, negative reactions to the teaching material concerned with the psychosexual development of the child. This had been anticipated, and the psychiatric instructors were prepared to deal with anxiety in this area by a variety of means, for example, by explicitly recognizing that all of us as adults have taboos in relation to these childhood interests. The indiscriminate application of what was being learned to oneself and one's family would most frequently lead to faulty conclusions, it was stated, and application was diverted to case material.

The seminars rarely became argumentative, yet the members acted freely in expressing their objections or criticisms or insistence on understanding. Concern about misapplying psychiatric knowledge and thereby upsetting a patient or the opposite belief that the application of psychiatric information would have no effect on a patient, were two of the general responses explored in a limited way to their irrational sources.

Some members consulted the psychiatrists outside of the teaching sessions on the meaning of observed behavior in their own children. The quality of these requests for help suggested that they arose primarily from a conviction that further information would be useful to them, rather than from anxiety stirred up by the course. This kind of consultation with the psychiatrists was practically nonexistent in this group of physicians before the teaching began.

The participants spontaneously discussed observations they made each day on their patients, and tried to understand them in the light of the psychiatric presentation. As the course progressed, the illustrations advanced became more and more appropriate to the material being discussed. This was another measure of the members' increased understanding and ability to apply what they were learning.

The psychiatric instructors had had contacts with most of the participants prior to the seminars in other teaching situations, at lunch, at hospital meetings or rounds. As these contacts continued, there was a noticeable change in the character of questions the surgeon and internist asked the psychiatrist about patients, first in the direction of supplying a psychologically richer picture of the patient, and secondly in the insistence on arriving at some comprehensible and useful picture of the patient. Besides these casual discussions, there were more thorough conferences between surgeon or internist and psychiatrist on individual cases that were presenting problems in medical management. Wherever possible, the material from these individual conferences was brought back to the larger group.

### Changes in the Teaching to the Students

The primary aim of the course was to assist the medical and surgical instructors in their teaching to the second year medical students, yet changes in this direction due to the psychiatric teaching were most difficult to evaluate. This has to be expected, and only several years of experience and observation will allow more definite conclusions.

As had been stated at the beginning of the course, and repeated throughout the seminars, the purpose of the teaching was not to give the members psychiatric information which they would in turn directly impart to the students, but rather to improve their own orientation, and thus affect their teaching to the students in more subtle ways. The changes that were expected, therefore, would not be gross or easily observed, but would probably consist in a shift of emphasis.

The psychiatric instructors (six, including four who had not participated in the teaching of this course) who taught the second year students in joint sessions with the surgeons and internists before and after the completion of the first year's psychiatric course, felt that there was increased attention on the part of most of the instructors to personality features of the patient. For example, a student's difficulty in obtaining an adequate history was quickly picked up and discussed by the medical instructor as a reflection of certain personality features of the patient, which in turn had implications in the approach to the patient and in the further management of the case.

One of the clearest kinds of change due to the course was the increased understanding on the part of the medical and surgical instructors of the anxieties of the students in their first contacts with patients. In this area, the instructors seemed not only more perceptive, but much more ready to give the students support in coping with their anxieties, for example, a student's undue concern over inquiring into intimate details of a patient's life. This had been discussed and understood as a problem that did not only trouble the young student, but also many experienced physicians and that could nevertheless be managed by other means than denial. One aid was to keep perspective on the purpose of the medical history and examination, i.e., on the essential function of the doctor in this specific situation. The good teacher of course has always helped students in such areas on the basis of his own inner freedom, yet many students at this critical point in their medical training are taught by instructors who, because they deny their own emotional reactions, unwittingly present this as a model to the students. The doctor certainly must not become overinvolved in his feelings for his patients. It would seem a significant improvement if he developed the freedom to become aware of his own feelings and those of the patient, and still retain perspective on his relationship with the patient. Instead the doctor frequently develops defenses that interfere with his useful sensitivity to the patient's feelings. We have observed with others the decreasing awareness of the feelings of patients in medical students and house officers during the period of their training. The first year student reports on a patient he has seen; the fourth year student discusses "a coronary" or a "liver."

The medical and surgical instructors' own evaluation of the effects of the psychiatric course on their teaching was reported at a conference of all instructors. The most general effect attributed to the course was that all of the teaching to the students had been much improved. They did observe that they were now more inclined to introduce personality features in discussing a case, and they especially stressed their increased understanding of the student's emotional reactions to his first contact with patients, and to his low position in the hospital hierarchy.

Another generally reported result of the course for the participants was an increased understanding of their private patients. Although this diverged from the primary aim of the course, it was a positive development that in turn re-enforced what had been learned in the course.

All participants felt, after the first year, that the course had raised questions without giving sufficient answers, and expressed a desire for more information in a similar course in subsequent years.

### Observations and Discussion

This is a transition period for the teaching of psychiatry in medical schools. It seems likely that in the future, the student will have a basic training in psychodynamics as thorough as his present training in anatomy or physiology. When this is achieved, it may no longer be necessary to offer special training in dynamic psychiatry to the student's clinical instructors. At present, however, the sensitivities to human behavior the student brings with him to medical school, may be dulled during his medical training rather than heightened. Under stress from his emotional response to the peculiar intimacy and responsibility that belong to the doctor's role, he turns for help (mainly in silence) to the doctors he can see managing patients, his clinical teachers. It seems unfortunate that these models for the student may omit from their teaching considerations they include in their medical practice, thus unintentionally providing the student with an inaccurate picture of how a doctor functions. The student, eagerness for help intensified by his anxieties, tends to identify with the model presented him and to develop some rigid and defensive type of bedside manner (which under favorable conditions he may be able to unlearn more or less successfully after he begins medical practice).

The student's anxieties and confusions with patients may be diminished if he himself receives early a thorough training in psychodynamics, and especially if he receives help with his own reactions. His clinical instructors will aways remain especially important models, whose influence may reenforce or weaken these gains.

This training of instructors is at least the solution of one part of the problem of teaching the student comprehensive medicine. The area of the student's use of his clinical teachers as models, deserves further study which may throw light on the other present-day concerns of medical education, e.g., the loss of interest in general practice during medical school training (from 92 per cent at the first year to 41 per cent of the fourth year students, in a 1954 poll by the Massachusetts Academy of General Practice). In an atmosphere of genuine cooperation, and with the common goal of improving the student's training, medical faculties might find it useful to clarify for themselves the subtler effects of their teaching methods.

### Summary

An experiment of one aspect of the problem of integrating psychiatry into the medical school curriculum is described. The medical and surgical instructors responsible for the physical diagnosis course to one group of second year Harvard students, attended an annual course in psychoanalytic psychology. These teachers were considered in the experiment as models for the student's attempt to master clinical medicine, and the aim of the psychiatric teaching was to assist the teachers toward a more explicit presentation of "comprehensive medicine."

Some of the special considerations that appear to need attention in teaching a course in psychiatry to a group of established and experienced doctors are discussed.

Observations made in the course of this study suggest that the student's first contact with patients is a crucial event, and that the circumstances surrounding this encounter may influence his further development as a doctor in a number of specific ways. This seems an area inviting further investigation. Such teaching in no way lessens the need for continued improvement of content and method in psychiatric courses for the medical students.

# Teaching Medical Psychology through Psychiatric Consultation

RALPH J. KAHANA, M.D.

OF THE POSSIBLE KINDS of psychiatric activity in a general hospital, consultation on questions of the management of medical and surgical patients is most frequently, perhaps, an immediate exercise in the integration of psychological thought in medical practice. In our experience, such consultation regularly presents special opportunities for the teaching of medical psychology to house physicians and medical students and can be effectively instructive when it is consistently based upon a comprehensive theory of personality. A discussion of some of the considerations that arise in consultative teaching and a delineation of the guiding principles of procedure concurrently evolved, may contribute toward a solution of the problem of usefully blending medicine and psychiatry.

The experiences of consultation that form the basis of this paper are drawn from the program of psychiatric teaching and training developed under Grete L. Bibring (1951, 1956) at the Beth Israel Hospital. The consultation service is one of a number of activities comprised within this program. Senior psychiatrists are regularly affiliated with the other major hospital services of medicine, surgery, obstetrics, and pediatrics. They serve as consultants and as psychiatric instructors to the house staff of their respective affiliated services. Psychiatric Fellows in advanced training act as consultants after they have gained experience in our methods. The assistance of our clinical psychologists and close co-operation with the medical social work program within the hospital are considered essential in the activity of the consultation service. There is no special

Reprinted from *The Journal of Medical Education*, 34:1003-1009, 1959.

ward set aside for psychiatric patients; although this limits the time in which we can treat people with very acute or persistent assaultive, suicidal, or other markedly disturbed behavioral tendencies, it has the advantage, from the teaching standpoint, of never permitting the house physician to relinquish to the psychiatrist all responsibility for the care of his patient within the hospital.

### The Integration of Medicine and Psychiatry

The growing modern integration of medicine and psychiatry has come about for many reasons. Almost all the patients who experience mild, transitory emotional reactions to physical illness, most of those who suffer from psychosomatic disorders, and many others with psychopathological states remain the responsibility of the general physician, internist, surgeon, or other specialist outside of the field of psychiatry. Even when symptoms of emotional disturbance are not apparent, the physician often needs special psychological understanding in order to secure the optimal co-operation of the patient for adequate history taking, physical examinations, or indicated treatment, or to determine the best way in which to discuss his medical findings with the patient. At the same time, the physician must frequently experience the emotional impact of exposure to difficult attitudes in people and extremely stressful and moving life situations. Another, less obstrusive but potentially valuable reason for developing, increasing, and systematizing the physician's psychological thinking lies in the area of mental hygiene or preventive psychiatry (G. L. Bibring, 1951). Because people turn confidently to their doctors and reveal themselves in times of physical stress, when their major emotional conflicts are intensified, the physician is frequently in a position to detect incipient psychopathology. His therapeutic activity, including his special relationship to the patient, can favor personality strength and mental health.

In the light of these considerations of the need for an integration of psychological thought into medical practice it is believed that the potential contribution of the psychiatric consultant should go beyond offering a specialist service. In addition to pointing the way to necessary care for mentally ill persons, the consultation service acts as a training resource to the staff of the general hospital. Each consultation becomes the means of exchanging information about diagnosis, interviewing techniques, problems of motivation and cooperation, other psychological aspects of medical management, and the physician's own emotional reactions as these affect the patient. Since questions arise in the care of people who are in the main well adjusted, the consultant must find a structured way to discuss normal personality. The diagnosis of personality type, as distinct from that of psychopathology, has particular importance in preventive psychiatry. Prevention not only requires the discovery of impending illness as early as possible, but also the anticipation of potential sources of mental stress and the strengthening of adaptive forces in the patient. The personality diagnosis includes knowledge of what is likely to constitute stress and of the patient's individual ways of coping with this. It must be mentioned that this discussion of psychiatric consultation focuses upon the medical care of adults, although much of it can apply in the treatment of children; among essential differences are the diagnosing of the stage of psychological development rather than of a more stabilized kind of personality in children, the emphasis upon working with and through the parents, and the using of special approaches in communicating with children.

## Theoretical Framework

The teaching and training program of which the consultation service forms a part was discussed recently with particular attention to the psychological approach utilized (G. L. Bibring, 1956). The essential psychological framework was defined as that of psychoanalytically oriented psychology. "This psychological system maintains that there is more to a person's emotional processes than appears on the surface and that his behavior patterns and attitudes are the result of conflicts between his deep strivings and his defensive methods against these strivings, developed in a slow adaptive process under the impact of environmental pressures and demands." The personality type is a summary of a person's principal and consistent ways of satisfying or warding off his deep strivings, and coping with the demands of the world around him. It depicts his leading attitudes and habitual behavior patterns, and the important needs, active conflicts, psychological defenses, skills, and values that give rise to his behavior. An awareness of different types including hysterical, compulsive, oral, and other kinds of personalities is very useful in teaching, but to describe them more fully would involve too great a departure from the main theme of this paper.

The physician's responsible activities in conducting an adequate examination, informing the patient (or his family, as necessary) of the findings in the interest of promoting health, and in recommending or carrying out treatment all have a potentially therapeutic emotional impact upon the patient. Beyond this, certain techniques having psychotherapeutic effect have been considered as being available to the physician who is not trained in formal psychotherapy (Levine, 1942). Some of these are directed toward the patient, while other methods aim to effect changes in the patient's environment. From the standpoint of psychological principles, following Edward Bibring's conceptual scheme, the major psychotherapeutic agent utilized by the physician who is not a psychiatrist is *suggestion* (E. Bibring, 1954). Suggestive techniques involve the induction by the physician of ideas, impulses, emotions, and actions of the patient on the model of a child-parent relationship; the patient unconsciously endeavors to gain the love and esteem or to escape the censure of the physician, as if the doctor were as important and powerful as a parent. Although some patients are more amenable to suggestion than are others, it is usually carried out without the physician having conscious knowledge of the patient's personality type. Thus it has a certain hit or miss quality. The physician's explanations to the patient of the meaning of symptoms and of the reasons for tests and treatment have the effect of *clarification,* a second psychotherapeutic principle. They enable the patient to view his illness with more detachment and to rely less upon fantasies, which are often very frightening. When the physician has made a personality diagnosis he will be able to employ selectively a third kind of psychotherapeutic procedure, that of adaptive intervention or *therapeutic manipulation.* In therapeutic manipulation "through our words or attitudes we may neutralize certain emotional systems in the patient, mobilize others, and utilize them for . . . curative aims; one can redirect existent emotional attitudes from neurotic toward adjustive goals, or one can intensify latent emotional systems favorable to readjustment which represent the patient's readjustive reserve; or one can, perhaps, establish 'new' attitudes." Adaptive intervention is especially useful in the area of medical management and will be illustrated in a clinical example of a consultation to follow. When correctly employed it means that the physician can help the patient to utilize the strength of his personality in co-operatively combatting illness, and that the doctor and his patient do not work at cross purposes.

### The Teaching Consultation

In the course of a psychiatric consultation special opportunities arise for the teaching of medical psychology. Careful consideration may be given to the ways in which the referring doctor formulates his request for consultation and introduces the psychiatrist to the patient, and to the method whereby the consultant organizes his impressions and recommendations. In every case the consultant will evaluate the existing doctor-patient relationship, take into account the effect of certain features of medical practice in a general hospital and pay particular attention to communication with the referring physician.

To the consultant the kind of question that is asked by the house doctor is an immediate indication of the doctor's relationship to the patient, his psychological training and perceptiveness, and his awareness of his own attitude toward the patient. By assisting the physician to formulate his questions the psychiatrist avoids a mutual misunderstanding of the nature and value of the consultation, and may stimulate the physician to a broader comprehension of the case. Usually the physician has been impressed by gross evidence of mental disturbance in the patient's current behavior or past history, has recognized an existing or impending problem in the management of a physically or psychosomatically ill person, or has a question of differential diagnosis. Problems in medical management have many forms: the refusal of recommended surgery; a threat to sign out of the hospital against advice; reluctance to leave the hospital, or a return of symptoms when discharge is discussed; the question of how to present a recommendation for surgery to an anxious patient; the question of what to discuss with the patient who has a neoplasm; the question of the effect of steroid drugs on a particular patient; the management of a colostomy; etc. Although they confront the physician more frequently than do frank psychiatric disorders, he may be less likely to ask for consultation on questions of management until he has learned what psychiatry may have to offer.

Sometimes the problem that occasions a request for consultation is resolved in the initial discussion between the consultant and the referring physician. More often the psychiatrist will proceed to interview the patient. The decision whether to introduce the consultant as a psychiatrist to the patient, whether beforehand, during the initial interview, or exceptionally (with certain apprehensive but unquestioning patients) after longer contact, and whether volunteered or in response to the patient's inquiry, is approached with the aim of not upsetting the patient or provoking his resistance. When it is feasible to have the house physician present during the psychiatric interview the consultant may be able to demonstrate ways of relieving some of the patient's anxiety and, at the same time, may teach interviewing technique. The consultant's appraisal will take into account the nature and course of the patient's illness, his familial, vocational, and other social relationships including those within the hospital, the clinical goals and problems of the referring physician, and the resources and limitations of the hospital. Although the patient's leading defensive reactions may be quickly recognized, it is usually necessary to correlate a variety of impressions of the patient's current behavior, childhood experience, ways of coping with crises, and so forth, in order to arrive at the personality diagnosis. For purposes of clear and concise formulation the consultant teacher may find it helpful to consider how the physical and psychological factors are related and what situational elements are inherent in the particular kind of physical illness or change: the patient may be coping adequately with his illness; he may have a physical illness with psychological repercussions; the course of the illness may be affected to an unusual degree by emotional factors as in psychosomatic disorders and some cases of advanced physical disease. Especially important situational elements may be those of acute illness, as such, hospitalization, special demands made upon the patient in the course of diagnosis or treatment (e.g., diabetic diet), chronic illness, rehabilitation, surgery, terminal illness, repeated minor illnesses, or a critical developmental period (e.g., menopause). In addition to questions of treatment and disposition of frank psychoses, behavior disorders and neuroses, the consultant is often concerned with distinguishing organic disease from states of anxiety and depression, conversion hysteria, hypochondriasis or malingering.

The psychiatrist may make recommendations to be utilized in continued management of the case by the referring doctor, or he may advise both medical and psychiatric treatment, or psychiatric care alone. The referring physician may find psychological terminology strange. He may be disappointed, at times, that the psychiatrist leaves him with a choice of possible measures and treatment goals rather than definitive recommendations. If he is sophisticated in psychological theory he may feel that the consultant tells him little more than what he already knows about his patient. Accordingly, the consultant will avoid psychiatric jargon, explain why he gives tentative recommendations, help the physician to make use of his psychological acumen, and specifically arrange necessary conferences for discussion and follow-up of the case. The observations and activities of nurses, dieticians and others who have close contact with the patient will be included and specified in the treatment plan. Thus, consultative teaching may reach many members of the medical team.

The effect upon the patient of the doctor-patient relationship is a central consideration in approaching every ward consultation. As far as possible the patient's conscious expectations of care are ascertained as well as his more childlike unconscious reactions to the doctor as a parental figure. The consultant's attention is, of course, focused upon the personality structure and situational problems of the patient; inevitably he must, to some extent, also take into account the personality and situation of the physician who has the greatest responsibility and activity in the care of the patient. When a relationship of mutual confidence and respect has been established, the house physician will more readily mention his own responses to patients and the consultation may become a means for him to increase his self-awareness, so valuable in work with upset and upsetting patients.

In the teaching hospital the doctor-patient relationship is influenced by the sharing of responsibility among the physicians of each service in a hierarchical organization and also among various medical specialists. The advantages of these arrangements in facilitating expert care of patients and the training of younger physicians are well known; some of the inherent problems often play an important part in management difficulties. The intern or resident may feel deprived of the responsibility and status that can facilitate his interest in the patient. At the same time his satisfaction as a helper of other human beings can be reduced. It is easier for him to withdraw from difficult patients in a general hospital than it will be later as a practitioner. Because of the division of responsibility and the rotation of house officers in a teaching hospital, there is the danger that patients lose the emotional support that they would receive if they had regular care by one physician. Often the patient may be unsure as to who is in charge of his case. He may feel, realistically or not, that he is uninformed or has been given differing medical explanations or recommendations. Certain patients utilize the authority structure in the hospital in a neurotic fashion for the unconscious reenactment of conflict experiences from childhood, for example, playing one person against another and disbelieving all of them. Hospital administrators and others who are aware of these difficulties are actively working to minimize the fragmentation and discontinuity of patient care (Lee, 1958). The psychiatric consultant will attempt to discover whom the patient regards as his doctor and to learn from the referring physician who it is that sees the patient most consistently. The consultant then tries to help achieve continuity of care for the patient. When it is not possible for one physician to make major decisions, it may yet be feasible to arrange a consistent plan of communication with the patient.

## An Illustration

Many of the clinical, theoretical, and procedural considerations that we believe to be important in teaching are illustrated in the case of a sixty-year-old, single man referred by the surgical service. He is representative of the large group of relatively well adjusted people who react to the stress of a physical illness with anxiety and intensification of behavioral traits.

The patient was referred for psychiatric evaluation because he repeatedly postponed surgical treatment. He had had an operation for biliary obstruction due to cholelithiasis almost seven months before, on a private surgical service. The complication of acute pancreatitis necessitated drainage of an abdominal abscess. Because of his financial situation in the face of his long illness, the patient was transferred to the ward service. Subsequently, a third operation for revision of the sinus was performed. Although it appeared that a fourth procedure to assist drainage would shorten his hospital stay, he had become anxious and talked of signing out of the hospital. The patient had discussed this important decision with his sister who lived in another city. Greatly concerned about him, she had contacted his former private attending surgeon and also a second senior member of the Surgical Service on several occasions. The psychiatric consultant noted that the interest of these two leading surgeons in the patient created in members of the surgical house staff a special determination to treat the patient very successfully. The difficulties which they encountered thus added to their feelings of frustration and led to definite tension between them and their patient.

When interviewed, the patient was friendly and polite in manner, very neat in appearance, and showed great consideration of others on the ward. He knew that he was upset and thought that the psychiatrist might help him to feel better. As the patient spoke of the grave fears about the proposed operation and then described his life and work, the picture emerged of a steady, reliable, responsible, planful, conscientious person who approached decisions gradually and strongly identified himself with the management at his job. The patient's positive appreciation of his former private surgeon contrasted with a feeling that the younger ward physicians were inconsiderate and "walked away" from him at rounds.

In succeeding discussions with the surgical house staff, the psychiatric consultant explained his impression ( based upon the foregoing observations) that the patient was a compulsive type of personality. The patient felt disappointed and anxious because of the stress of his prolonged illness, and he characteristically reacted to pressure with indecisiveness and obstinacy. His transfer to the ward service had deprived him of the direct care of his private surgeon and he had found it difficult to establish a close relationship with the ward "management" in his accustomed manner. The consultant believed that it was important to approach the patient in such a way as to permit him to use his careful, planful method of proceeding in order to deal with his anxieties adequately and to minimize the chance of his developing a paranoid attitude. Thus it was decided that the patient should not be pushed, but rather be allowed further time in which to make up his mind about the operation; his questions were to be answered carefully, in thorough detail, repeatedly as necessary, and as unhurriedly as possible; the doctor would try to establish clearly that the patient understood the surgical recommendations and took an appropriate amount of responsibility in accepting or rejecting them. The patient was to be told that his present anxiety at the prospect of a relatively minor surgical procedure could be understood in light of the strain and discomfort of the long illness (which he had actually borne in good spirit). It was to be suggested that if he felt that anyone tried to avoid answering his questions, he did not have to accept this as final; perhaps it would be possible for him in such circumstances to make an appointment with the doctor to see him at a convenient time after the rounds were completed. Finally, the doctor planned to explain his recommendations similarly to the patient's sister. The psychiatrist was to be available for further consultation and planned at least one additional talk with the patient.

Following discussion along these lines between the surgical house officers, the patient, and his sister, the patient decided to permit the operation. Afterwards, he expressed appreciation of the talks with the psychiatrist and the surgeons because they had shown him how he could be strong. The house officers regained their positive regard for him even though he continued to be mildly critical of the attitudes of the younger doctors. On their own initiative, the physicians made a special point of enlisting the patient's active help in the finer details of caring for his dressings; this confirmed that they had gained a deeper understanding of him. The patient's subsequent course was one of rapid healing.

In this clinical example, one may see how the personality diagnosis has directed an adaptive intervention, with the result that the patient was enabled to use his characteristic modes of adjustment in a constructive, co-operative way. Management of the case remained the responsibility of the house physicians, and the consultant served as an advisor and teacher. Comparable consultative approaches with some differences in emphasis have recently been described in the outpatient department of a teaching hospital (Adams, 1958) and in general practice (Balint, 1957).

### Summary

A delineation of the guiding principles of procedure evolved in teaching medical psychology through psychiatric consultation is offered as a contribution to the useful integration of psychological thought in medical practice. Special opportunities for teaching may arise when discussing the initial formulation of the request for consultation, in introducing the psychiatrist to the patient, and in the presentation of the consultant's formulation. A case is presented to illustrate how personality diagnosis based upon psychoanalytic psychology may permit the house physician to employ psychotherapeutic measures in a specific, purposeful way.

# Personality Types in Medical Management

RALPH J. KAHANA, M.D.

GRETE L. BIBRING, M.D.

IN THE COURSE OF our efforts to implement and study the integration of medicine and psychiatry within a general hospital, the diagnosis of personality structure has become an important element in the psychological management of the physically ill patient (G. Bibring, 1951, 1956; Dwyer & Zinberg, 1957; Kahana, 1959). We have found it convenient to delineate seven basic categories of personality types and attitudes: (1) *the dependent, overdemanding personality;* (2) *the orderly, controlled personality;* (3) *the dramatizing, emotionally involved, captivating personality;* (4) *the long-suffering, self-sacrificing patient;* (5) *the guarded, querulous patient;* (6) *the patient with the feeling of superiority;* (7) *the patient who seems uninvolved and aloof.* The first three types especially bear the direct imprint of specific developmental periods in childhood (S. Freud, 1905, 1908; Abraham, 1921, 1924, 1925). In the following four, the leading attitudes represent certain defensive reactions directed against impulses stemming from these early phases of development (Fenichel, 1945; A. Freud, 1946; S. Freud, 1905; Jones, 1913; Loewenstein, 1957; Reik, 1947). The above diagnostic categories do not designate personality disorders. They refer to the psychologically normal, well-functioning person and are especially applicable to the individual in any stressful, anxiety-producing situation. Physical illness invariably represents an emotional crisis which may be very intense but will be transient if well handled by the patient and the environment. A psychopathological diagnosis in a given case may be warranted if there is marked accentuation of character traits, neurotic or psychotic symptoms, serious difficulty in dealing adequately with social relationships, limited capacity for work, and even impaired ability to gain satisfaction and enjoyment in life.

As with much of our fundamental psychological knowledge, the recognition of personality structures has been derived in part from the study of the abnormal. These types and attitudes became familiar to psychiatrists first in their pathologically exaggerated forms, and were named respectively *oral, compulsive, hysterical, masochistic, paranoid, narcissistic* and *schizoid* personalities. We have not used the psychiatric terms because they seem to blur the important distinction between health and disease, but we shall include them parenthetically in the headings of the descriptive subtitles, to indicate the pathological correlates. These personalities are paradigms and, as with other models such as a "classical" example of a disease, few actual patients will represent one of them in pure culture. As we describe each category, we shall formulate briefly the meaning of physical illness to the particular kind of person in terms of his basic needs, the threat that he is trying to cope with, and the kind of defensive and adaptive behavior that has become intensified under this stress. Some general inferences for medical psychotherapy—the employment of psychotherapeutic measures in medical management (G. L. Bibring, 1956; E. Bibring, 1954; Kahana, 1959) will be drawn.

### The Dependent, Overdemanding (Oral) Personality

This type of person often impresses the physician with the urgent quality of all his requests. He seems to need special attention or an unusual amount of advice. He may reach out quickly and impulsively, putting himself in the hands of the doctor with an optimistic and naïve or self-assured expectation of limitless care. Even when he appears generous and concerned about others, he expects manifold repayment and becomes strongly resentful if this does not materialize. It becomes easily apparent that this sort of patient is very dependent upon others to protect him and to help him feel accepted and secure. His frustration tolerance is reduced, and unfulfilled needs may lead him to intense anger, depression, the feeling of helplessness, or apathy. If his formative childhood experiences were marked by feelings of disappointment, then revengeful, nagging, and demanding attitudes may prevail; the patient comes with a chip on his shoulder, expecting that the doctor will not make any effort to help him. The craving for satisfaction or stimulation through overeating, drinking, smoking, and taking medicine may be prominent, and a tendency toward addiction may be observed. These personality traits stem from the earliest period of childhood when the helpless infant's biological needs for food and protection become linked up with his growing awareness and interest in the outside world through the attention, affection, and care provided by his mother. For this patient, being given food or medicine or special consideration has persisted as an equivalent to being loved.

## The Meaning of Illness

We may say that for this person the anxiety accompanying illness tends to be transformed into the wish for boundless interest and abundant care, and into a deep fear of being abandoned, helpless, and starving. Thus sickness presents the temptation to return to an early, blissfully secure, infantile state, but it is also perceived as the consequence of a lack of concern and protection on the part of others. In the struggle over these intense fears and wishes, we may see any of the following responses, representing attempts to re-establish equilibrium: the patient may become extremely demanding or overdependent upon what his doctor prescribes; he may react strongly against his unconscious wishes and overindependently fight any need for care; he may become depressed, apathetic or withdrawn, perhaps feeling as small children often do, that if he suffers it must be because nobody loves him; he then may blame others for his discomfort in a complaining, vengeful, or spiteful way.

When the physician understands the meaning of illness he can decide to what extent it is possible to help the patient by attempting to satisfy his needs for special attention, whether or not the setting of certain limits is indicated, and how to facilitate or modify the patient's defensive efforts. Many elements of psychological management suggest themselves. Directly or implicitly, by word, action, or attitude, the doctors, nurses, and other medical attendants should convey their readiness to care for the patient as completely as possible. For the many acutely ill in whom dependent tendencies have become temporarily active, simple undemanding nursing care directed to physical comfort is not only a basic part of professional help, but is specifically important in meeting their psychological needs. If limits have to be set because the patient's demands have become excessive and self-perpetuating, great care must be exercised not to introduce them as if they were the expression of impatience or punitiveness. Setting of limits should not take the harsh form of a withdrawal of interest and consideration, but rather should be presented through thoughtful explanation. This patient may be willing to accept necessary restrictions if the doctor offers some form of concession as compensation. Such concessions may be of a minor nature, simply expressing the friendly interest of the physician, like a desired change in the diet, or helping his family to visit by providing transportation to the hospital, etc.

## The Orderly, Controlled (Compulsive) Personality

This person offers an example of excellent self-discipline. When under stress, he relies upon having as much knowledge as possible about his situation, not only as a basis for dealing with problems rationally, but also as his preferred way of handling his anxieties. Alongside of his logical approach, we can often observe a ritualistic tendency as a clue to diagnosis: he may keep to a set order of procedure even in small matters in daily life. The woman who spends a major amount of time eradicating the last speck of dust in her house, and the man who takes special pride in the exact fulfillment of obligations, including the most minute ones, are often of this type. This kind of patient tends to be remarkably orderly, tidy, punctual, conscientious, and preoccupied with right and wrong. With his rectitude and careful way of proceeding, we are not surprised to find that he can be quite obstinate. He places great value upon collecting and retaining possessions and is frugal in money matters. The formation of an orderly, controlled personality appears to be related to factors operative in the period from ages two to four years. Precocious development of motor and intellectual abilities and increased strength of aggressive impulses in the child play a part. Strong early insistence by the parents that the child be clean and good may have an intimidating effect, or the parents' excessive preoccupation with control of body functions and behavior may achieve a like result through intensifying the child's inner struggle between compliance and rebellion. Similarly, overindulgent disregard of the child's need to achieve a comfortable balance between expression and suppression of these tendencies may lead eventually to excessive and inflexible self-restraint. Early-maturing intellectual abilities are brought into the service of curbing impulsive behavior. Thinking tends to become a substitute for action, rather than a preparation and guide. Characteristically, impulses are warded off by the development of rigid opposite attitudes. The leading traits of orderliness, obstinacy, and frugality represent overcompensation against childhood tendencies to disorderliness, dirtiness, impulsively aggressive behavior, and pleasurable indulgence.

### The Meaning of Illness

Sickness threatens the individual with loss of control over these impulses. It may impair or interfere with his capacity to master aggression and to satisfy his conscience through accomplishing "good" constructive hard work. He tries to cope with the danger by redoubled efforts to be responsible and orderly, and to suppress uncontrolled emotions. There is often an intensification of self-restraint, formalized behavior, and obstinacy so that the patient seems inflexible and opinionated. His increased striving for intellectual control, with the need to be certain that he understands and has taken into account every aspect of his problems, may lead to hesitation, doubting, and indecisiveness over the question of whether he knows all the essential facts. At times we might be startled to see the breakthrough of disorderliness and anger, but generally his self-control predominates.

The orderly, controlled person usually finds the scientific medical approach a congenial one. He responds well to the precise and systematic efforts that characterize the doctor's careful, rational method of procedure in history-taking, physical diagnosis, laboratory studies, and treatment. He values highly the emphasis upon sympathetic efficiency and cleanliness in nursing care. In fact, these qualities are so important to him that he may evince unexpectedly strong disapproval of any lapse of routine or contradictory statement which he cannot fit into his logical framework. When his equilibrium becomes taxed under the stress of illness, perhaps leading to anxiety and intensification of characteristic reactions, an explicit therapeutic approach is indicated to facilitate his adaptation to the threatening situation. He should be informed methodically and in sufficient detail about his illness and the appropriate steps in diagnosis and therapy so that he can establish intellectual control over his anxiety. In doing this, one proceeds cautiously, carefully considering the risk of introducing new sources of anxiety, and not feeling bound to discuss all of the upsetting possibilities and unpleasant minutiae for the sake of "completeness." The patient's active participation in decisions is welcomed and, whenever it is feasible, he might be encouraged to carry out details of his actual medical care—for example, exercises or changing certain dressings, or carefully calculating his caloric intake. The physician will do well to give him recognition for his discernment, comprehension, sound reasoning, and high standards.

### The Dramatizing, Emotionally Involved, Captivating (Hysterical) Personality

The physician usually finds himself interested, charmed, fascinated, and challenged with this kind of person. However, at times he might feel mystified and suspect the patient of not really being sick, or even of malingering. The patient tends to react to the doctor in an eager, warm, very personal way, and to expect a similar response from him in return.

He or she may be imaginative, dramatic, flighty, teasing or inviting, and characteristically strives for an intense, idealizing relationship with the doctor. This type of person may have an accentuated need to be noticed and admired as attractive and outstanding, and may show jealousy of the doctor's interest in any other patient. A man may repeatedly attempt to prove and even exaggerate his manliness and courage, especially before nurses and women doctors. In turn, with a male physician, a woman of this personality type may bring out in an inviting way her defenselessness and need for gallant support and protection. She will dress and make up in an attractive manner, notwithstanding rather severe physical conditions. This colorful, lively personality readily develops anxiety in connection with even minor medical procedures. The patient will avoid frightening situations if possible, but sometimes, in an attempt to overcome the fear, will rush into danger. A tendency toward denial or not remembering previous upsetting experiences may be apparent, so that the doctor may feel that this patient is not the most reliable informant. These personal traits are most typically derived from a period of development between three and six years of age, in which the child forms a strong attachment to the parent of the opposite sex. In his or her warm, colorful response, the adult of this type gives emotional expression to impulses stemming from this early affection. Guilt over hostile urges toward the parent of the same sex who is seen as a rival by the child, and fear of punishment and retaliation, form the basis for the later characteristic anxieties of the patient.

### The Meaning of Illness

To the dramatizing, emotionally involved kind of person a sickness may feel like a personal defect; it means being weak and unattractive, unappreciated, and unsuccessful. It is often taken unconsciously as a punishment for forbidden childhood wishes. In men, the major fears are of bodily damage and loss of manly accomplishment and power: exertion of physical strength, competitiveness or pugnacity in order to deny these anxieties may dominate the picture, and amorous fantasies involving nurses or other attending women may be actively pursued. Women of this type feel threatened with the loss of their attractiveness: they may become flirtatious or dress up on the ward as for a special occasion. The struggle against anxiety in both men and women may be marked by increased efforts to gain admiration, dramatic bids for attention, or even an attitude of indifference to serious implications of disease if the illness is used by the patient to secure the attention and sympathy of the environment. Under intense anxiety, these reactions can go a step further and lead to a paradoxical condition in which the patient pushes for those very events that he fears the most. For instance, he may show an inappropriately light-hearted readiness to venture into a serious operation, without truly appreciating and accepting its necessity and consequences. Such "foolhardiness" in an otherwise intelligent and realistic person is reminiscent of the stunts of anxious adolescents who carelessly expose themselves to dangers in order to cope with anxiety by proving that they are not "chicken."

Since these patients seek appreciation of their attractiveness and courage, it would be an error for the doctor to be too reserved. At the same time the physician should remain aware of the patients' readiness for emotional involvement and anxiety, and should proceed with a measure of calmness and firmness to avoid stirring up these reactions. If anxieties are intense, reassuring explanations about the illness and the medical procedures will help the patient to distinguish reality from alarming fantasies. These discussions need not be as comprehensive and systematic as they should be with the orderly, controlled personality. It is often useful to allow the patient of this type a chance to discuss his fears repeatedly, if necessary, and in this way discharge some of his pent-up feelings.

### The Long-suffering, Self-sacrificing (Masochistic) Patient

Physicians frequently see patients with a history of repeated suffering whether from illnesses, disappointments, or other adversities and failures. These people often regard their difficulties as a sign of bad luck. Upon closer examination of their experiences, we can discern that among those patients there is a group with a strong unconscious tendency to precipitate their own misfortunes—perhaps by placing themselves in difficult positions or by reacting too sensitively to the unpleasant aspects of life situations. They are inclined to disregard their own comfort and be of service to other people. Despite their apparent humility and modesty, we usually observe in such patients a tendency to display suffering in an exhibitionistic way. They evoke sympathy and praise from most people but also may arouse in them uneasiness and a guilty intolerance.

The desire to seek suffering is difficult to understand since it is contrary to the prevalent notion that pain can only be unpleasant. Though we cannot here do justice to the complexity of this attitude, it may be helpful to discuss this problem more extensively. The picture may become less puzzling if we consider the relation of pleasure to pain and the dynamic function of suffering and self-sacrifice. Pleasure and pain are often closely associated both physically and psychologically. For example, we are familiar with the co-existence or fusion of pleasure and pain in athletic exertion and in bitter-sweet states of experience such as love-sickness or the adolescent *Weltschmerz*. In women, menstruation, intercourse, and childbirth are intimately associated with discomfort and yet also with the most deeply gratifying feminine experiences. Furthermore, as children we may have frequently encountered painful situations which were linked with satisfaction. Children repeatedly discover that when they become ill they can receive more than their usual share of love and attention from their parents. Beyond this, looking at the seeking of suffering from a dynamic point of view, we find in some individuals a search for punishment in order to expiate and relieve the pressure of a deep feeling of guilt. We are familiar with people who consciously or unconsciously believe that they do not deserve to succeed in life. They expect that when things go well something bad has to happen, and sometimes they bring about their setbacks, so that this suffering may temporarily atone and pacify the guilty worry in them. The extreme instance of this type of personality is exemplified in the martyr who finds glory and resolution of his guilt by achieving his social, political, or religious ideal through severe self-sacrifice and suffering. The co-existence of pain and satisfaction in the biological function of the woman, the young person with *Weltschmerz*, the child who is cherished and forgiven because he is ill, the person who atones unknowingly for guilt, and the martyr—all are models that demonstrate involuntary self-victimization.

Among the early experiences that appear to contribute to the development of this attitude we find severely repressive upbringing in which the child was made to feel excessively guilty, was not permitted to show anger even in a harmless manner, and was given corporal punishment, which in some children provokes excitement that is tinged with pleasure. An attachment to a parent who was aggressive toward the child may have shaped later relationships to important figures in life according to this pattern, or the child may have unconsciously modeled himself upon a suffering parent. In the youngster who felt especially favored and loved when he was sick, this satisfaction may take over as an end in itself and become established as a pattern that is carried throughout life.

### The Meaning of Illness

The basic striving of this personality is to gain love, care and acceptance, although he feels too guilty and anxious to expect this without self-sacrifice and suffering. The dangers and discomforts of illness may be elaborated by the patient in intensified attitudes of submission and suffering, complaining, or self-effacement, and feeling martyred. For the doctor, the most frequently encountered form of this attitude is the childlike expectation, "you have to love me because I suffer so terribly." But when he tries to comfort a patient of this kind, perhaps a pitiably distressed elderly lady, he discovers a paradoxical phenomenon. He is confronted with a person who seems to work against his encouragement and above all to deny any improvement. As he offers helpful suggestions or comforting reassurance, her complaints increase. She disregards evidence of progress toward recovery and accentuates those aspects of her illness which have not improved. Very understandably, this may lead to feelings of disappointment and irritation on the part of the doctor if he does not recognize her reaction as fitting into a special pattern of behavior. When a person of this type says, "it's not easy, doctor," he is not asking for encouraging remarks but for acknowledgement of his pain and sacrifices. Accordingly, the doctor should express his appreciation of the difficulties of illness as they are experienced by this patient. The long-suffering, self-sacrificing person is better able to co-operate in a medical regimen out of a readiness to add to the "burden" that he must carry, than for the personal relief that health would bring to him. The physician may have to present the recovery to the patient as a special additional task, if possible for the benefit of others. For example, an older woman of this type who repeatedly refused a rehabilitating operation when it was urged as essential to preserve her well-being and comfort, was able to accept it only when it was pointed out that she could not continue to be of help to her children unless her physical condition was corrected.

### The Guarded, Querulous (Paranoid) Person

This patient is openly or covertly watchful of other persons, inclined to be suspicious of their intentions, or querulous and blameful of their motives. He may nurse grievances, especially a deep sense of having been let down by people. He particularly fears being placed in a vulnerable position in which he could be unexpectedly hurt or taken advantage of. Patients who consistently expect the worst are oversensitive to slights and to hints of negative feelings in other people. They easily feel oppressed and even persecuted and are likely to react with a self-righteous counter-attack, exaggerated out of all proportion to actual insults. This excessive sensitivity to criticism and expectation of being assaulted reflects a deeper concern with their own faults and weaknesses. They deal with their inner problems and self-reproaches in a very interesting way, by disclaiming them entirely as if they had no place within themselves, and reading them, with indignant disapproval, into the attitudes of other people. We can understand this kind of reaction in an adult better by referring back to the behavior of small children. In its simplest form, we see the youngster who hurts himself by running into a table and then blames the "bad, nasty table." At a somewhat older age, we may observe the little girl who, when chided for misbehaving, says with guilty defiance that her naughty doll did it, not she. An echo of this childhood cry of "I didn't do it— he did it" is found in those adults who have to get rid of whatever is painful, dangerous, or intolerable within themselves by attributing it to others. By thus freeing themselves from what seems unworthy, they both elevate their self-regard and perceive other people as threatening and bad. We are familiar with the individual of this type who does not want to acknowledge in himself impulses to infidelity but is hypersensitive and very critical when he has any possibility of finding and fighting these urges in his marital partner.

## The Meaning of Illness

The guarded, querulous patient tends to blame others for his illness. During periods of sickness, his tensions and aggressive tendencies and his expectations of being harmed may be intensified. He becomes even more fearful, guarded, suspicious, quarrelsome and controlling of others. In medical management, it is essential to let this kind of person know, as far as foreseeable, the strategy of diagnosis and treatment so that his suspicions may be kept in abeyance. The frequent oversensitivity to slights of individuals of this type should be respected so as not to create a conflict between patient and doctor. A friendly and courteous attitude on the doctor's part, that avoids getting too close to or excessively involved with the patient, is often indicated. If the physician goes beyond this, there is the risk that the patient will feel he is either being forced or manipulated. Arguing with him or ignoring his suspicious attitude does not help, and if as his doctors we try to convince him that everyone has the best of intentions, he is unable to believe it and it might lead to further mistrust.

In the case of a man with these personality traits who had undergone a very serious cancer operation and who complained bitterly about any inconvenience or irregularity in the hospital routine, we could observe two different reactions of the people attending him. Some were drawn into agreeing with him, sharing his irritation over the coldness of the food, the slowness of the nurses, and the inaccessibility of the doctors. This had the effect of increasing his acrimonious discontent. Others tried to point out how exaggerated his reproaches were, or, becoming provoked, told him in effect that he was asking for too much and was ungrateful for the care that he had been given. He responded with recriminations against them as well as undiminished anger at the hospital. We were able to lessen his preoccupation and mitigate his querulous response by taking a third approach. He was assured that we could appreciate how upsetting these inconveniences and delays can be for a person of his sensitivity who had gone through such a trying illness. By acknowledging and giving him full credit for his feelings as his way of perceiving and encountering the world —without disputing his complaints, but especially without reinforcing them—we could help him to detach himself and reduce the intensity of his reactions. Only then was it possible to take the next step: to appeal to his tolerance regarding these experiences in the hospital which, although very distressing to him, were less significant compared with the lifesaving surgery and rehabilitating postoperative care. Thus we were able to regain his co-operation.

### The Patient with the Feeling of Superiority (Narcissistic)

Among our patients, we find people who have to see themselves as powerful and all-important. This need may lead to an attitude of self-confidence so exaggerated that a person of this type appears smug, vain or grandiose. Or his basic frame of mind may be covered by an artificial, patronizing humility. Frequently, associated characteristics include a kind of arrogance (he looks down on most other people), the tendency to surround himself with an aura of mysterious knowledge, and sometimes a fondness for holding forth—mainly in monologues. A considerable amount of every adult's interest centers around his own self. If this attitude is not excessive we speak of self-respect rather than a feeling of superiority. As we have discovered with so many exaggerated tendencies which serve the purpose of counteracting doubts, the patient who feels superior has an urgent need to surpass everyone else, coupled with an underlying uncertainty about his own transcendence. When he falls ill and must turn to a doctor, this person deems only the most eminent or senior physician worthy of serving him, choosing someone who will reinforce the sense of his own grandeur. Even in a large teaching hospital where he is cared for by a medical team, such a patient may only acknowledge that he is being treated by the Chief of Service. His attitude toward the younger physicians is frequently that of a benevolent supervisor who tolerantly aids them in their quest for education. In spite of his need for a doctor who has the utmost competence, the patient is bound at the same time to vie with him and outdo him. He may allow that he himself is not a medical expert (if this be the case), yet he might feel free to reject his doctor's counsel on the basis of his own conclusions and considerations which he believes to be of greater moment. This patient tends to search constantly for weaknesses in the doctor and is inclined to lose confidence in him, dwelling upon his faults and belittling him at the slightest provocation.

### The Meaning of Illness

The person with the feeling of superiority is likely to react to a sickness as if it threatened his self-image of perfection and invulnerability. His characteristic behavior becomes intensified, often in the direction of a defensive grandiosity. Accordingly, he will feel most comfortable and secure if the doctor fulfills his need of being implicitly acknowledged as a person of achievement in his own right. Of course, this does not mean that the physician can or should deny his own expert knowledge and skill. In fact, this kind of person, in spite of all his effort to find weaknesses in the doctor, is at the same time deeply afraid of discovering that he might be in the hands of an incompetent physician.

### The Patient Who Seems Uninvolved and Aloof (Schizoid)

This person gives an impression of remoteness, reserve, and lack of involvement with everyday events and concerns of people. His emotional expression may be reduced to a minimum and he may appear quiet, distant, seclusive, and unsociable. He may pursue his own way of life, seemingly with little need for emotional ties with others, appearing quite independent and not easily impressed. Beneath this surface such a person often is oversensitive, fragile, and lacking resilience, so that his inner equilibrium is too easily upset in the course of the ordinary difficulties of human relationships. His aloofness is a protective denial of these excessively painful experiences. The life history of such a person reflects solitary interests. He gravitates to noncompetitive jobs that require a minimum of contact with others. Within this group, we find eccentric persons engrossed individually with dietary and health fads, religious movements, and social improvement schemes. The aloof, eccentric patient may exhibit an unusual manner of dressing or behaving without concern for the reactions of conventional people.

We often find in the childhood history of this kind of patient that his earliest efforts to form a loving attachment to another person led to repeated disappointments, with the result that the child could invest feelings in others only in a tentative and limited way. This might be the consequence of repeated separations from mother, or of a lack of consistent responsive, empathic care by the environment. The infantile experience then is carried into the patient's later relationships, leading finally to the type of personality who impresses us as uninvolved and remote. There are also indications that constitutional factors may play an important role in the genesis of this kind of personality, especially in its most pronounced form.

## The Meaning of Illness

The aloof person tries to remain undisturbed by life, seeking solace and satisfaction within himself. Illness intrudes into this system, threatening to upset this careful equilibrium. The patient frequently protects himself against this by intensifying his denial in proportion to the increase in underlying anxiety and thus seems to remain strikingly unperturbed and even more seclusive and distant than usual. Foremost in the psychological management of this patient, his "unsociability" has to be understood and accepted. We should make as few demands as possible upon him for personal involvement with others, yet he should not be permitted to withdraw completely. This may be achieved by trying to maintain a considerate interest in him, quietly and reassuringly, without requesting a reciprocal effort on his part.

## Clinical Application of Personality Diagnosis

We have taken up only major aspects of personality diagnosis. Clinical experience reveals a wide vista of possible shades and combinations of characteristics in the make-up of different individuals. In practice, one must avoid the premature and rigid use of a diagnostic classification of personality since this involves the hazard of becoming limited in one's perception of the patient's structure. This will happen if "typing" a patient becomes a shortcut, replacing the natural development of a relationship and full observation of the distinguishing qualities of the person. Moreover, it is not always easy to establish quickly the correct personality diagnosis. The problem of perceiving the leading personality traits is complicated by the fact that in some degree everyone has passed through similar phases of early development and, therefore, in his adult personality tends to show an admixture of all modes of behavior. Nevertheless, each person has his particular means of adjustment and should be judged by his predominant psychological organization. But while the basic personality structure of an adult remains relatively stable, under special stress shifts between a variety of defenses and needs may occur (G. L. Bibring, 1961; Prange and Abse, 1957). With these pitfalls in mind, let us now take up a clinical example illustrating the task of managing flexibly the medical psychotherapy of a patient whose leading attitudes varied in the course of his illness.

A thirty-nine-year-old man with an acute, severe myocardial infarction, the fourth within nine years, was extremely apprehensive during his first days in the hospital.[1] Fully aware of the nature of his disease, he was terrified that he might die. Yet, despite his desperate desire to live, he frequently refused to rest or take medication. This handsome, physically powerful man regarded any request by the nurses as arbitrary and refused to be "commanded" by them. He was also aggressively seductive towards them. His previous pattern of reaction to illness suggested that a tendency toward hyperactivity might interfere with his recovery. Though he had been advised to return to only moderate physical activity after his earlier coronary thromboses, he had vigorously pursued water polo, handball and wrestling with his children. We discovered that these attitudes had a long history.

He had run away from home at the age of thirteen, shortly after his father had died of a malignant tumor. His flight had followed a quarrel in which he felt that his oldest brother had tried to order him around. He was a big youngster and passed himself off as sixteen or seventeen when he got a job with a traveling carnival. In subsequent years, he worked as a roustabout and rigger of amusement "rides," a bulldozer operator, a truckdriver and a two-fisted bouncer in a penny arcade—nothing was too difficult for him to take on. In his marriage, he immediately established his position as the master of the household. Both in the home and at work, he felt that challenges and fights gave meaning to his life. He boasted about his manly prowess, yet, in listening to the account of his many successes, one had the definite impression that he exaggerated. All of this indicated his need to see himself as prepotent.

[1] Dr. Arthur R. Kravitz and Dr. Robert E. Eisendrath have contributed their observations of this patient.

It was evident that this colorful, lively man had many features of the dramatizing, emotionally involved personality. Typically, he responded to his life-endangering illness as if it threatened his masculinity. Because he suffered from this anxiety and, therefore, might jeopardize himself by premature and excessive exercises, it was necessary to give immediate attention to help the patient re-establish his psychological equilibrium. It was found that he accepted the nurses' care with more comfort and appreciation when all medical recommendations were given to him personally, as far as possible, by his male doctor. At the same time it was considered essential to permit him to apply some initiative and strength. Thus, even while he had to remain strictly on bed rest, he was encouraged to carry out his own schedule of simple leg exercises and rest periods and to help in dietary planning. As an essential part of the therapeutic program, he did some light work with the occupational therapist. His physician repeatedly acknowledged the great discipline which the patient applied, and expressed his appreciation of the difficulties this illness may create for an active, vigorous man. Information about his illness was offered with the aim of reducing some of his uncertainty about the outcome of his condition, and to prepare him to cope with the illness in a more rational way. In responding to his questions about the future, emphasis was placed on his improved chances of survival with collateral coronary circulation, if he maintained his activities within limits under continued medical observation.

With this approach the patient was helped to make the shift from displaying his strength by muscular activity to exercising it through intelligent self-control. He became less quarrelsome and more optimistic, and was full of high praise for his house physician who had explained thoroughly some of the medical problems to him. However, as we have seen in similar cases, this patient who had dealt with the acute, critical, and life-threatening situation by the protective mechanism of denying his weakness, in the convalescent period displayed different attitudes and needs in dealing with his underlying anxieties. This in turn required modification of the psychological management. When the patient returned home, he became very apprehensive whenever he went outside of the house. He had to lie down and complain to his wife that she did not realize how sick he was. He would ask whether he looked pale; his pulse seemed fast and weak to him. Pains occurred in his upper abdomen and chest which were not relieved by nitroglycerine but were helped by sedation. It was apparent that he needed special care and attention at this time in a dependent, anxious way. In response, his physician took a definitely protective attitude. He told the patient that his doctors were willing and able to take full responsibility for his treatment, and could be trusted and depended upon. With this assurance the patient's anxiety lessened. When he returned to work he felt better on the job than at home because he could be more active there and was less prone to yield to his dependent wishes. He was able to relinquish his bid for extra attention from his family and knew that he could be a well-functioning man in his own right. He came to the clinic less frequently, but kept a solid, confident relationship with his doctors and was able to adhere to the medical regimen.

### Summary

In a long-term program aimed at blending psychological understanding with medical practice in a general hospital, it has been found that a knowledge of personality structure is an important basis for the physician in order to employ appropriate psychotherapeutic principles in the management of physically ill patients. A paradigmatic classification of personalities is described that is useful as a guide for medical psychotherapy. It includes the following "types": *the dependent, over-demanding personality; the orderly, controlled personality; the dramatizing, emotionally involved, captivating personality; the long-suffering, self-sacrificing patient; the guarded, querulous patient; the patient who feels superior; the patient who seems uninvolved and aloof.* For each type a brief formulation is made of the essential psychological meaning of physical illness and inferences for medical management are drawn. The classification is particularly applicable to the normal personality under stress. A case illustrating medical psychotherapy is presented.

# Psychiatric Rounds on the Private Medical Service of a General Hospital

NORMAN E. ZINBERG, M.D.

REGULAR PSYCHIATRIC ROUNDS on the private medical service of the Beth Israel Hospital were introduced in September, 1955, as a logical continuation of the extensive teaching relationship which had been developed between psychiatry and medicine over a period of eight years (G. L. Bibring, 1956; Dwyer and Zinberg, 1957; Kahana, 1959). Because there had been so much useful interchange between psychiatrists and internists at Beth Israel, the experiment of teaching psychoanalytic psychiatry to medical house officers with private patients was begun under favorable conditions. Nonetheless, from the first, both the inherent difficulties of teaching so complex a theory as psychoanalysis, and the issues raised by that theory which do not pertain to its intellectual content, presented serious problems.

Because psychoanalysis is more than a form of psychiatric treatment, theoretical and emotional problems continually arise in the teaching situation. As a theoretical system which seeks to understand human motivation, inevitably, it is concerned with human values. The psychodynamic model of personality constructs the psychological characteristics of the individual from his sexual and aggressive biological drives, his defenses against those drives, and his capacity for successful adaptation. As the individual grows up, in his family and in his culture, he develops the complex set of attitudes, goals, values, and standards of thought and behavior that comprise his character and personality. The difficulty of teaching so complex a theoretical system simply and effectively is complicated by the skepticism of many physicians about psychoanalytic theory, or their sharp disagreement with it.

The development of a systematic concept of medical psychology by Grete L. Bibring (1956) has made the task of teaching easier. She has constructed a classification of personality types based on habitual behavior patterns which become more marked under stress. Further, she has outlined a style of therapeutic intervention which attempts to maintain the structural equilibrium of the patient's personality (manipulation[1]) without involving the patient in a prolonged exploratory attempt at understanding his troubles. Although Bibring's concepts solve a considerable part of the difficulties of teaching psychoanalytic theory, there remains a most difficult technical teaching problem, the application of general principles of psychoanalytic psychiatry to individual patients. While making the floor rounds, attending physicians would like the psychiatrist to make a definitive diagnosis of various patients, even if he sees the patients for just a few minutes. For the purposes of teaching, however, the psychiatrist wishes to point out how these patients illustrate theoretical issues. My efforts to surmount this difficulty, as the Assistant Director of the Psychiatric Service and the person who conducts the rounds on the private medical service, form the subject of this paper.

# I

To begin, it is necessary to understand the special problems of teaching on a private medical service which do not usually arise on the wards. All teaching hospitals with both ward and private services find it difficult to maintain the same high educational standard in the private service as on the ward. On the ward service, one senior physician visits almost every day for a month and is consulted about all the patients. This arrangement permits him to plan and, hopefully, to execute a comprehensive teaching program for his period of supervision. A comparable approach is impossible on a private service because no matter how interested in teaching the staff physicians are, they have access only to those patients they themselves have admitted. Wards are peopled increasingly by elderly patients, and

---

[1] "We do not use the term 'manipulation' . . . to describe the undesirable attempt . . . to force concepts and plans on the patient. We use the term in a more positive sense. After listening to and observing the patient we may use our understanding of his personality structure, his patterns, his needs and conflicts, and his defenses . . . to modify our attitude and approach to his problems; or we may purposely activate relevant emotional attitudes in the patient for the sake of adjustive change" (G. L. Bibring, 1949).

it is only on the private service[2] that the house staff has the opportunity to see and, to a degree, treat large numbers of young patients. For some years, many teaching hospitals have tried to ameliorate this situation by improving the quality and variety of the teaching on the private service. The need for these efforts has been intensified by the increasing number of people who would once have been ward patients but who now have medical insurance which pays for private care.

Several attempts have been made to institute medical teaching rounds on the private service at Beth Israel. Understandably, when the proposal was first made, some of the visiting staff were opposed to major extensions of teaching which would use their private patients as subjects. Hospitals are difficult enough for patients, they agreed, without increasing the number of medical visitors, examinations, and other inconveniences to the patients, and thus intensifying their discomfort and anxiety. There was also some feeling that the private side rounds might meddle in the patient's treatment and in the doctor's relationship with his patient. A number of physicians felt that, because of their thorough and lengthy study of their private patients, they were best able to see a current illness in perspective and to know if consultation were needed. Others were concerned with the possibility that the physician on rounds would, for purposes of discussion, raise relatively obscure issues that called for a multiplicity of tests and procedures. Of course, many private physicians agreed that a colleague's fresh response to a patient might be of value. Any physician could, of course, refuse to accept a suggestion he did not agree with. Nevertheless, the proposed changes in the hospital atmosphere might well result in the private physician's feeling that someone was looking over his shoulder. A few physicians also objected openly to the possibility of competition. They did not like the idea of their patients being seen by another physician who would be followed, like a sage, by a retinue of house officers. These visits might undermine the patient's faith in his own doctor.

In 1955, when the Psychiatric Service was included in the proposal to

[2] It is not only the inconsistent nature of the teaching that makes the private service unpopular to the house officer, but also his anomalous position on this service. He is asked to take a history, leave orders, and in general care for a patient who is not his. Supposedly, the extent to which he is asked to assume responsibility varies with each staff doctor, but, because he is there all the time, in practice the house officer has a basic responsibility for the well-being of the patient that occasionally takes precedence over the wishes of the private physician. The patient, although aware that the private doctor is responsible for the medical regimen, frequently turns to the house officer with requests or questions that are difficult to answer, postpone, or side-step without affecting, at least, the psychological management. House officers become impatient with this situation.

reorganize and intensify the teaching program on the private side, many staff doctors objected strongly, even though it was clearly stated that the doctor's permission would be required before any private patient could be seen. These physicians overlooked the fact that G. L. Bibring had given lectures to the house officers, using patients as clinical illustrations, from 1946 to 1953, and that since 1952 I have been conducting regular ward meetings similar to those proposed on the private side. Both the lectures and the ward rounds were considered valuable by the house staff and never disrupted optimum patient care. Other worries raised against psychiatric rounds on the wards were resurrected: the psychiatrist would upset the patient; he should be permitted to see the patient only after the anxiety of illness had entirely abated; he should see only certain patients, those who were considered "neurotic" by their own physicians. These objections, which were usually expressed in ideological or moral terms, revealed many common misconceptions about psychoanalytic psychiatry, such as the belief that an interest in the emotional reactions that exist below the surface of the mind implies a lack of respect for consciously expressed motives. It was also assumed that the psychiatrist would only be interested in what was wrong with a patient and would search for defects and faults.

However, the need for the improved teaching program was so great that it was instituted as proposed despite the objections. It was agreed that the house staff assigned to the private service would meet twice a week with internists, once a week with me, and once a week on rotation with various other medical subspecialties.

I recognized that, although the objections raised to my interviewing private patients were irrational, they represented an important body of medical opinion which must be considered in the content and method of my teaching. At grand medical rounds, in an attempt to meet these objections, I explained to the medical staff how I planned to conduct psychiatric rounds on the private medical service. First, I pointed out, the psychiatrist is trained in the principles of interviewing and in recognizing the anxiety level of the person being interviewed, and is, therefore, less likely than other interviewers to upset the patient. Only brief psychiatric interviews were planned, and they would follow the standard medical history-taking procedure, rather than any psychiatric interviewing technique.

Secondly, I indicated my awareness of the necessity for the psychiatrist, as well as the other staff doctors, to disturb the patient as little as possible, and made certain specific suggestions which might make the rounds more acceptable to the internists. Some physicians asked whether, when they gave permission for me to see patients, they could have the option of specifying that I present myself merely as another staff physician.[3] I agreed as long as this arrangement involved no outright deception, because it fitted with my conception of the purpose of the rounds, which was to teach psychoanalytic psychiatry in the form of medical psychology, that is, to teach the basic psychiatric principles necessary to enhance knowledge of patients and of medical management for internists. It was not intended to train the house officers as psychiatrists. Medical psychology applies to all patients, not only to those who suffer from emotional difficulties. As for the objections which seemed to me to represent misconceptions about psychoanalysis, I decided not to answer them directly but to allow experience with the teaching procedure itself to provide the answers.

## II

The procedure set up for the rounds calls for the medical resident in charge of the private service to obtain permission from the private physician to visit the patient, to see that the patient knows about the visit, and to let the psychiatrist know where to meet the house staff. When the rounds began, the medical resident often asked me to help him choose the patients to be seen. I told him I was willing to see any case that the house staff was interested in. At first the house staff chose patients they considered to be emotionally disturbed, but after a while, they learned to select patients whose medical management was a problem.

After the case is selected, the house officer assigned to the patient presents a resume of the patient's history and hospital course, stressing whatever makes this patient interesting. From the start, this step in the procedure always raised an important teaching difficulty. If the discussion emphasized the patient as an individual, the house officers tended to overlook the general psychological principles involved. But if I was inconclusive about the problems of the individual case, they would lose interest in the broad principles of personality diagnosis and medical management which are the principal matter of the psychiatric teaching program.

I know very well that the information available to me from the resumé and my ten- or fifteen-minute interview with the patient limits the possibility of precision about the personality structure and medical management of the particular patient. However, what the house officers have

---

[3] In fact, on two occasions, internists requested that I wear a stethoscope so that the patient would not even suspect that I was a psychiatrist.

heard about a particular case, and especially what they hear in my interview with the patient, interests them in that specific case. If I can sustain this interest, a lively discussion usually follows in which many participate, but in which general psychiatric principles can easily be lost sight of.

To avoid this pitfall, I urge the group, before we see a patient, to speculate about the particular problem raised by the case, using only the information given in the history. Since the patient himself has not been seen, we are free to speculate about the case, and we can plan what questions might verify or eliminate various possible diagnoses. In the course of this planning, we often discuss the important question of how psychological understanding, both in general and about individual cases, is necessary and worthwhile for the general physician. I make a point of asking if any other house officers have patients with similar problems. Occasionally, if the discussion is lively and constructive, we discuss general problems the entire time and do not see the patient at all. The purpose of teaching rounds, which is to provide general education about personality and not psychiatric consultation about individual patients, is thus reaffirmed convincingly.

When I do offer specific suggestions for the management of individual cases, I emphasize that these manipulations will not solve all future management problems and will certainly not help long-standing personality difficulties. The aim of the system of medical psychology developed by G. L. Bibring is to select from what we learn about a patient the pertinent emotional conflict. In a curious way, what we believe to be a general human response to illness aids us in this teaching procedure. Illness is always accompanied by fear, and as a result, especially in a hospital setting, all patients are deprived of their characteristic ways of behaving. Also, importantly, people behave differently toward them. This interferes with the individual's usual concept of himself; one could say that his dignity or identity suffers. This point can be brought out in an interview with a patient, when I can demonstrate how characteristic defensive maneuvers intensify. Therefore, the stress of illness makes the selection of whatever emotional responses or conflicts are pertinent for medical management easier.

In a sense, the fact that illness often simplifies an individual's emotional responses is corroborated when patients I have first interviewed on these rounds consult me after they have left the hospital. Usually it requires several interviews before I can make the same educated guess about the patient's central emotional conflict and his defense against it that I was able to make in a few minutes when the patient was hospitalized. Of course, a conflict which is stirred up by illness and hospitalization may not be the same one that might be activated by another kind of crisis.

Occasionally, I will use a meeting to report to the house officers about my later interviews with a patient we had previously seen together, to show this difference. However, even when reporting a psychiatric interview, I ask them to remember the same general principles as in the interviews that we share. That is to say again, a patient's behavior, a patient's comments, and the inferences derived from these about his less conscious feelings, supply sufficient information for appropriate management. What we try to emphasize is that this information can be obtained by any doctor who knows how to direct the standard but elastic medical interview toward obtaining it.

## III

A brief clinical example will illustrate how this procedure functions on the rounds.

Mr. A., fifty-nine years old, had been admitted with subacute glomerular nephritis. He improved rapidly according to his laboratory tests, but continued to feel sick and had a fresh complaint every day. The house officer felt that the patient reacted with an intensification of symptoms to assurance from his private doctor that he was improving and would soon go home. There was no material in his history to indicate neurosis. I chose to ask the house officer, Dr. C., to repeat in some detail his apparently typical exchange with Mr. A. that morning. Dr. C. had gone in, said good morning rather cheerily, and asked how Mr. A. was. Mr. A. said that he had had a bad night and was very worried because he still had pain. Dr. C. was quickly reassuring and told Mr. A. of his improving tests. Instead of responding with the pleased smile that Dr. C. had hoped for, Mr. A. gave a grimace of pain and expressed doubt that he was getting better. Dr. C., still reassuring, told Mr. A. that clinical improvement should follow the proved remission of the disease, and that he would surely be feeling better by the morrow. Dr. C. left the patient's room feeling dissatisfied with the interview, but with no clear idea of what he could have done that would have been more helpful.

There seemed to be enough evidence in this exchange to indicate masochistic trends in Mr. A., so we went over the history again for corroborative data. Two things came to light which could easily have been overlooked. Dr. C. remembered that he had been impressed by Mr. A.'s excessively detailed description of his suffering during a previous operation. Also, when Mr. A. had been asked about his family history, instead of answering succinctly, which was usual for him, he had described elaborately how he had borne the responsibility and done much of the actual nursing during his father's long terminal illness.

Slender threads indeed these were, but with them I led the group to discuss the nature of reassurance. It was generally conceded that what Dr. C. had done was to be reassuring in his own terms without sufficiently taking into account Mr. A.'s possible conflicts. Reassurance is only reassurance if it reassures the patient about what is worrying him, not about what the doctor thinks should be worrying him. On the basis of other patients they had seen, two house officers offered suggestions about Mr. A. One resident thought that Mr. A.'s relationship with his father might be important, and wanted to know more about Mr. A.'s father's illness, particularly at what age it had occurred and what the symptoms had been. Another resident suggested that Mr. A. might feel threatened by getting better. Perhaps if more were known about his reaction to his acute illness or about his entire life situation, one of these possibilities would be supported. All agreed that Dr. C. could not effectively reassure Mr. A. until some of these questions were answered more specifically.

When the group went in to see Mr. A., it was not specified that I, as the visiting doctor, was a psychiatrist. The interview began by my apologizing for the intrusion. The apology was waved off weakly by the patient, who lay slumped in bed looking wan and waiting for questions. When asked how he came to be in the hospital, Mr. A. replied by asking if he had to go through the story again. Instead of answering directly, I commented on what a hard time Mr. A. was having. This invoked a flood of speech from him about his difficulties and fears. I mentioned how co-operative Mr. A. was to see all of us, feeling as sick as he did. For the first time in the interview, the patient brightened. Mr. A. was then asked what his doctors had told him about his illness and, after his obviously mistrustful answer that he was supposed to be getting better, I pointed out how little such protestations helped when one still felt sick. With Mr. A. becoming more and more vigorous with each exchange, I continued on the tack that the doctors could really do only so much and that after that the patient had to do the hard job of bearing the aftermath and fighting his way through convalescence. Mr. A. was now sitting up in bed and speaking with animation. He talked about his fears that the illness had taken so much out of him that he would never be his old self again. I only replied that it was a painful struggle, and asked if there was anything that Mr. A. felt about himself, or that he had been told about his condition, that indicated that he would be unable to make it. Mr. A. thoughtfully said no, and his goodbye was infinitely warmer than his hello.

The group reassembled and agreed that Mr. A.'s change of manner had been a result of my allowing him to be ill and giving him some credit for and some part in the struggle back to activity. There was a general recognition of how easily the house officer and the visiting staff member could have been drawn into trying to reassure this patient by telling him he was getting better. They then commented, somewhat complainingly, that they still could not answer the questions raised before the interview. That was the opening that permitted them to see the rounds as a teaching situation and not as a psychiatric consultation. From there I asked them how Mr. A.'s house officer could go about getting more evidence for one or the other of the hypotheses, what that evidence would mean about Mr. A. in particular, and what it would mean about personality types with a conflict about strength and weakness in general. Mr. A.'s house officer, Dr. C., agreed to report to the group the following week.

It is true that not every patient's response is as direct as was Mr. A.'s. In fact, as much as the psychiatric service on these and other rounds wants to convey to a physician of another specialty the practical use of understanding personality structure and adapting his approach to the patient's struggle, they also try to see patients whose management problem is clearly not going to be easily resolved. In Mr. A.'s case the practicality of an approach using the patient's habitual personality responses was demonstrated, but at the same time the need for more information to maintain an effective relationship with the patient was clear to everyone. Moreover, the groundwork had been laid for a more theoretical discussion of people's fears of being strong, turning a feeling into its opposite, anxiety in general, and many more such topics. So often, when psychiatry or medical psychology is taught, other physicians are quick to say, "Show me what is valuable for me and my patients without my having to spend hundreds of hours learning it." Translated, this means no ivory-tower theories, but practicable, relatively quick techniques. However, once the logical relationship between personality conflict and behavior becomes apparent, these physicians invariably want more theory.

In fact, requests for more direct theoretical discussions during the rounds rather than the interview of a patient are a regular yearly sign that the teaching has had effects. There are others, the most consistent and significant of which is the type of patient selected for the rounds. Early in the year, as mentioned above, patients with overt emotional difficulties are selected. Later, when a psychiatrist is no longer seen as a busybody poking his nose in where it doesn't belong, that is, assessing nonneurotics, patients are selected for rounds because of a problem of medical management caused by an interaction of personality and illness, not by neurosis. Sometimes, at this stage the house officers suggest foregoing the excitement and concreteness of seeing a patient in favor of just talking about a psychological concept such as the character structure of addicts, the factors in the differential diagnosis of ambulatory psychosis, psychosexual development, symptom formation, and countless others. The house officers seem to have greater objectivity about patients on the private service than they do about patients on the ward service with whom they are more directly involved. This permits a freer discussion, especially of the vicissitudes of the doctor's management of the patient, than is possible on the ward rounds where the house officer has a prime responsibility and an emotional commitment to the patient.

At about this time, another ever-present aspect of this complex teaching situation comes to the fore, that is, the intricate three-cornered relationship among the psychiatrist, the house officers, and the visiting staff whose patients are the subject of discussion. To treat this in detail would require a separate paper, but any presentation of teaching on the private service without some consideration of its effect on the visiting staff would be incomplete. As the house officers get to know me better and feel easier, the atmosphere of the rounds becomes less formal. As mentioned, this helps show the group a clearer picture of the relationship between patient and doctor, and to know where the doctor's personal values seem to clash with what is being taught. But this freedom can make it difficult to limit discussion, especially concerning the visiting staff. A degree of freedom encourages the house officer to mention that, for instance, he has been angry at the demanding patient being presented. This expression of feeling makes it possible to show how this patient tends to annoy people and how the doctor's complying interferes with medical management. Furthermore, the question of whether it is "right" for the doctor to feel or express anger with a patient, and the difference between feeling and doing, are discussed. Almost inevitably, the relationship between the patient and the visiting doctor will come up.

Such a discussion is a mixed blessing. It is a help to the teaching effort because it is not a psychiatrist but the visiting staff of internists with whom the medical house officers identify (Dwyer and Zinberg, 1957). Showing that a visiting doctor has used the principles of medical psychology in managing a case is more likely to make a lasting impression than a psychiatrist's expressing the same idea.

The less desirable side of it is largely the result of the stage of professional development that being a house officer represents. Typically, the house staff divides the medical world into Olympians who practice medicine absolutely correctly and local medical doctors who know practically nothing. This intolerance for differences and shades of opinion could easily turn, in the relative freedom of the psychiatric rounds, into harsh criticism of some of the visiting staff. With house officers, it takes very little to begin a gripe session that could extend from a general criticism of the private practice of medicine to the hospital administration, the clinical laboratories or nursing, or almost anything else, expressed with the exuberance that characterizes students everywhere.

Consistently, I ask them to remember that it is possible to approach many problems, psychological and other, in different ways, and that there is no place in these discussions for personal criticisms of the visiting staff or others. The visiting staff has become aware that they are not being "analyzed" or their medical practice examined, that their patients are not being upset or seen as "neurotic" on these rounds. The automatic reduction of their objections to the psychiatric rounds has led to greater interest in the content. The visiting physicians have begun to ask the house officers assigned to their patients whether the discussion has yielded anything that might be useful to them. Although refusing to write an official consultation, I often informally—at lunch, on the stairs, in the hall, on the telephone—convey information to the visiting staff member concerned. The visiting physicians have become less reluctant to have their patients seen, and their more positive attitude is conveyed each year to the new house staff who, in turn, are less inhibited by their intellectual and emotional disagreements with dynamic psychiatry.

The variety of problems encountered on these rounds seems infinite. However, certain ones inevitably recur and lend themselves most naturally to discussion, both practical and theoretical. The use of placebos, techniques of dealing with irrational arguments against a necessary procedure, the role of and relationship to the patient's family, the mutual influence between organic and functional disturbances, and the differential diagnosis of a transient reaction to illness and the more permanent institution of a neurotic response, are some of the subjects that appear again and again. Tact, thoughtful attention to teaching techniques, and a solid nondeviating theoretical base are the standards followed throughout the psychiatric teaching. A greater knowledge of the psychoanalytic theory of personality is shown to augment and enhance the use of logic and common sense to achieve effective medical and psychological management of patients.

# Teaching Medical Psychotherapy in Special Clinical Settings

EDMUND C. PAYNE, JR., M.D.

THIS PAPER DESCRIBES an experience of teaching medical psychotherapy in two special clinical settings, a Tumor Clinic and a Home Care Program. The discussion is divided into two sections, the first devoted to the orientation of the teaching problems and the areas chiefly concerned, and the second to a detailed description of the settings and how they influenced the teaching. Each of the programs presented a teaching situation which offered both distinctive opportunities and particular problems for the psychiatrist; thus it seems worthwhile to describe them in some detail. The work began as part of the broad program of the Psychiatric Service at the Beth Israel Hospital of teaching psychotherapeutic principles to physicians of other specialties and to medical students. Many of the principles of teaching that had been developed from the experience gained in this broad program could be carried over into the new settings. For instance, the form of therapeutic intervention which Edward Bibring (1954) called manipulation, signifying those activities by a therapist that permit a patient to use his existing psychological structures in a more constructive and adaptive manner, retained a central position as the psychotherapeutic technique which could best be taught to and utilized by these other physicians. But it was also found that certain modifications in this approach and certain special emphases were necessitated both by the structure of the settings in which the teaching was done and by the nature of the clinical problems that were encountered there.

The Tumor Clinic at the Beth Israel Hospital is responsible for the diagnosis, treatment and follow-up care of all the hospital's outpatients with malignancies. It is staffed by internists, surgeons, and representatives

135

of other medical specialties who are particularly interested in the problems of malignant tumors. In addition, surgical residents and interns serve the clinic in rotation, and social workers work actively with many of the patients and their families. The task of the psychiatrist was to work out a position for himself, in relation to the other physicians and to the patients in a busy clinic, which would enable him to transmit his point of view in the most effective way. An unusual feature of this setting was that the psychiatrist was able to be present with the other physicians during the examination and treatment of their patients and thus could orient his teaching to the processes actually observed in the patient and to the doctor-patient interaction. He could thus participate with the doctor in the care of his patient, a participation which helped to overcome some of the difficulties in teaching psychological medicine in ways which will be described in detail below.

Another special aspect of the teaching in the Tumor Clinic stemmed from the fact that the patients who come to such a clinic have serious illnesses which raise emotional issues of an urgent and dramatic nature. These issues include the intense anxieties generated by the diagnosis of cancer, the patient's reactions to the disruption of bodily functions that results from the mutilative surgery often necessary in the treatment of a malignant process, and the special psychological problems faced by a dying patient. The impact of these issues on the physician makes it easier to demonstrate convincingly the usefulness of his acquiring skill in understanding the emotional reactions of his patient.

The Home Care Program presented a teaching situation of a different sort. This program was organized by a group who were interested in extending the facilities of a modern hospital beyond the confines of the hospital itself. It was undertaken with the explicit goal of providing comprehensive medical care to those patients who are too sick or disabled to be treated at home under ordinary circumstances, but who could be maintained outside of the hospital, either at home or in a nursing home, if optimum treatment were offered by a team that could draw on all the resources of the hospital. From the beginning, the personnel of the program was organized as a group, with positions planned for representatives of medicine, surgery, physical medicine, psychiatry, social work, and the nursing services, and the emphasis was always on a co-ordinated team approach. In this setting the psychiatrist had a varying degree of direct acquaintance with the patients, but in most instances he did not have extensive personal contact with them, nor was he present at the time of the physician's examination and treatment as was possible in the Tumor

Clinic. Instead, he worked chiefly in a consultative capacity, and participated in the weekly conferences at which all patients were regularly discussed. Thus the opportunity of interviewing the patient with the doctor, which often permits material to emerge in a more convincing way, was lost, and the psychiatrist usually had to rely on the material that was presented by other members of the group. However, there were also important advantages deriving from the nature of the Home Care Program. These advantages arose chiefly from the fact that the Home Care team had a much more highly organized structure than did the personnel of the Tumor Clinic. The weekly meetings at which problems were extensively discussed made possible a more consistent presentation of a psychological point of view over a long period of time. In addition, and more important, the Home Care group became a group in a dynamic sense. This development, which will be considered in detail below, facilitated the acceptance by each individual member of the point of view contributed by the others. All of the members of the team helped to forge a common group ideal for the care of patients, in which the psychological point of view played an important part. This group ideal was then incorporated into the professional standards and approach of each member.

The nature of the problems encountered in the patients influenced the teaching in this setting, as it did in the Tumor Clinic. In the Home Care Program these problems included not only chronic, eventually fatal illnesses, but also the complex interactions between the patient, his family, and the doctor and other personnel which arose because medical care was based in the patients' homes. Anyone who was seriously interested in working in the program thus necessarily committed himself to trying to increase his knowledge of these emotional issues. The result was one of the highest sustained levels of interest in psychological problems that has been encountered among nonpsychiatric personnel.

**Orientation of the Teaching**

The basic concepts that are utilized in this approach to teaching psychological medicine are derived from psychoanalytic principles. Psychoanalytic theory provides a broad basis of observations, hypotheses, and principles that are consistently applicable to the understanding and explanation of a patient's relationship to his physician, and of his reaction to the crises posed by disease, hospitalization, surgery, aging, and dying. Edward and Grete Bibring and their co-workers have developed a comprehensive method of medical psychotherapy based on psychoanalytic principles which can be taught to and applied by physicians of specialties other than psychiatry (E. Bibring, 1954; G. Bibring, 1947, 1949, 1951, 1956; Dwyer and Zinberg, 1957; Kahana, 1959). This method requires that physicians be taught to utilize their understanding of the existing structures and forces in the personality of a patient in such a way as to enable the patient to adapt in the most effective way of which he is capable to the stress of his illness, to co-operate realistically in his medical management, and to utilize the doctor-patient relationship in the most constructive manner. In the application of this psychotherapeutic approach the physician must recognize that the patient responds to his illness and to the physician with habitual patterns of adaptation that he has developed throughout his lifetime. In order to understand these reactions, the physician requires some knowledge of the course of normal personality development, including the important areas of conflict encountered in this development, and of the patterns of defense that are utilized in dealing with these conflicts. He must develop skill in communicating with his patient and in eliciting and recognizing emotionally important material so that he can identify the patient's leading personality patterns.

The teaching of psychological concepts and of psychotherapeutic methods encounters certain problems that are not present, at least to the same degree, in the teaching and learning of other medical disciplines. Three broad and overlapping areas of problems have been selected for closer inspection. The first set of problems results from the fact that most physicians and medical students lack a systematic knowledge of psychological principles that in any way compares with their knowledge of other areas of medicine. Most doctors in the course of their training acquire a professional understanding not only of clinical medicine, but of pertinent areas of physiology, pathology, biochemistry, and other related basic sciences. But, in general, they possess only the most superficial grasp of pertinent psychological theory. One of the several reasons for this deficiency may be that most of the other courses in medical school are complementary to each other; the principles taught in one course reinforce what is learned in another course. Psychiatry unfortunately does not share this advantage, at least in most medical schools of today. The hiatus may result in difficulties of communication between the psychiatrist and other physicians. When a cardiologist discusses with another physician the cardiac decompensation that complicates the management of a patient, he can rely on a common comprehension of the underlying pathophysiological mechanisms. When, however, the psychiatrist discusses the complications resulting from the decompensation of a patient's normally adaptive obsessive-compulsive personality structure, he cannot necessarily rely on a common understanding of the implications of even the diagnostic term, "obsessive-compulsive." This lack of systematic knowledge limits the physician's application of psychotherapeutic approaches to empirical, unsophisticated, or idiosyncratic maneuvers, and limits also his ability to understand his patient's emotional reactions. Thus the psychiatrist should feel a special responsibility for including some discussion of basic concepts in whatever teaching approach he employs.

A second source of difficulty in teaching psychotherapeutic principles stems from the fact that the material being discussed may evoke emotional responses in the listener which create resistances to its being understood and accepted. This difficulty is easily understandable, since the subject matter of dynamic psychology deals primarily with basic, universal human conflicts, some of which the physician may share. Thus, emotionally charged concepts that touch on areas that are personally unacceptable to the doctor may arouse anxiety and therefore be misunderstood and disbelieved.

A related area of difficulty involves the characterological structure of the physician himself, which strongly influences the particular manner in which he perceives and responds to different types of patients. This structure affects the way in which he deals with the emotional problems that arise in the patients' medical management. Thus a physician will react differently to a dependent patient, to a paranoid patient, to an obsessive-compulsive patient, or to a hysterical patient, depending upon his own personality makeup. His own needs will affect the ease or difficulty with which he can adapt new psychological knowledge to his work with any particular patient. It is, for example, much easier for a physician to learn and apply a new impersonal medical or surgical technique than it is for him to adopt a new approach to a type of patient whom he has previously found frustrating, gratifying, or difficult to understand.

The difficulties that are created by unconsciously determined resistances to learning psychodynamic material have been discussed by many authors, and perhaps even stressed too heavily by those who have suggested that such learning must be preceded or accompanied by insight into and resolution of personal conflicts. This demand seems extreme, and experience shows that if sufficient motivation is present, a genuine appreciation of basic concepts can be taught, although greater motivation is required than with less emotionally charged subjects. When interest is not already present, the psychiatrist must link his teaching as closely as possible to the pre-existing commitments of the physician of another specialty. A clinical setting in which such a physician is already deeply involved is an admirable base from which to forge such a link. If, in addition, the setting can be utilized to help the physician recognize the ways in which his personality characteristics facilitate or hinder his work with patients, even though he may still not appreciate the underlying reasons for them, he may achieve greater flexibility in medical-psychological management. In both the Tumor Clinic and the Home Care Program it was possible to structure the presentation of psychological concepts around issues created by medical problems that affected the patient's welfare in an obviously vital manner. Both settings contained elements that helped to overcome the difficulties created by unconsciously determined negative attitudes toward psychological concepts. In addition, each program, in different ways, embodied aspects that helped the physician to become aware of some of his attitudes toward patients, and made possible some modification in his attitudes.

A third area of problems encountered in teaching medical psychotherapy arises from a subtle difference between the attitude of the psychiatrist and that of other physicians toward patients. Although attitudes vary widely from physician to physician, most of them tend unconsciously to see a patient as a more or less passive object, on whom they act by means of their special training and equipment. The psychiatrist, to a much greater degree, sees his patient as a complex organism pursuing a historically determined course, oriented and directed by individual needs and unique personality, who reacts to events, including disease and medical treatment, in specific ways that are determined by his needs and characteristics. The psychiatrist "tunes in" on the patient in order to understand him, and attempts to adapt his therapeutic interventions to the patient's psychological make-up. A physician who is not also a psychiatrist sees a therapeutic effect as resulting from what he has done to the patient; a psychiatrist, even when he intervenes quite actively, sees an impetus for change as still coming from the patient. If the physician who is not also a psychiatrist is to apply his psychodynamic understanding to the fullest and to work most effectively with the emotional reactions of his patients, he must modify his wish to act directly upon the patient. When a physician changes his attitude in this direction, he usually does so through an identification with the psychiatrist's approach to patients. In the Tumor Clinic, direct participation of the psychiatrist with other physicians in joint interviews of patients provided an opportunity to demonstrate the way in which the psychiatrist works. The latter's attitude could then be conveyed even by simple maneuvers, such as his tendency to elicit routinely the patient's attitude toward his illness, or to ask the questions that permit the patient to express his fears rather than to "reassure" him immediately on the basis of preconceptions entertained by the physician. In the setting offered by the Home Care Program, this attitude is more difficult to convey because it is more difficult directly to provide a model of how to work with a patient in a particular way. This disadvantage is partially offset by the opportunity of working together in a cohesive group over a long period of time. Factors, which will be described in more detail, are active in this group that promote the participants' identification with each other's points of view. The program thus encourages recognition of the necessity of understanding the particular style of each patient and of working within the individual framework of his life. This recognition is powerfully augmented by the close contact between the personnel of the program and the family life of the patients.

An effective method of teaching psychodynamic principles must fulfill certain criteria determined by the problems discussed above. Since a method adapted to one need will often slight another, some degree of choice must usually be made as to what particular aspect of the problems is to be emphasized. The advantages of giving a systematic presentation of psychological theory must be balanced against the necessity of conveying it within a framework that will combat the tendency to isolate the material. It must be presented to the physician in such a way that he will accept it as important and significant. Teaching in a clinical setting does not provide the same opportunity for comprehensive presentation as do more didactic approaches, nor does it offer to the physician the kind of personal insight attempted by some approaches based on group psychotherapy (Balint, 1954, 1957), but it does meet some needs in a uniquely satisfactory way. Most nonclinical settings require an already strong motivation in the physician. Teaching in a clinical setting can reach a wider group of physicians because it can make use of important pre-existing motivations and commitments. A doctor who is caring for a sick patient has a strong personal and traditional commitment to the welfare of that patient. In the setting of the Tumor Clinic or the Home Care Program, the psychiatrist can often demonstrate that powerful emotional forces do affect the well-being of the patient, and can show that it is necessary to understand these processes in order to provide adequate care to the patient. The involvement of the psychiatrist in an enterprise that physicians of other specialties regard as important promotes bonds that further the acceptance of information and of new points of view.

There is a special difficulty encountered by the psychiatrist working in a clinical setting, especially in an outpatient clinic. Other physicians, such as the internist, the surgeon, and the radiologist, assume a central and major responsibility for those particular aspects of a given patient's care which are appropriate to their specialties. But the psychiatrist is not in the same position. The recognized problem that brings the patient to the doctor is a medical or surgical one, and the psychiatrist does not assume primary responsibility for the decisions relating to such a patient's illness. On the other hand, he must avoid falling into the role of a specialist who treats only the neurotic patient or the patient with "psychological problems"; that role would give him a more definite clinical status, but it would involve a vital loss to his teaching. The central thesis of his work is that what he has to offer is potentially applicable to every patient in the clinic, and that what he can teach is useful to every physician. If he permits himself to be placed in the role of a specialist who treats only a particular group of patients, further separation of the emotional and physical aspects of illness and further fragmentation of patients' care will result. In avoiding restriction to psychotherapy or to consultations with neurotic patients who come to the clinic, he risks isolation because of a too ambiguous status in the clinic. The most important factor in overcoming his possible isolation or restriction will, of course, be his demonstrating that what he has to offer is of importance to the clinic. But, before he can so demonstrate this, he must first be admitted to participation, and for that the support of the physician in charge of the clinic is essential. Thus the initial step in such a teaching effort is to reach an explicit agreement with the director of the clinic that the function of the psychiatrist will be to teach and demonstrate, with sufficient freedom of movement to allow him to participate in whatever aspects of the clinic work he feels will be the most productive. Unless such an agreement can be reached, the prognosis for his program is usually poor.

## Theoretical Considerations

A psychiatrist who works in a specialized clinical setting such as the Tumor Clinic or the Home Care Program will usually be confronted with special problems, often of profound emotional significance, which are characteristic of the patients in that particular setting. In a pediatric clinic these special problems might be aspects of the mother-child relationship, or the determining influences exerted on a child's reaction to illness by his current developmental phase. In an obstetrical program the central focus might be on the psychological processes of pregnancy. Three important areas of problems encountered in the Tumor Clinic and the Home Care Program were those of the dying patient, of aging, and of the emotional impact of mutilative surgery.

As stated above, the teaching of psychological concepts is greatly facilitated if they can be presented in a manner that closely links them to pre-existing clinical interests of the physicians from other branches of medicine. In order to teach well, the psychiatrist must first understand the problems with which the other physicians are confronted, and must then formulate them in terms of his own theoretical concepts. When he has done so, the psychotherapeutic interventions that he demonstrates are more precise, and the relevance of his concepts is more apparent.

The following discussion concentrates on the three areas of problems mentioned above, dying, aging, and mutilative surgery. The presentations are condensed and at certain points rather sketchy, since the intention is to illustrate an approach to teaching rather than to discuss exhaustively the problems themselves. As an introduction to the discussion, however, the psychoanalytic concept of regression must be considered. It is a concept of a higher order of abstraction, but one that is essential to the understanding of all three areas.

The concept of regression is useful in explaining many of the otherwise puzzling attitudes that a patient shows in response to illness. By regression we mean the replacement of more complexly organized and more recently acquired aspects of the functioning of personality by more primitive and chronologically earlier modes of functioning. Human personality develops by changing and integrating simple forms of behavior into more highly organized patterns that possess a broader capacity for adaptation. Libidinal aims, ego structures and functions, and the complex patterns used in relating to the external world and the people in it exhibit this development. Many of the earlier patterns, however, persist in modified form in a hierarchically ordered relation to the more highly developed and usually controlling systems. In the face of stress, whether caused by internal conflict or by external danger or frustration, a person may give up the more mature aims and ways of functioning and again seek gratification and attempt to cope with his problems in ways more in accordance with these earlier patterns. A simple example of regression is seen in the toddler who is gaining increasing independence and self-reliance, but who periodically turns back to his mother's lap for comfort and security when the world is temporarily too much for him. When a person falls ill, some degree of regression invariably occurs, induced by a number of factors. Illness interferes with bodily functions that are necessary for the maintenance of important aspects of the personality. The patient who comes to the hospital loses freedom of movement, is deprived of his clothes, and must literally put himself into the hands of other people and depend on them to care for many of the needs that he normally attends to himself. His passive dependent needs are increased, his usual patterns of adjustment are disrupted, and he often suffers intense conflict. Illness is a threat to the integrity of his body and to his life, and consequently generates feelings of anxiety. Since he may be unable to cope with these dangers himself, his anxiety is usually accompanied by a feeling of helplessness. Thus he is forced to rely on the physician for security in ways that resemble his dependence on his parents when he was a child. All of these factors encourage regression. When regression occurs, conflicts that were important in childhood but that may have subsequently become latent tend to regain their intensity, and the old defenses that were associated with those conflicts may be mobilized again. In many cases these unconsciously determined defensive reactions are not appropriate to reality, to the requirements of dealing with the present illness and of adapting to the necessary medical procedures; in some cases they may be diametrically opposed. The regressive process not only adds a burden of irrational anxiety to the difficulties created by the illness, but may also distort the patient's relationship with his physician. Under the pressure of regression, the patient frequently attributes to the physician characteristics that really belonged to people who were important in an earlier period of his life. In some patients this attribution will increase their confidence and trust in the doctor and thus augment the doctor's effectiveness in providing support and allaying anxiety. In other patients it may produce a negative reaction that can prove both baffling and frustrating to the physician.

Regressive processes in the patient can be utilized for teaching. By bringing characteristic defensive patterns into prominence, they may facilitate personality diagnosis; the genetic roots of these patterns are often more evident in the regressed patient. An opportunity is thus available for demonstrating the influence of early primitive modes on the patient's present-day reactions, and also for enabling the physician to increase his skill in dealing with one of the most troublesome areas of patient management.

### The Dying Patient

Death and dying are obviously of central concern to both physicians and patients in a Tumor Clinic and in a Home Care Program, where most of the patients have chronic or incurable diseases and belong to the older age groups. The process of dying represents a situation of maximal emotional stress for the patient and for his family. The psychiatrist can contribute both knowledge and skill to the physician's management of this difficult phase of his relationship with his patient, and can also utilize it as a dramatic demonstration of the importance of the physician's acquiring psychological understanding.

It is important to recognize that a patient does not necessarily use the same mechanisms throughout the course of his terminal illness. The defenses that a person is compelled to rely on initially may not be as essential to him later. Therefore, the physician must be flexible and must be prepared to modify the type of support that he gives to the patient as the patient's needs change.

The recognition of approaching death induces fears in most people, fears which in some persons reach the extreme of terror or panic. On close examination, these fears are seen to be related to the anxiety situations which have been most important in a person's life, and in important ways they seem to be closely connected with the most significant situations of danger that confronted the infant in his development. The significance of previous experience is emphasized by the observation that these fears often diminish in the final stage of a terminal illness, when the physiological processes of dying take over. This period frequently seems relatively peaceful, although physical discomfort is usually greater at this time.

A significant component of the fear a dying person experiences is his anticipation of separation from the people and things in the world that he has loved and depended on. This element can be clearly seen in the panic felt by those patients who cling desperately to their homes, resisting terminal hospitalization, although the nursing problems may be almost impossible to manage at home. The psychiatrist is reminded of the infant's earliest fear of the loss of his mother, on whom he must rely for the satisfaction of all of his needs, and indeed for survival. This fear is usually most manifest in those individuals who have remained relatively dependent throughout their lives, but it is important in most dying patients.

The anxiety that some people experience when they are dying is intensified because their conception of dying is colored by fantasies in which they are the victims of hostile and aggressive forces. These fantasies focus on the helplessness, the damage to the body, and the extinction of the self that is involved in dying. The most tormenting aspects of these fantasies may originate in the conflicts that surrounded aggressive impulses directed toward parents or siblings in early childhood, impulses which resulted in fears of retaliatory aggression.

Often a sense of guilt resulting from unresolved sexual or aggressive conflicts plays an important part in a person's fear of dying. Death is then seen as a punishment, and thus as a confirmation of the feeling of being a bad person. This conception of one's self as being unworthy and unlovable can intensify the feeling of isolation and the fear of abandonment which so often are part of dying. These fears will be illustrated by examples from case histories of patients in later sections of this chapter.

When faced with the reality of dying, a person reacts in a characteristic manner and attempts to cope with his fear by means of his own unique characterological defenses. In addition, however, a special mechanism of defense, that of denial, often appears. The defense of denial originates in the tendency of the infant to accept and recognize that which is pleasurable and to ignore and reject whatever produces displeasure. In normal development this tendency is gradually replaced by an increasing ability to recognize and adhere to that which is "real," and the prominent and habitual use of denial is usually a sign of severe psychopathology in the adult. However, in times of great stress and danger, especially when the person is in reality helpless to avert the danger, he frequently reverts to the use of denial. Most people with a fatal illness, after the initial shock of recognition, tend to repudiate the reality to some extent. The denial may be complete, blocking all recognition of the truth, or it may be a partial denial of some of the implications of the danger. The subsequent manifestations of this defense vary according to individual character structure. Some people may need to use denial prominently throughout the course of terminal illness. Others may gradually relinquish it and develop an increasing acceptance of the true state of affairs as they are able to find ways to reconcile themselves to the fact of death.

One of the mechanisms involved in the defensive use of denial is the withdrawal of the cathexis of attention from perceptions. When the symptoms of a disease increase in severity, especially when there is increased pain, stimuli that indicate the nature of the disease press into awareness with greater insistence. At this stage the patient will usually increase his efforts to deny the significance of his illness, but he will probably not be able to ignore his fears as completely as before. When the physician discusses the patient's anxiety with him, as he usually should in order to give effective reassurance, he is more likely to be confronted with questions concerning the nature of the illness. Generally the patient is in search of support for his denial. Especially at such a time, the physician must carefully evaluate the character structure of the person he is dealing with before deciding how to answer his patient's questions. The physician should always remember that most people show great capacity to reinstate their denials when some relief of their symptoms can be given. Thus, even with a patient who he feels may be able to face the reality of death, he will usually find it wise to proceed very cautiously, postponing any confirmation of his patient's suspicions until a more stable period has been reached.

Regression, like denial, plays an important adaptive role in the emotional reactions to dying. Most, if not all, patients with a fatal illness correctly interpret the significance of their symptoms, even though this knowledge may be excluded from full awareness by the mechanism of denial. Thus faced with the threat of extinction, they often experience a sense of helplessness. In particular, the feeling of standing alone to meet the danger may be very strong. Under these conditions a special pattern of regression frequently appears. This pattern is based on a longing for an earlier time, in infancy and in childhood, when a feeling of helplessness was often experienced, but when protection and security were provided by the parents' care, and dangers were dissolved by the comfort of the mother's presence. In his regression the dying patient reinvests the memory of these early times with emotional significance, and to some extent revives the associated attitudes. Dreams, vivid memories of people and events from childhood, and especially the relationship with the doctor all provide evidence of the process (Eissler, 1955; Deutsch, 1936).

The patient with a terminal illness may transfer to his physician his longing to be comforted and protected as he was by his parents. He then attributes to the doctor the wisdom and the magical power to help and to hurt that as a child he believed his parents to possess. When his feelings toward the doctor are positive, he can feel a security that helps to mitigate the sense of isolation and dread that so often accompany dying. On the other hand, a patient with negative attitudes transferred from his parents, attitudes which are augmented by his inevitable disappointment, can place a severe strain on the relationship and challenge the skill and knowledge of the physician.

The physician's special position enables him to exert a powerful and beneficial influence on his patient's reaction to a terminal illness. In order to realize this therapeutic potential to the fullest, and to deal successfully with the crises that threaten the relationship, he needs to understand in some detail as well as intuitively the concepts sketched above. This organized understanding can guide him in planning many aspects of medical management, in giving skillful reassurance, and in knowing when and to what patients he should offer protection from knowledge too painful to face and when he should encourage a patient to face fears more openly. The psychiatrist can use his formulations to link closely the teaching of medical psychology to these central issues of medical practice.

## Aging

The patients in the Tumor Clinic and especially in the Home Care Program are predominantly older patients; the Home Care patients, for example, have a mean age of over sixty-five years. Therefore, the psychological issues involved in aging assume considerable importance in medical management and in psychiatric teaching in these settings.

Many losses occur in aging. Loss of health is one of the most important. This loss is especially evident, of course, in the group seen in a general hospital, where illness is the primary motivation for seeking help. But even in the absence of specific disease, aging involves loss of activity, of functional reserve and of various capacities. These losses lead to restriction of functions, to inability to engage in important habitual pursuits, and to a generally more sedentary life. Restriction of function and loss of activity promote regression, increased dependency, and vulnerability to depression, and these effects are accentuated by other losses that the elderly may sustain. Retirement, often forced, results in loss of status and of a role that may have been important in maintaining self-esteem. It means the loss of important opportunities for the sublimation of otherwise conflict-producing impulses. In addition, for many people retirement results in more concrete deprivations: loss of income, a reduced standard of living, and an enforced dependence on children or on the community. As people age, they are faced with the increasing probability of losing through death the people in whom they have made important emotional investments: parents, siblings, relatives, friends, and spouse. With aging there is also an increasing rigidity of the personality, and a decreased ability to reinvest emotional interests in new people. Thus this loss of important people also results in an increased susceptibility to depression, a decrease of interest in the environment and an increased preoccupation with one's self. Furthermore, this series of losses and restrictions greatly increases the significance of the emotionally important people who remain. Psychiatrists have repeatedly observed a complex interdependence between husband and wife, in which two exceedingly frail and vulnerable people are able to function at a relatively high level in the face of great difficulties because of the support that each derives from the other. They have also observed that after the death of one partner, the other often quickly succumbs to ill health or regresses to a much lower level of functioning. Physicians can be led to see in such a situation an impressive and effective demonstration of the importance of understanding the nature of the patient's object relations and of his place within the family structure.

Increased dependency and the narrowing of the elderly patient's range of interest in other people increase the importance of his relationship with the physician. As a doctor works with such a person, he comes to appreciate the importance of skillful manipulation on his part for maintaining the stability of the patient's adjustment. This realization has been especially important in the Home Care Program, where the Home Care team serves the patient primarily in his own home. The team almost always has access to adequate information about the relationship of the family members to each other. In almost every case, the success or failure of their efforts to maintain the elderly patient at an optimal level of functioning outside of the hospital has depended on understanding the personality structure of the patient and of the person who assumes primary responsibility within the home, and on accurately assessing the nature of the relationship between them.

In teaching in the Tumor Clinic, the psychological issues involved in aging arise in the discussion of the reactions of this primarily elderly group to their disease and treatment, and in planning for their long-term care. These issues appear and can similarly be utilized for teaching in the Home Care Program, but there their impact is much greater because of the physician's more intimate involvement with the family. For instance, he can see clearly the effect of changes in one spouse on the other. Examples of this kind enable the psychiatrist to discuss medical psychology in meaningful terms. Equally important, the psychiatrist is himself exposed to an invaluable opportunity to learn.

### Reaction to Loss of Bodily Functions

The patient's reaction to a disease or surgical procedure that results in a loss of the integrity of his body presents another important opportunity for teaching psychiatric principles in a general hospital, and especially in a Tumor Clinic or Home Care Program. Illnesses such as rheumatoid arthritis or cerebrovascular disease can interfere drastically with important bodily functions. In the surgical treatment of malignancies, or vascular complications of diabetes and of other diseases, extensive mutilation and the loss of highly cathected parts of the body may result. The body and its functions are of central importance in the developing structures of the personality. Experiences with the body form the core of an awareness of the self as distinct from the environment. The interaction of the infant with the need-satisfying and life-preserving people in his environment, which is vital for the differentiation of complex personality structures, is mediated through basic bodily modes and organs. The psychosocial development of the child is closely integrated with and paced by his genetically determined biological development. Much elaboration and modification occur with maturation. Those aspects of his self-image and his self-esteem that are related to the successful mastery of the tasks demanded at various stages of his maturation are still, in the adult, rooted in the bodily functions. If a significant conflict surrounded the functioning of an organ in childhood, the person will be more vulnerable as an adult to any threat to this organ. As an illustration, let us consider a man with strong compulsive needs for order, cleanliness, and control. Struggles around the mastery and control of his anal functions in childhood were important in the development of these traits, and the functioning of his anal sphincter in the present is important for their continued maintenance. If such a man develops a cancer of the rectum that requires the surgical removal of his rectum and anus and the establishment of a permanent abdominal colostomy, he will have great difficulty in continuing to see himself as a clean, controlled person. He will be faced with the danger of unexpected, inopportune fecal discharges and will thus be forced back to renewed preoccupation with excretory functions.

Some aspects of the reaction to the loss of bodily functions and organs are universal. The most important of these aspects are decrease in self-esteem, grieving for the lost part, and varying degrees of depression (Sutherland and Orbach, 1953). Other aspects are determined by the patient's particular personality structure, by the symbolic significance of the organ involved, and by the conflicts that surround its functioning. For the man with a compulsive personality structure and a special emphasis on cleanliness, tidiness, and control of himself and of his environment, the loss of bowel control is a crucial problem. If these character traits have become autonomous and firmly established, his self-esteem is less vulnerable and his functioning may not be grossly or permanently impaired. However, if these attitudes are primarily reaction formations that defend against a still active instinctual conflict, a severe disruption of his ability to function may result.

It is obvious that organs such as eye, leg, arm, or breast, and functions such as tasting, walking, or sphincter control, as well as other bodily parts and functions, may have an emotional significance that extends beyond the important reality purposes that they serve. Thus, the loss of a tooth or a toe or damage to an arm may symbolically represent the damage to the body that was feared in childhood as punishment for forbidden wishes, and lead to disability that far exceeds any actual loss of function. An orally dependent person who relies on supplies both concretely and in his relations with other people can experience intense frustration when his pleasure in eating, speech, and other oral activities is interfered with by the treatment of a cancer of his mouth with a mutilating operation or with radiotherapy. A woman's feminine narcissism may be importantly represented by her breasts. A radical mastectomy can deeply disturb her image of herself, damage her self-esteem, and lead to depression.

Teaching that focuses on reactions to mutilative surgery can be effective. A surgeon is highly motivated to rehabilitate his patient as fully as possible after an operation. Emotionally determined disabilities of the kinds described above often explain the failure to achieve this goal. Once this connection is demonstrated, interest in medical psychotherapy often increases. The physician is encouraged to look beneath the surface of his patient's reactions and to discover the highly personal and varied nature of the fantasies that dictate the form of those reactions, which differ greatly from what superficial observation or "common sense" would lead him to expect. When he does so, he may well develop a new appreciation of the complexity of an individual's personality and a greater respect for the importance of understanding a particular patient's character structure.

### The Clinical Settings

The first section sketched three of the special areas of clinical problems that are encountered in a tumor clinic or a home care program. In different clinical settings, other important problems will undoubtedly emerge. A careful formulation must be made of the specific clinical issues if they are to be fully utilized in teaching as a source of illustrative material and as valuable aids in enlisting the interest and motivation of physicians. The following section describes teaching and its application in the Tumor Clinic and the Home Care Program in more detail.

### The Tumor Clinic

When a psychiatrist first begins to work in a clinic as a teacher, his initial activities are quite likely to be met with a rather distant politeness. This reaction is not surprising, since the situation is one in which he invites himself to tell the doctors about the patients whom they are treating. With the individual physician in the Clinic, he is in the position of being a consultant of whom no consultation has been requested. In the Tumor Clinic this initial chill was somewhat alleviated, and the psychiatrist's integration was facilitated by the Chief of the Clinic's active interest in emotional problems of patients and in the contributions to their solution that could be made by a psychiatrist. This fortunate situation made it easier for the psychiatrist to adopt, from the very beginning, a role that permitted maximum flexibility.

A procedure was adopted of circulating informally with the doctors as they examined their patients. This practice proved of importance in a number of ways. In the first period of the work it permitted the psychiatrist to become familiar with the structure of the Clinic and to test and experiment with the ways in which he could function most effectively. In addition it contributed importantly to his own education. Teaching in a clinical setting is a two-way process. In successful teaching not only does the internist or surgeon learn from the psychiatrist, but the psychiatrist also needs to understand the medical problems with which they are dealing so that he can integrate his contribution to the patient's management in a specific and sophisticated way. This procedure of accompanying the other physicians during their examinations of the patients permitted him to become familiar with the problems of cancer patients, while, at the same time, he was able to take part in the interviews with the patients to whatever extent seemed most appropriate. The interest shown in the psychiatrist's contributions, of course, varied widely from physician to physician. In some instances the psychiatrist was primarily a spectator; at other times it was possible for him to take an active part in the interview. A few physicians remained completely uninterested, and when it became clear that their lack of interest would in all likelihood persist, the psychiatrist dropped his efforts at direct participation and maintained further contact through general discussion. A few physicians met the psychiatrist's initial efforts with keen interest. The usual response, however, was a mild but friendly interest, which frequently increased with further contact.

In his initial participation with a particular doctor, the psychiatrist usually attempts to bring to light some significant aspect of the patient's reactions that is readily accessible. The approach may consist simply of demonstrating that the patient is frightened or of interjecting a question or comment into the interview that will permit the patient to express some of his anxiety or depression. From even such slight participation, the psychiatrist is often able to pick up some obviously important area for medical management which had been overlooked previously. An illustration is the case of a patient whose illness and treatment had estranged her from her husband.

A small, apprehensive, fifty-six-year-old woman was seen in the Tumor Clinic by the surgical resident and the psychiatrist four months after her discharge from the hospital, where a radical vulvectomy had been performed because of a carcinoma of the vulva. She did not refer to the vulvectomy directly, and indeed seemed deliberately to ignore the whole area of her genitals. Instead she complained intensely and inconsolably of discomfort which she said resulted from a simple pimple on her thigh and from lymphedema of her upper legs. A few simple questions elicited the information that she had been living with her daughter since leaving the hospital and was still postponing her return to her own apartment and to her husband. It became clear that she had never been able to discuss with the doctors the extent of her operation and its effect on her sexual functioning, and had never been able to bring herself to tell her husband that her genitals were now damaged. She was afraid that if she returned to live with him he would demand sexual relations with her and reject her if she were unable to comply. This easily attainable information, which had clear relevance for this woman's adjustment and for her management, had not previously come to light.

The demonstration of such material often stimulates the physician's interest and curiosity, and may lead to further discussion of such issues as unconscious motivations and a patient's character structure, issues which it would be unproductive to attempt to discuss before his interest is engaged.

As work in a clinic progresses, changes occur in the relationship with the other physicians. Physician and psychiatrist establish an increasing familiarity with working together and, through casual contacts and conversations, they can exchange information much more freely. The range of what can be taught is thus expanded. For example, as the psychiatrist and the surgical resident continued to see the woman described above at her subsequent clinic visits, a deeper understanding was gained of her reaction to the illness and operation. The mutilation of her genitals had been a numbing blow to her, damaging her image of herself as a woman and consequently her self-esteem. Her belief that her husband would reject her had resulted chiefly from the projection of this devalued picture of herself. This reaction was intensified by the reawakening of a strong sense of guilt connected with sexuality. She had always felt that there was something shameful and wrong about her sexual impulses, and as a result had been quite inhibited in her sexual behavior. As she came to feel more at ease with the physician and was able to discuss her feelings more openly, her embarrassed questions and remarks indicated that she had a persistent nagging fear that the cancer was the result of her sexual activity, and that she interpreted the cancer and the operation for it as a punishment for sexuality. This interpretation served to confirm her feeling of guilt, since in her view she must really have been a bad person to have deserved such a punishment.

Under the impact of the trauma of the operation and of this conflict she had regressed, and her need to be taken care of had become increasingly strong. In addition, she felt resentful because of what had befallen her, a resentment that was directed in part at her doctors. However, her personality structure was such that she was not able to make demands or to give vent to her anger openly. The only way in which she could express her dependent needs was to present herself as a damaged, suffering person, and the only way that she had of expressing her anger was to nag the doctor with unremitting complaints of discomfort. The physician's initial response was to feel a strong sense of sympathy for her and a wish to help her, but as all of his efforts proved of no avail and her complaints continued unabated, he began to experience a growing sense of irritation and a reluctance to see her. By this time, however, the relationship between the doctor and the psychiatrist had progressed to the point where it was possible to discuss with him the reaction that she induced both in him and in the psychiatrist, and to use this personal response to gain a further understanding of the patient. Her behavior could then be discussed as typical of the way in which the patient with a masochistic character structure responds to a stress-induced increase in instinctual pressures. An effective therapeutic plan for this patient could then be formulated. When the surgical resident recognized that his patient had to complain and that he could not expect to hear an admission of improvement from her for a long time, he was able to work successfully with her once more by modifying his immediate goals, setting some limit on the amount of time that he spent with her, and by giving an open and explicit recognition of her suffering instead of minimizing it, while at the same time encouraging her to use her strengths to function in spite of her disability. The resident was also better able to appreciate masochism as a significant rather than an abstruse concept after he had himself struggled with these problems in his patient.

In working jointly with other physicians in this way in a busy clinic, the psychiatrist must usually modify the customary pattern of a psychiatric interview. He often has to be able to elicit pertinent material in a considerably shorter period of time than is available to him in purely psychiatric practice. With experience, however, and especially with familiarity with the particular types of problems that are likely to arise in the setting in which he is working, he can still often demonstrate a patient's central anxiety or the necessary evidence for the leading personality pattern. Sometimes, as with the patient discussed above, an adequate formulation may be made over the course of a number of relatively brief interviews. The resulting formulation is certainly not as complete as that which can be arrived at in insight-oriented psychotherapy. What is lost in this way, however, is more than compensated for by the opportunity to demonstrate an approach that the physician in another specialty can use successfully in his everyday practice.

The work with this patient permitted the psychiatrist to demonstrate the use of some simple interviewing techniques, to show the disrupting effect that illness and operation can have on a patient's adjustment, and to illustrate how an understanding of a patient's personality structure can be used to manage more effectively the patient's rehabilitation and the relationship with the physician.

The treatment of a woman with an obsessive-compulsive personality further illustrates how a patient's reaction to a particular operation is determined by her personality structure, and how an understanding of her personality can be used in restoring her to effective functioning.

A fifty-eight-year-old woman was seen in the Clinic following the treatment of a carcinoma of the rectum with abdominal-perineal resection. The operation had left her with a permanent colostomy. After discharge from the hospital, she was tearful, hopeless, and utterly distraught. She stated that she had always been "crazy clean." After a hard day's work she used to return home and devote hours to cleaning her apartment, whether it needed it or not. Now she felt so disorganized that she could not co-operate with her doctor in learning to care for her colostomy. Whenever he attempted to discuss it with her she began to weep helplessly. She had withdrawn from her friends because of her fear that she might "have an accident," or emit a fecal odor in some social situation. Her depression persisted until it was possible to find a way to use her compulsive personality patterns in the service of her rehabilitation, i.e., by arousing her interest in cleaning up her "dirty" colostomy. With a great deal of support from the doctor, she began to feel some tentative interest in this project, which paralleled the former interest she had shown in eliminating all dirt from her house. As she progressed, she began to feel some pride of achievement. Instead of seeing herself as a dirty, helpless person, she was able to strive with increasing gratification toward the goal of having the cleanest, best controlled colostomy in the Clinic.

The work with this woman involved explaining and using concepts from several important psychological areas. It led to a consideration of some of the factors important in the regulation of self-esteem, and of the importance of guilt, shame, and a sense of helplessness in the development of depression. The important role of early developmental conflicts in the formation of her characteristic personality patterns could be reconstructed. The break-down of her character defenses could thus be related to disruption of the functioning of the organ system that played an important part in the evolution of these defenses. Both the psychiatrist and the physicians he was working with gained a more detailed appreciation of the concept of the compulsive character, and also of the significance of diseases of the anus and rectum.

The case of Bertha C., a woman with a terminal illness, further illustrates the way in which clinical situations encountered in the Tumor Clinic were used for teaching personality diagnosis.

Mrs. C. was a stout, energetic, chronically anxious woman, somewhat past middle age. She had a capacity for a quick and warm involvement with the doctor that was accompanied by a nagging, complaining quality, stemming from the fear and depression produced by her disease. Her manner was somewhat controlling and showed a curious mixture of denial and a pessimistic conviction of impending disaster. Several years before the psychiatrist's first encounter with her, she had undergone a radical mastectomy for cancer of the breast. Later, metastases to the bones had been discovered, but had undergone a temporary remission following oophorectomy. Now she was experiencing pain from a recent exacerbation of the metastases. When asked how she felt, she described, in a flood of words, the discomfort and disability produced by her "arthritis," and told how it interfered with running her small, women's apparel shop, which she was sure she would soon have to close. When tacit permission to speak more freely was given by asking her about her fear, she asked, with great anxiety, "Do I really have cancer?" The doctor was under great pressure to answer her questions and to find some way to help her deal with her anxiety, but at this point too little was known about the patient to do either with any assurance. It was not clear whether she was in reality seeking knowledge that she could use to achieve greater stability, or whether her questions represented the breakdown, because of her increased pain, of a denial that was a necessary defense. We could not even be sure at this point what the concept "cancer" meant to her, and thus could not know for what question she was actually seeking an answer. Rather than having her questions answered directly, she was asked further about her reactions to her disease, and the following story emerged in this and subsequent interviews.

When she had discovered a mass in her breast three years ago, she had thought at once of cancer, but had delayed consulting a doctor because she was convinced that she would die during the operation, and that even if she did not, the cancer would certainly recur. In her conception, cancer was a painful and, most frighteningly, a weakening disease that made its victims helpless. She had attempted to deny the reality of the mass in her breast for a long time, but finally her increasing anxiety forced her to seek medical advice. During her convalescence after radical mastectomy, her greatest burden was the passivity imposed by her hospital stay, and she had felt a tremendous impatience to return to her responsibilities at home. She had continued to suffer from a moderate depression precipitated by the loss of her breast during the ensuing years, but had buried this and a persisting fear of the recurrence of her disease by throwing herself into her work in her little dress shop. She had no assistant there except her diabetic husband, and the business was consequently a precarious one, dependent upon her continued ability to work. Since her symptoms had increased in severity, the shop was always on the edge of bankruptcy.

Mrs. C.'s greatest fear was that she would not be able to remain self-supporting and would thus become a burden to her husband and her married son. She regarded both of these men as weak, her husband because of his diabetes, and her son because of emotional difficulties. She was especially concerned that the responsibility for her care would break down their physical and emotional health.

The history of her earlier life added to the understanding of her personality pattern, and helped in the formulation of a plan for her medical-psychological management. She had spent her childhood in an atmosphere of financial and emotional privation. Her father was a warm but passive and unsuccessful man, for whom she felt affection but little respect. Her mother was the dominant member of the family, strong but always tired, and mildly depressed by the responsibility of maintaining her family of several children with inadequate means. Her mother relied on Mrs. C., the oldest child, for assistance. She subordinated her feelings of anger toward and jealousy of the youngest siblings, resulting from the frequent frustration of her wishes for nurturance from her mother and of anger and disappointment with her father, to her more conscious feelings of affection for her parents. The anger and jealousy were partially resolved through an identification with her hard-working mother. In this role she assisted her mother by working with her and helping her to take care of the younger children, albeit in a compulsive, controlling, and overprotective way. When she grew up, she married a passive man, and carried on the overprotective pattern with him and with her son. When her husband developed diabetes, she made him even weaker by encouraging him to quit his job and bcome her assistant in the store, thus expressing both her aggression and her leading defense against aggression, which consisted of taking care of others.

With the development of her illness, Mrs. C.'s defenses were threatened. A situation in which she could not remain strong and independent placed her in the hated position of losing control and of being helpless and dependent on others. No longer able to compensate for her aggression, to maintain her self-esteem, and to promote a feeling of security in her usual way, she became afraid that her husband and son would be harmed in some way through her. On a deeper level, when her mechanisms for compensating for conflict-producing impulses were threatened, the resulting guilt gave rise to a fear of abandonment, the fear that her husband and son would not really want to take care of her if she became totally dependent.

On the basis of this formulation it became apparent that the most important issue in this woman's medical-psychological management was not what to tell her about her cancer, but rather to find some way of helping her to deal with the fears aroused by the threatened loss of her important defenses of control, activity, and independence. She both knew and at times did not permit herself to know the truth. She could speak of cancer, and at the same time talk of getting well. In part the doctor followed her own lead, using the term arthritis as long as she clung to this fiction, and then talking with her in terms of her cancer when she herself had adopted this term. Even when she spoke of cancer, however, the denial to some extent remained, and almost to the end of her life she continud to speak of what she would do when she was well. For the most part the doctor bypassed the issue of the diagnosis entirely, and talked with her about her fears of being helpless. He supported her attempts to remain active with all the means that he had at his disposal. He used a variety of medication to attempt to produce a remission of her disease or at least to give symptomatic relief; he used his medical judgment to help her plan her activities for maximum utilization of her strength. Most important, he conveyed to her, both explicitly and through his total attitude, that he would stand by her and would work with her in such a way that she would not become completely dependent on her family. She developed a strong attachment to her doctor, and was able to let herself lean on him and feel protected by him in a way that she could never have permitted with any of her family. She derived a sufficient sense of security from this relationship to continue functioning by overseeing her store with relative stability until terminal hospitalization became necessary. She was then able to transfer some of the trust that she had felt in her doctor to the hospital to which she was admitted, and to see it as a protecting institution. By accepting hospitalization she also was able to avoid successfully her fear of becoming an intolerable burden to her husband and son.

The joint work of the psychiatrist and the surgeon with this patient helped to realize some of the goals of teaching medical psychology. From the point of view of teaching psychological concepts, this case provided an opportunity to show what is meant by a compulsive character structure. It could be used to illustrate convincingly the dynamic point of view which holds that overt behavior and conscious concerns are the reflection of an interplay between deep and vital needs and the defensive and adaptive patterns developed to deal with them. It demonstrated a method of eliciting a pertinent psychological history, and of using what was thus learned to improve significantly the adjustment of the patient within the framework of medical management. Furthermore, these concepts could all be taught in relation to a problem that the physician felt was very much within his area of responsibility, so that his already existing motivation to provide the best possible care for his patient gave him an additional incentive to learn what was offered. He was not only learning a psychological approach; he was becoming aware of a new dimension of the disease process and of his patient's reaction to it. In understanding his patient's fear within the context of her life history and individual personality structure, he was learning to adapt himself to the patient's pattern, rather than to impose a stereotyped approach of his own on the relationship with her.

One final comment on the work in the Tumor Clinic is in order. The effect of this teaching on the work of individual physicians varied widely.

Even when the physician had insufficient interest to permit much effective, direct work with him, some influence may have been exerted on him indirectly. Some modification in the atmosphere of the clinic occurred as a result of the psychiatrist's presence. This modification in turn affected the work of each physician. The presence of the psychiatrist serves as a reminder of the point of view that holds that the feelings of the patient are always important and must always be taken into account. In time, the effect of the psychiatrist himself is reinforced by the adoption of this point of view by other members of the clinic staff, and this orientation gradually becomes one of the characteristic features of the clinic. An attitude of sympathetic interest in psychological matters in the clinic and in the hospital is especially important in its impact on new staff members and on incoming house officers. The resident physicians find it easier to incorporate such an attitude into their approach to patients when it is displayed by the internists and surgeons who already form their models rather than when it is represented almost solely by the Psychiatric Service.

### The Home Care Program

Teaching in the Home Care Program differed in several important ways from teaching in the Tumor Clinic, although the aim of the psychiatrist was the same in both programs. The aim was to provide the physicians and the personnel from other specialties with a background of basic psychological knowledge closely integrated with the problems encountered in actual medical practice, and with appropriate psychotherapeutic approaches to medical management. The psychiatrist drew on the same basic formulations and psychotherapeutic system for the material he used in both settings, but the methods available to transmit this information and to cope with obstacles to teaching dynamic psychology were different.

In the Tumor Clinic considerable reliance was placed on joint interviewing with the doctor, and the preceding section has illustrated the way in which the resulting material was used. In the Home Care Program most of the material from the patient was obtained by the internist, the social worker, and the nurses who were working with the family. The psychiatrist was often able to see the patient once, upon referral to the Program or during a subsequent hospital admission, and infrequently worked more intensively with a patient. There was seldom an opportunity to demonstrate facets of the patient's personality directly, and most of the material on which he based his formulations was obtained by others. These data differed in several respects from those obtained in Tumor Clinic. They were often richer, in terms of social history and interpersonal relationships within the family, because of the opportunity for observation of the patient in his home environment over a long period of time. On the other hand, they were less likely to include information concerning fantasies, wishes, or personal preoccupations, and some important areas of the patient's developmental history were inaccessible. Thus formulations regarding preconscious or unconscious factors in the patient's reactions and diagnoses of personality structure were sometimes less specific and consequently less convincing. When a specific personality diagnosis could be made, it was discussed with the group. Even when a diagnosis could not be made with assurance, however, other dynamic issues could be used for the teaching. For example, the patterns of dependency that are important in work with the elderly, the issues of ambivalence between marital partners or between parents and children, and the manifestations of guilt and of grief were prominent in various cases. Certain typical anxiety situations, such as the crisis that arises after discharge of a markedly disabled patient from hospital to home, could also be studied and discussed.

In addition, two factors in the Home Care Program were helpful in overcoming the difficulties encountered in learning dynamic concepts. One factor was the extensive contact and intensive involvement of the personnel of the program with the patients and their families. This close contact created a keen awareness of the importance of emotional issues in all aspects of the medical management. The special viewpoints of both social service and psychiatry helped to keep the broader social and emotional issues in focus.

The other factor, which existed in the Home Care setting to a much greater extent than in the Tumor Clinic, was the development of a cohesive group with strongly cathected, albeit sometimes ambivalent bonds between the members. Various factors contributed to this dynamic group formation. The group was of stable composition, with regular weekly meetings over a long period of time. All members had an equal voice in all decisions made by the group, with no hierarchical stratification along professional lines; for example, the nurse's vote carried equal weight with the physician's in deciding to accept a new patient into the program. The group forged a common ideal of patient care.

Each member played a specific role within the group, although as time went on identification with each other's point of view occurred, so that an uninformed observer might not recognize at first glance who was the internist and who the psychiatrist. The director of the program had a background primarily in public health and hospital administration. He provided a long-term sense of direction to the group, served as mediator between different points of view within the group, and promoted co-ordination between the program, the hospital, and community agencies. Two internists provided the medical care that is the heart of the program. They saw each patient at intervals of two or three weeks, or more often if indicated. In addition to practicing careful preventive medicine, they were explicitly responsible for evaluating the strengths and weaknesses of the patient's family, and for planning the most efficient utilization of the efforts of the family in the care of the patient.

Most of the patients in the Home Care Program suffer from some loss of physical functioning. A physician trained in physical medicine contributes his special knowledge to their rehabilitation. His effect on the other members illustrates the way in which the personnel of the Home Care team tend to adopt each other's points of view. As a result of the many discussions of the factors that make for the success or failure of the management of a disabled patient at home, the physicians, the social worker, and the nurses tend automatically to measure the width of bathroom doorways, note obstructing door sills, and evaluate other obstacles in the homes of patients who must rely on wheelchairs.

The social worker, who devotes full time to the program, carries several important responsibilities. Her initial interview with the family of a newly referred patient supplies data that are necessary for determining whether the family possesses sufficient strength to take care of the patient at home. She also does supportive casework with patients and especially with their families, and from these contacts furnishes important material which the group uses at the weekly conference in coming to decisions about the care of the patient. A nurse evaluates the nursing needs of the patients, and provides liaison with the Visiting Nurse Association. The team is completed by a senior medical and surgical consultant, and by the psychiatrist.

The patients on home care represent varying degrees of helplessness and dependence on outside support. A deficit exists in the physical, psychological, or socioeconomic sphere for which they are not able to compensate themselves. In the hospital these needs can be met almost totally. Many patients in the hospital recover adequate function to permit them to become self-sufficient once more, but others remain almost completely dependent, and require continued care in a hospital for chronic cases or in a nursing home. Some patients are intermediate between these two groups. A case in point is that of an elderly man whose congestive heart failure has progressed to a stage where frequent systematic medical supervision is necessary to prevent an incapacitating decompensation, and his activity is compromised to such an extent that the assistance of another person is required to meet his basic needs of living. Such a person may be too sick to come to the outpatient clinic of a hospital, and since he can no longer work, he is unable to afford the many services necessary to provide medical care at home. His wife is available to fulfill his essential nursing needs, but because of her own anxiety about his illness she is unable to assume this role without receiving adequate emotional support, carefully attuned to her particular personality pattern. If the needs of this family are not adequately met, the situation will collapse, and the result will either be repeated hospital admissions for the patient or, eventually, permanent hospitalization. The ensuing separation of husband and wife is often followed by a depression in the remaining partner, which may result in the loss of whatever autonomy remains. Such a patient is ideally suited for the Home Care Program, which can meet both the medical and the psychological needs of this family through the use of its own services carefully co-ordinated with the resources of the community. In so doing the Program maintains the family as a more independent unit, preserves the dignity of the family members, and forestalls the deterioration to which the elderly are so vulnerable.

The patients in the Program are suffering from a wide range of diseases which include chronic cardiovascular and cerebrovascular diseases, amputations, terminal malignancies, severe chronic respiratory diseases, and many others. In all cases the disability is so severe that several important areas of living are affected, and for some patients the usual pattern of life has been completely disrupted. Such was the case with Mrs. K., who was referred to the Program from the medical ward of the hospital.

Mrs. K., aged sixty-two, was admitted to the hospital with a massive myocardial infarction. For the first two weeks of hospitalization she was not expected to recover and, even after her progress became well established, she continued to have anginal pain and mild congestive heart failure. Even more limiting was the fact that she was afraid of the slightest exertion, to the extent that she would not attempt even to wash herself. Because of her vulnerable medical condition and her extreme apprehension about returning home, she was referred for Home Care. The initial evaluation by the social worker disclosed that she had many obvious dependent needs which, however, produced strong feelings of guilt and which she found it very difficult to express directly. She was afraid of being a burden to her husband after her return home, and he in turn was frightened of her coming home because of the possibility that she might die.

At the Home Care meeting at which her referral was discussed, these issues were carefully considered by the group. It was felt that without the support that the Program could offer, her management at home would collapse because of the anxiety of both husband and wife, and that a rapid rehospitalization would almost inevitably occur. Therefore she was accepted in the Program. Both were considerably reassured by the knowledge that careful medical supervision would be provided for the transition from hospital to home and for her subsequent care.

The psychiatrist was not able to interview Mrs. K. before her acceptance for home care, although he did see her later at home when complications arose in her management. In the initial discussion his chief contribution was to help assess the magnitude of her anxiety and of her dependency on the basis of the material that was available. In view of her obvious guilt over needing to be so dependent, he helped to devise an approach of giving as much reassurance as possible without minimizing the great difficulties created by her illness.

Mrs. K.'s initial adjustment at home was accomplished without incident, but difficulties very soon became evident. As the doctor and social worker were able to observe the interaction between her and Mr. K., they recognized that an intense mutual ambivalence existed. Mr. K. infuriated his wife by minimizing her complaints and through his controlling, overprotective attitude, which was usually expressed in his restriction of those of her activities that would have given her the greatest satisfaction. Her despondency gradually developed into an agitated depression, in which she tormented both herself and her husband with her complaints and with her insomnia. She began to hint that she entertained thoughts of suicide, and the possibility of maintaining her at home seemed increasingly unlikely. Because it was deemed necessary to evaluate the risk of suicide more carefully and to study a deteriorating situation more closely, a further psychiatric evaluation was made at home. From this and from the data furnished by the internist and social worker, the following picture emerged.

From her earliest years, Mrs. K. had had an insecure relationship with her mother, whom she described as a very nervous and demanding woman. When she was twelve, she was sent to live with her older sister in a distant city. She resented this separation from her family, which confirmed her fear that her mother did not really want her. This belief was further strengthened two years later when she was sent from Russia, her native country, to the United States to live with other relatives. These experiences left her with a strong unsatisfied longing to be taken care of, and with unexpressed feelings of biting hostility, but also with the dimly recognized fear that the direct expression of these impulses would cause the significant people in her life to desert her. She had found marriage and motherhood trying, but made a fair adjustment until she underwent a hysterectomy at the age of thirty. Afterward, she had developed a number of somatic complaints and diffuse fears. However, she had still been able to maintain a certain balance and to find a channel for the discharge of many of her impulses through a demanding, compulsive program of housework and by working for long hours in her garden. The relationship between her and Mr. K. had been strained, but so long as she was active each could satisfy some of the other's needs and also maintain enough distance to make their mutual hostility bearable. Now that she was so restricted by her severely damaged heart and her fear of another heart attack, she lost her necessary sublimations, and was forced into an unbearably close and dependent relationship with her husband.

At first the Home Care group tended to attribute Mrs. K.'s somatic complaints and marked limitation of function primarily to her damaged myocardium, but this attitude steadily changed to an increasing appreciation of the role of her emotional conflicts. One of the earliest indications was the mounting frustration of the internist and social worker in direct contact with this family, and indirectly of the total group, as they felt the impact of her disguised hostility and control. As the hostility between Mr. and Mrs. K. and his role in maintaining her disability became apparent, some of the anger of the group shifted to him. One of the valuable functions of a psychiatrist in this type of group is to increase its sensitivity to the meaning of such countertransference reactions.

Initially the social worker contributed all of the information about this family, and the psychiatrist helped to interpret it in the group meetings. However, a sufficiently precise formulation could not be made to answer all the questions raised by Mrs. K.'s increasing depression and the threatened collapse of the family situation. One of these questions stemmed from the fact that Mr. K. was semiretired and currently unemployed. Should he remain at home with his depressed wife, giving her the support and protection of his presence, or should he be encouraged to take a part-time job, giving each some time away from the other? The psychiatrist interviewed the patient in her home. After exploring some areas of her history more fully and observing her interaction with him, he could integrate the total picture more exactly.

These issues were discussed at the meetings of the Home Care group, with all of the members participating. A number of important general issues and specific problems were considered in evolving a program of management.

As the various facets of the case were discussed, the factors that play a role in the development of a depression were thrown into relief. These factors included the assessment of the part played by aggressive impulses and by guilt, and also the importance of the feelings of hopelessness that result when customary patterns for resolving conflict and obtaining gratification are rendered inoperative and no satisfactory substitutes are found; the role played by illness in disrupting the psychological patterns was evident as well.

The vexing problems posed by the complex interaction of Mr. and Mrs. K. provided a continuing illustration of the importance of the central people in a patient's life both for maintaining a satisfactory adjustment and for perpetuating maladaptive patterns of functioning. In attempting to solve these problems, the group found it necessary to correlate the patient's life history, the dynamic formulations of her personality structure and of the structure of the family, and the pathology of her cardiovascular system. The resulting plan of management had to balance the medical need for restriction of activity against the psychological need for the restoration of the important activities that had served as stabilizing sublimations. It was necessary to steer between her great need for reassurance and the danger of antagonizing her, and thus increasing her depression, by minimizing her suffering as her husband did. The application of this plan was primarily the job of the physician, who reassured her by being available to her, and by confidently supporting the activities that were possible for her and yet acknowledging seriously her complaints of constant discomfort. The social worker saw her in regular interviews, in which her emotional problems were dealt with more directly. The psychiatrist acted as an advisor in the group, where the work with the family was regularly reported. He helped to determine the role each member should take with the family, and the specific psychotherapeutic maneuvers that could be employed. He was also available to consult individually with the social worker from time to time about the more complex psychotherapeutic problems that arose in her casework.

Both the doctor and the social worker had to take account of Mr. K.'s envy of the attention his wife was getting and of his resentment of the extra demands now being made on him. He was given abundant recognition for the responsibility that he now carried. Attention was paid to his own somatic complaints. At other times, when he was behaving too childishly, the physician took a sterner attitude toward him to help maintain a balance in the marital relationship. He was supported in leaving his wife for half of each day in order to take a part-time job, and this separation proved useful in diluting the irritation that constantly being with his wife produced in both of them.

A difficult and frustrating couple such as the K.'s inevitably produced a strong emotional response in those members of the team who worked directly with them, and to a lesser extent in those who were involved only through the group discussions. These highly charged personal responses were expressed in the meetings, sometimes directly and with vivid affect, and sometimes through opinions and value judgments supposedly determined by objective considerations. They were expressed by group members who worked together, were familiar with each other, and among whom primarily positive bonds had been established. In this setting it was often possible for other members of the group, who were not so involved, to assist in making these attitudes more explicit by means of a joke, a clarifying comment, or by presenting another, more objective, point of view. The members of the group thus helped each other to become aware of prejudices and sensitivities in relation to patients, thereby increasing the range of problems that could be worked with successfully.

These experiences in understanding the responses of patients and their families in dynamic terms took place not as psychological exercises, but as a vital part of the care of seriously ill people. The psychiatrist did not serve ostensibly as a teacher, but as a participant with special knowledge, whose presence helped catalyze many of the processes that took place in the group. The motivation for grasping psychological concepts was a direct derivative of the wish to give superior medical care under especially difficult and challengng circumstances, and the application of this knowledge was regarded as one aspect of the special medical practice in which the whole group took pride.

This process of learning medical-psychological management through work with families was repeated as various aspects of personality structure and of the reactions to illness were seen in the other patients in the Program. A young woman with severe diabetes and an infantile, hysterical personality structure, who was followed through the conflicts of post-adolescence, marriage, and motherhood, presented some fascinating contrasts to the predominant number of patients who were in the older age group. A man who was blind, who had lost both legs as a result of peripheral vascular disease, and whose wife had withdrawn because of the anxiety stimulated by her husband's mutilation, impressively demonstrated the extent to which illness could induce a regression. As he learned to walk again on short, artificial legs, he showed how a man, with skillful support, can struggle against such disabilities. Many other patients presented equally striking examples of psychological factors in medical management.

As mentioned in the foregoing discussion, the Home Care team's transition from a group of people doing a job to a group that functioned as a unit, with important emotional ties between the members, played an important part in overcoming the difficulties usually associated with learning psychological concepts. The formal aspects of having the same individuals meet for discussion around a table at the same time and place at frequent intervals contributed to the group's development. But probably the most important determinant was the enthusiasm that each participant brought to the work, and the conviction that the group's task was of the highest importance. Each member helped to define the purpose of the group, and so was prepared to identify himself with the standards and approaches that resulted. The work was successful; the care given to the patients in general met the most exacting standards of all the participants. Morale was high, and an almost cocky attitude of "If it can be done, we can do it" developed. A number of areas of friction developed from time to time between the members of the team, but the cohesiveness of the group was strong enough to permit these to be worked out.

The medical-psychological approaches developed in the Home Care Program not only affected the personnel of the team, but had an impact on a much wider group. Physicians from the community, from schools of public health, and from other countries, as well as social workers and nurses, attended the meetings to observe the functioning of the program. Medical students serving their clerkships in medicine at the hospital also observed some of the meetings, and accompanied the physicians on home visits. The resident physicians who presented the histories of the patients whom they were referring for home care were drawn into an even greater involvement as they were required to think through plans for the post-hospital management of their patients in discussions with the Home Care group. For them this participation constituted one of the most effective antidotes to seeing patients in the relative isolation from the patients' accustomed environment that the hospital so often creates. Thus the Home Care Program became an articulate and effective representative to the medical community, both within and outside of the hospital, of the psychological point of view in comprehensive medical care.

# Teaching Principles of Medical Psychology to Medical House Officers: Methods and Problems

JOHN F. REICHARD, M.D.

ONE OF THE MOST difficult problems for a psychiatric teacher is to teach physicians of other specialties about the psychological aspects of illness. This opinion is widely shared, and it is borne home to young psychiatrists at the Beth Israel Hospital in a directly personal way. One of their important duties is to serve as consultants to the other inpatient services in the hospital. The assignment has often proved frustrating. In many cases the psychiatrist has found that he had information or a point of view that should have been of value to another physician, but that much of the value was dissipated because of the extreme difficulty he encountered in conveying this information to the other physician. In a moment of despair one of the psychiatrists remarked, "It is like watching a man dig a hole with his bare hands and offering to lend him your shovel, only to be told that he does not feel he needs a shovel."

The author's frustration stimulated a wish to learn more about this puzzling state of affairs. If the psychiatric teacher could establish a close and prolonged relationship with the physicians he was teaching, he should be better able to observe and comprehend their reactions to psychiatric consultations. Accordingly, the author was made the permanent psychiatric consultant to the Male Medical Ward for a period of two years. He spent every afternoon from one to three o'clock on the ward, the time of day when the house officers were most free from rounds and conferences. While on the ward, the psychiatrist was available for consultation with the house officers and medical students. As they became

This study was supported by a Career Teachers' Grant from the National Institute of Mental Health.

more accustomed to working in close contact with a psychiatric consultant, he was gradually able to become more active as a teacher. If consultations were slow in coming, he might ask the nurses if there were any patients they felt he should talk to, or might select certain patients who appeared to be having psychological problems. Much of the time he and the house officers discussed matters which were not directly related to medical psychology. They talked about sports, politics, books, hospital gossip, new medical developments, and psychoanalytic theory. Informally, the house officers brought up their gripes about the visiting staff, discussed their own family difficulties, and aired their emotional problems and conflicts with their colleagues. As a result of these chats with the house officers, the psychiatrist gradually became accepted as a "member of the family" on the ward.

In this fortunate situation, the psychiatrist was able from time to time to obtain sudden glimpses into the house officers' thoughts and feelings. Three cases which afforded such glimpses will be described in this paper. They offer insight into some of the problems encountered by house officers in their dealings with patients and in their efforts to understand psychiatric methods which are intended to help them.

Before proceeding to the specific cases, however, it will be well to assess the importance of a general problem that is encountered in teaching psychiatry to nonpsychiatric house officers: the question of lack of time.

It is often maintained that house officers are so busy that they do not have the time to devote themselves to the psychological aspects of medical problems. In the beginning it seemed that this factor might well be genuine, although it was clear from the first that on some occasions the house officers used lack of time as a rationalization to justify their ignoring some of their patients' feelings. However, rapidly accumulating evidence showed that lack of time was far more rationalization than reality, and was not the basic obstacle which kept the house officers from investigating the psychological complications of medical illness. The fact is illustrated by a series of events which recurred regularly whenever a new group of house officers began their work on the ward. During the first few days the house officers and the psychiatrist would chat about whatever they found of common interest. This talk might go on for as much as twenty minutes, with everybody chatting comfortably and showing no signs of pressure to be doing something else. But if the psychiatrist remarked, "Well, about this patient we were discussing . . ." everyone would find that suddenly he was very busy. After the house officers had gotten more accustomed to the psychiatrist, they enjoyed talking to him about patients at great length, but his slightest suggestion that they should go to interview a patient would once again scatter them to urgent duties. Still later, when a group, or part of a group, had come to enjoy watching him interview patients, he would try to get one of them to do the interviewing while he observed. This attempt brought the same reaction: they would all invariably discover that they were *really* pressed for time.

This reaction was so gross that frequently the house officers commented on it themselves. Once, for example, one of the house officers said that he did not have time to interview a patient with the psychiatrist and then spent the next twenty minutes discussing the patient. At the end of that time, he laughed and said, "My goodness, in the time we spent talking we could have had time to do an interview," a piece of insight that the psychiatrist was delighted to reinforce.

Even though the observed facts do not bear them out, it is important to realize that there is a kind of subjective truth to the house officers' feeling that they do not have enough time. They feel that they are sitting on a powder keg. At any moment an emergency may erupt, or several severely ill patients may be admitted, and since they are on duty for long periods of time, there is little respite from this pressure. Thus when the psychiatrist appears on the scene and says, in effect, "You have faced only half of your responsibilities; here is the entire area of the patients' emotions which you have been neglecting," it is not surprising that the house officers shrink from accepting this statement. It cannot be expected that people who are already heavily burdened with anxiety can accept an additional load of anxiety, unless they are given substantial help.

The first case to be discussed focuses attention on some of the conceptual difficulties a house officer encounters when he attempts to understand the psychological aspects of illness.

The patient, Mr. M., was a 58-year-old Jewish man who was hospitalized because of his second myocardial infarction. He presented a problem in medical management that is familiar to everyone who has answered requests for psychiatric consultations from the medical service. He refused to stay in bed, he insisted on walking to the bathroom or the television room, and he took his medication only when he chose to. When the doctors cautioned him about his behavior, he brushed aside their recommendations with jokes and boasted that he knew how to take care of himself.

When the psychiatrist discussed this patient with the house officer, she seemed to have a good understanding of his personality. She said that two weeks before admission he had suddenly developed severe angina. Since he had had a previous myocardial infarction and occasional mild episodes of angina, he presumably knew the significance of this pain. Even so, he had not contacted his physician, he had not decreased his activity, and he had not even taken the nitroglycerin that he had been given to relieve his pain. When she asked him why, he said that he was finishing his work on a large furniture order and had found that he could "get the better of the pain" if he just rested a few minutes and then continued working. When the patient gave his history on admission to the hospital, he described a previous hospitalization as if it had been a trivial affair, but when the house officer consulted the old record she found that he had had acute peritonitis caused by a foreign body which had perforated his intestine. It had involved several operations and had been complicated by a pulmonary embolus which had almost been fatal. He also concealed the fact that a sister and brother had both had myocardial infarctions and two other brothers had died of myocardial infarctions.

The house officer saw clearly that this man had a desperate need to deny that he was sick, and she also saw that his behavior in neglecting his treatment and ignoring his doctors was a result of that denial. On the basis of this appraisal, she decided that the critical element in the management of this patient was to avoid a direct challenge to his denial of illness. Any effort to convince him that he was sick would be frightening and might push him into even more extreme displays of imprudent activity. Thinking back to his comments that he "could take care of himself" and that he knew how to "get the better of the pain," she decided that the most promising approach was to appeal to his wish to master his illness and to give him extensive responsibility for managing his own treatment.

As a teacher, the psychiatrist was delighted by the house officer's understanding of this patient. She had only recently joined the ward service, so that Mr. M. was one of the first patients she had discussed with him. Her excellent understanding of Mr. M.'s personality was evidence that she was psychologically perceptive and had a firm grasp of the principles of medical psychology which were formulated by Edward and Grete Bibring. These fundamental principles are intended to guide the physician in his attempt to deal with the emotional complications of illness, and int his case, the house officer had applied them intelligently. She had accurately observed Mr. M's characteristic pattern of behavior and she had understood how it affected his reaction to illness and medical treatment. Then, following the method of medical psychology, she had evolved a plan for treating the patient that would enlist this behavior pattern in the service of medical treatment. The psychiatrist watched the case with a feeling of interest and satisfaction.

Ordinarily, when a house officer understands a patient's personality, even a difficult problem in medical management will quiet down fairly quickly. After a day or so it was obvious that something had gone wrong. The patient continued his willful ways. The house officer was annoyed at the patient, at psychiatry, and at the psychiatrist, and the psychiatrist in turn was puzzled. He suggested that he should talk to the patient and then observe her interview with him to see if he could make any helpful recommendations.

Mr. M. was a plethoric, bull-necked, heavy-chested man. When the psychiatrist talked to him, he was cheerful, active, and full of jokes. He poked fun at the doctors who were telling him to stay in bed and asked if they had sent the psychiatrist to scold him. He described his arrival in Boston when he was seventeen. He and three older brothers had been offered a chance to leave Russia and come to the United States to live with a distant cousin until they could make a start for themselves. His brothers had decided to stay at home, but he had jumped at the chance to emigrate. Three months after he arrived in Boston, his cousin was hospitalized with tuberculosis and he was left completely alone in an alien land, unable to speak more than a dozen words of English. He wrote to his father, who told him he had better come back home; but he decided to stick it out. With some help from a rabbi, he got a job and learned English. He taught himself to be a carpenter and eventually became a furniture maker. He said he could still do the job faster and more skillfully than much younger men who worked in the same shop. He said with great satisfaction that he had eventually saved enough money to send for his brothers and his sister. He began to talk about his wife and, when he described her death some thirty years before, his rather strident exuberance began to fall away from him. He had two children, whom he described with tears in his eyes as "all I have left of her." He went on to say with bitterness that his son had married against his strong objections a girl who had no character and was not Jewish. His daughter was going with a man who did not meet his approval. Behind these remarks lay the definite hint which did not quite come out into the open, that his children's disobedience had brought on the heart attack and that if anything happened to him, it would serve them right.

When the time came for the house officer to interview Mr. M., she started off well. The patient complained that he was not sleeping well at night. The house officer asked if he would like a sleeping pill. He said no, the reason he wasn't sleeping was that he was not active during the day. But even so, he did not like to take pills. He thought that if he could get himself into a relaxed frame of mind he could get to sleep by himself. She adroitly took advantage of this opening to observe that he liked to do things for himself. She added that she thought it was fine for the patients to do things for themselves and she liked to give them responsibility for managing their own treatment. At this point he interrupted to tell her in his boastful manner that when he was first married he had gotten a second job working weekends on the fish pier so that he could buy his wife a special birthday present. His wife couldn't understand why he was away from home every weekend and suspected that he might be carrying on with another woman. The house officer seemed to experience this prolonged interruption as a threat to her control of the interview, which it was in part. The presence of a psychiatrist probably increased her discomfort. A more seasoned and flexible command of interviewing technique might have enabled her to use this anecdote as a means of developing more rapport by accepting the patient's view of himself as a bit of a devil, albeit a soft-hearted one. However, she was obviously thrown off stride, and she attempted to recover the situation by becoming firmer and more serious. At the same time, she appeared to feel ill at ease acting in this stern manner and gave the impression that she would have liked to plead with him to behave himself and act like a nice person. Her confusion seemed to provoke him into an attempt to get her completely rattled. He said, "You're such a nice little girl, but you're always giving me lectures. You always look so serious. You don't have to worry about me. Look, I'm strong like an ox" and he flexed his biceps. She was exasperated by this behavior, and shortly afterward the interview was broken off.

Later, in their discussion of this case, the psychiatrist suggested to her that perhaps they had not placed enough emphasis on Mr. M's difficulties with his children. He told her what the patient had said about them. Then he pointed out that the patient apparently felt that his children were defying his authority, and he was venting his anger and wounded pride on the house officer. Since this anger had nothing to do with her, it was necessary to find a way to get her disentangled from it and at the same time give the patient what he wanted. The psychiatrist suggested that they retain their original approach but add to it an appeal that the patient follow her recommendations because she was concerned about him. She could say, for example, that even though *he* was sure he could handle his illness without limiting his activities, it caused her a great deal of distress to see him taking risks. So would he please follow her recommendations even though he felt they were silly. By now the house officer had recovered her poise, and she agreed to talk to the patient again that afternoon without the psychiatrist, and to approach the problem from this new point of view.

When the psychiatrist came on the ward the following day, the nurse, an exuberant person, greeted him by asking "What did you do to Mr. M? He is so much more pleasant today." Feeling pleased that the patient seemed to be behaving better, the psychiatrist sought out the house officer. At first she denied the change in Mr. M's behavior, but in response to questions she observed that he *was* staying in bed, that he *was* taking his medication, that he *had* stopped his teasing, unpleasant behavior. She concluded by agreeing that he had made a dramatic change in his behavior, and added spontaneously that the change had taken place after her second interview with him on the previous day. The psychiatrist then asked if she thought there was any connection between her interview and the patient's subsequent change of behavior. She said she doubted it, and wondered if the apparent relationship between the two events might merely be a coincidence. The psychiatrist suggested that a scientific way to test this hypothesis was to go and ask the patient. She agreed, and as they approached the bed, Mr. M. greeted her with: "Here's my darling." He said, "You know, doctor," turning to the psychiatrist, "I would do anything for this little lady. She is such a marvelous doctor and takes such wonderful care of me. The only thing is that such a nice girl should raise a family. I promised her that when she has her first baby, I'm going to get her a wonderful present."

In discussion with the psychiatrist following this interview, the house officer could not believe that the patient's change in behavior was related to his changed feelings toward her. It was also difficult for her to see that her remarks had helped the patient to respond to her and to hospitalization in a way which was quite different from the way he was currently responding to his children. She fell back on the disappointing idea that the patient had "just decided to change." She felt it was only a coincidence that the change had occurred after she had changed her approach toward him.

One of the most interesting aspects of this case is that at the end of this episode the house officer had less understanding of the case than she did at the beginning. This is a startling turn of events, and to explain it we have to try to perceive how she organized and understood the psychological data at her disposal. At the beginning, she was guided by an excellent concept. She understood that the patient had an unconscious fear of being weak and concealed it by overactivity. This concept explained his refusal to follow medical advice, and it also indicated the appropriate way to deal with the problem.

As she worked with this patient, however, new and confusing data began to emerge, particularly in the area of the patient's reaction to her. He insisted on treating her like a little girl toward whom he should behave in a flirtatious and domineering manner. At this point, the psychiatrist was struggling to fit the patient's behavior into some plausible conceptual scheme, but his attempts in this direction were incomprehensible to her. As time went on, she became increasingly confused and her understanding of the case diminished. Finally, she was left with the idea that the patient just decided to change his behavior, which is another way of saying "it just happened," or in effect of completely abandoning any attempt to find a psychological explanation for these events. A significant point is that, as she abandoned her effort to understand those events in psychological terms, she also lost her ability to "see" what was happening. In the end we are left with the extraordinary situation that she was unable to "see" that the patient's behavior on the ward had changed. The change was too obvious to overlook, once it had been pointed out, but she was still unable to "see" that his change in behavior had been directly caused by her altered method of dealing with him. It is unfortunate that she was unable to comprehend the changes in the patient's behavior as they evolved, for she could have enlarged her understanding of the case and increased her ability to deal with this difficult patient.

Why should the new developments which clarified the case for the psychiatrist have been meaningless to the house officer? An important part of the answer is that she did not possess a conceptual framework which would have permitted her to assimilate and use the new data as they emerged. In particular, she lacked a firm understanding of the concepts of transference and psychic determinism. It is instructive to follow out in some detail how a solid grasp of these two principles might have increased her understanding of the situation.

The patient's attitude toward her was so totally inappropriate that it obviously was a transference relationship that was largely uncorrected by reality. Anyone accustomed to thinking in terms of transference would recognize immediately that these feelings had nothing to do with the house officer, and he would begin to wonder what past object relationship had served as their source. On the other hand, it is understandable that to someone relatively unfamiliar with transference, the patient's attitude would seem so embarrassing and personal that it would be difficult to think about it in an objective, scientific way.

The concept of psychological determinism states that every psychological event must have a cause. A corollary is that under favorable circumstances, one can draw a patient out and learn useful clues which point to the past causes for current events. In the case of Mr. M., anyone who was familiar with this principle would begin to suspect that this man had a highly eroticized relationship with his daughter. His behavior with the house officer certainly suggested the situation of a father being very flirtatious with his daughter. His hurt and resentment at his daughter's forthcoming marriage indicated that he was having more than normal difficulty in giving her up to another man. He told us that, after his wife's untimely death, he had transferred all his affection to his children, making it likely that his relation to his daughter had become highly libidinized. From these clues a hypothesis can be constructed which begins to make some sense of past and present events. This man had always had an excessive need to assert his virility. After his wife's death he used a flirtatious relationship with an adoring daughter to buttress his masculine self-esteem. When he was faced simultaneously with the loss of this daughter and with a life-threatening illness, he was under terrible pressure. He not only clung to his relationship with his daughter, but transferred this whole set of feelings to the young woman doctor who was caring for him. Admittedly, after such a brief acquaintance with the case, the evidence for these suppositions was not overwhelming, and the psychiatrist had no idea that they were going to produce such dramatic results. However, it was a perfectly plausible hypothesis and worth subjecting to a clinical trial.

Accordingly, the house officer was asked to change her approach to the patient. This altered approach was meant to say several things. First, it said that the limitation on his activity was no reflection on his masculine strength. Secondly, it said, "Look, I am not a rebellious, unfaithful daughter. Quite the contrary; my only reason for making these requests is that I am deeply concerned with your welfare." The patient responded to this change with dramatically altered behavior, suggestive evidence that the hypothesis was correct. At the same time he developed a paternal, affectionate relation to the house officer with the erotic elements thinly disguised. To a psychiatrist, this development is unequivocal confirmation for the hypothesis; yet the house officer did not see these events as they unfolded. Even after the episode was over and the psychiatrist went back and tried to point out step-by-step what had occurred, she was unconvinced. Her explanation was that he had been behaving badly but really knew better. She had asked him to behave himself and he had complied. That was all that had happened. The events required no elaborate explanation and justified none. It was clear that she considered the psychiatrist's explanation to be rather far-fetched.

The psychiatrist, working from well-established principles, was able to perceive a certain order in the psychological data. The house officer, because she did not share the psychiatrist's conceptual framework, was unable to perceive this order. For her the situation remained a jumble. This contrast illustrates the important point that to perceive a psychological event, an observer must have an adequate conceptual framework in which an event can be placed. The reference here, it should be noted, is not to the *use* of psychological data but merely to their *perception*. Without a suitable conceptual framework, an observer cannot even perceive psychological events as they occur. The problem is thus unfortunately circular: without a conceptual framework one cannot perceive psychological events, yet the repeated observation of psychological events is the only method of acquiring the conceptual framework which one needs. Finding a way of breaking through this impasse is one of the most frustrating and difficult problems encountered in the teaching of psychiatry to nonpsychiatrists. Referring back to the case of Mr. M., we can see that if the house officer had grasped what was going on, it would have enriched her understanding of transference and the other psychological concepts involved in the case; yet, a prior understanding of these very concepts was what she needed to enable her to perceive what was occurring.

In discussing the case of Mr. M., we have examined only two psychological concepts, transference and psychological determinism. It should be noted, however, that they do not exhaust the concepts which contribute to our understanding of the case. For example, there is the concept of instinctual impulse. From his daily work, a psychiatrist knows that an instinctual impulse is a powerful force that strives incessantly toward expression and resists any attempt to deflect it. The remarkable urgency of Mr. M's wish for a dominating, flirtatious relationship with the house officer reveals the hidden presence of especially powerful instinctual impulses. Impulses as strong as these do not disappear abruptly. This fact adds support to the opinion that the patient's behavior did not change spontaneously. It helps to confirm the conclusion that the change in behavior occurred because the house officer altered her attitude and permitted some appropriate gratification of his instinctual impulses. In this way, the expression of these impulses could be converted into a form which would facilitate rather than obstruct the course of medical management.

Or, to state this in another form, the patient began to act like a loving and indulgent "daddy" rather than a neglected and angry one.

The same brief series of events which we examined above in the light of the concepts of transference and psychological determinism can thus be considered from a slightly different point of view by introducing the concept of instinctual impulse; moreover, there are other important psychological concepts which can be related to these events. In fact, to be complete, it would be necessary to go on for many pages describing basic concepts and how they influence our understanding of what occurred. These three concepts can, however, serve as illustrations. Each of them affects our understanding of what happened in this case. If we compare the separate discussions of these concepts, we see that there is a good deal of overlap. In fact, to isolate any one concept and discuss its relation to the case is a highly artificial process, only justified by the fact that it is necessary in order to achieve clarity in the discussion. The three concepts are not at all independent of each other. In this particular case, each concept describes a somewhat different aspect of the same process. Each concept complements, modifies, and qualifies the others. Each also modifies and in turn is modified by related psychological concepts which have not been introduced.

The interrelationship of concepts presents a special difficulty in understanding the conceptual basis of dynamic psychiatry. The concepts are difficult to understand if they are isolated from one another; to a considerable degree, the conceptual system can only be understood as a whole. Acquiring an understanding of this conceptual system can be compared to moving an intact house. When one moves a house, no part of it can be moved abruptly or for any great distance. To do that would mean tearing the part away from the main house and destroying the very unity which one wishes to preserve. Instead, each corner is moved a few inches at a time so that its relationship to the whole house can be maintained. Then, the next corner is moved a few inches and in this way the whole house gradually changes position.

The psychiatric teacher thus faces a constantly recurring dilemma. To explain a given situation he must go back to the pertinent psychological concepts, but if he discusses a single concept in isolation, he robs it of part of its meaning and its ability to compel conviction. On the other hand, in teaching persons who are unfamiliar with psychological theory he cannot discuss all the concepts which are relevant to a single event for fear that the students will be overwhelmed.

A further difficulty is that a medical man is accustomed to a very different mode of thinking from a psychiatrist. In medicine, the relationship between data and concept and the relationship between different concepts are generally clear and self-evident. The relationships may, of course, be quite complex, as for example in the mechanism of blood clotting, but when a hematologist describes his theory of the process of blood clotting, what he says is generally clear. He may be mistaken, or another hematologist may disagree with him, but there is usually no confusion about what he means. Contrast this situation with the case we have been discussing. Here the psychiatrist was completely unable to make his view of this case clear to the house officer. It was not that she disagreed with him; she could not really understand what he was talking about. She could not see how the concepts related to the data or how the concepts could be fitted together to form an over-all description of the case. This lack of communication is no reflection on either of them. It has to do with the nature of the material that was being communicated.

To return to the example of blood clotting, it is fair to say that if a student does not understand the process of blood clotting, he *knows* that he does not understand it. Furthermore, he can identify the aspects he does not understand and can study them until he does understand them. The situation with psychiatric concepts is different. Basic psychiatric theory can be stated fairly briefly, and to a beginner the relation of the concepts to the clinical data and to each other may seem clear. But after five years' experience, he has a wholly different understanding of the same concept stated in the same words. After ten years' experience, he may find himself working with a concept that has long been familiar and suddenly see it in an entirely new light. His subjective feeling is that he has never really understood the concept before. In every branch of medicine one continues to learn, but in organic medicine one extends one's knowledge by including new ideas and discoveries. In psychiatry, on the other hand, knowledge generally increases not through new information but through deeper understanding of the known.

This difference causes grave difficulties. We are faced with the situation of two groups of people who work side by side and yet are separated by a conceptual abyss. When two groups do not share a common conceptual scheme and a common vocabulary, communication between them is seriously obstructed. The medical profession, of which psychiatry is a part, will have to find a way to cope with this frustrating problem. An important first step toward its solution would be to admit candidly that this conceptual abyss exists. Psychiatric and medical doctors should recognize that their thinking stems from two quite different intellectual systems. As a consequence, communication between them must necessarily be limited and difficult. The current tacit assumption that psychiatric and medical doctors share a common conceptual system has caused unnecessary mischief. When communication collapses, as it inevitably must, it gives rise to uneasy suspicions that one party is "resisting" or that the other is talking "hot air." The case of Mr. M. illustrates the problem clearly. For the psychiatrist, it was an unnerving experience to be going along in the belief that he was communicating with a colleague and then to find suddenly that his words were meaningless to his colleague, while his colleague's seemed preposterous to him.

The problems involved in teaching psychiatry to a colleague who is not versed in the concepts of dynamic psychology are closely analogous to the problems encountered in the children's puzzle of "Find the Hidden Fox." This puzzle presents a drawing of a landscape. Certain of the lines in the drawing, if taken together, represent the outline of a fox. Initially, however, the fox is hidden because the observer's eye naturally follows the outline of trees, bushes, rocks, and other objects in the drawing, and he does not realize that some of the same lines can also be seen as forming the figure of a fox. It is instructive to pursue this analogy in some detail. It can readily be seen that if one is familiar with the size, shape, and anatomical details of foxes, the figure will leap much more quickly to the eye than if one had never seen a fox and had no idea what one looks like. Furthermore, in the drawing, the eye of the fox is really just a leaf and the ear is really two twigs which cross. They only become an eye and an ear when you realize that if there *were* an eye here and an ear up there, then they would be in the correct relationship to be parts of a head. Then you reason that if there is a head here, there should be a snout down there. When you search, the snout suddenly leaps out of the picture, and then there is no difficulty in tracing out the forepaw, the body, and the tail. It is psychologically interesting that once the fox is seen, it can never be "unseen" again, and it becomes difficult to comprehend how another observer can look closely at the picture and not see the fox.

The same situation exists when a psychiatrist tries to delineate a patient's personality structure for a house officer. The psychiatrist has an extensive and detailed familiarity with the shapes of different kinds of foxes. As he looks at the picture, he begins to see objects which can be eyes and ears. He searches further for the parts which would complete the picture, and suddenly the fox leaps to the eye. The house officer, however, has never seen a fox, so that the particular spatial arrangement which seems so convincing to the psychiatrist makes little impression on him.

He stares at the picture and sees only foliage. The psychiatrist must continually retrace the outline of the fox, carefully describing the details. If the picture suddenly clicks together and looks like a fox, then the house officer has taken another step toward the understanding of dynamic psychology. If it does not click together for the house officer, then the psychiatrist can only drop it and go on to the next picture.

A special kind of relationship must exist between the house officer and the psychiatrist before this sort of teaching can go on. The house officer must have confidence that if he continues to reflect on the psychiatrist's description of the patient's personality, the picture may suddenly click together as an insight. He must also be prepared to accept the possibility that it might not click together, and still remain willing to try again with the next case. The psychiatrist has to have the patience to go over the details repeatedly, realizing that until the house officer can put the whole picture together, he will probably learn relatively little. It is often difficult for the psychiatrist to determine what aspect of the case is confusing the house officer. The better he knows the house officer as a person, the more cues he will find that may suggest the nature of the house officer's difficulty in understanding the case. An incident involving the house officer who treated Mr. M. illustrates this point well.

This particular house officer was an attractive young woman who was perceptive and sympathetic with her patients. Just a day or two before Mr. M. was admitted to the hospital, she had taken part in an event whose relevance to Mr. M's case had passed unnoticed at the time. She and the psychiatrist had been discussing an adolescent patient of hers who had taken quite a liking to her and who had obviously blossomed under her care. The psychiatrist had commented that it was nice to have a woman on the service. To his surprise, she had abruptly replied that she "did not think that female doctors should take advantage of the fact that they were women." It had not been a propitious moment to discuss this issue further, but to keep the door open in case it came up again, he had merely asked in an off-handed manner, "Why not?"

Thoughtful consideration of this brief incident might have enabled an observer to surmise that this house officer had the capacity to form a good, close relationship with a male patient and yet needed to deny defensively the value of this relationship when attention was called to it. As later events were to show, this set of attitudes had a significant influence on her relationship with Mr. M. At the time, however, the psychiatrist was unaware of the significance of her comments; he merely noted them as important remarks which, hopefully, would become more understandable in the future. It is worthwhile pausing to consider the importance of this incident. If the psychiatric teacher has a close relationship with the house officers, he will discover many clues similar to this one which will show him why a house officer may be having difficulty dealing with a particular patient or understanding a particular psychological principle. In many cases, these clues may be so subtle that they will not be explicitly recognized by the teacher, even though he may gain considerable information from them. Without a close relationship to the house officers, however, these clues cannot be observed and teaching is thereby made much more difficult.

It is a curious teaching relationship, and one that puts considerable strain on both parties. There is a certain "lumpiness" involved in learning dynamic psychiatry. One goes along learning very little, until suddenly a fairly large portion of interrelated ideas becomes clear. There is an unfortunate tendency to ascribe the lumpiness to the students or to the teachers, but it should be recognized that the lumpiness is inherent in the material itself.

The preceding section has discussed the house officer's difficulty in bringing together enough data so that he can see the patient's personality as a coherent, intelligible whole. The case of Mr. M. also illustrates another difficulty that the house officer must guard against, and that is reaching a final conclusion too quickly and then closing his mind to new information which might alter his view of the patient. One of the causes of this tendency is that medicine and psychiatry approach clinical material from profoundly different points of view.

When a patient is admitted to a medical ward, the admitting physician generally lists half a dozen possible diagnoses. During the patient's stay in the hospital, various diagnostic tests are performed. With few exceptions, all the possible diagnoses can be foreseen early in the case. Therefore, the doctor's thinking is directed toward narrowing the list of possibilities and focusing attention on the one or two most likely diagnoses. Once a diagnosis is established, the house officer's interest and curiosity generally drop off sharply. The patient is then started on a course of treatment which is in most cases routine.

The situation in psychiatry is markedly different. After a patient has been in psychotherapy for a year, new material may alter the view of the patient which the psychiatrist has previously held. As the psychiatrist treats the patient, he is constantly putting together what he knows of the patient up to that point. But he can never make a final decision. He must constantly keep his ear open for new experiences of the patient which will force him to revise his previous conclusion.

The case of Mr. M. illustrates this difference of approach nicely. The house officer made a psychological "diagnosis" of this patient and knew how to "treat" him. When her "treatment" produced no results, she assumed there was something basically wrong with her "diagnosis" or "treatment," and had no idea how to proceed from that point. This attitude conforms well to the accepted medical approach to a patient. If a physician makes a diagnosis of cardiac failure and the patient shows no response to digitalis, it is time for him to suspect that he has committed a blunder. However, the psychiatrist approached Mr. M's problem from quite a different point of view. He realized that focusing on the patient's counterphobic and counterdependent defenses had arbitrarily limited attention to a single aspect of a complex situation. When the attempt to deal with these defenses produced no results, it seemed likely that some other, unrecognized problem was putting pressure on the patient. This other problem turned out to be his oedipal feelings for his daughter, which he had transferred to the house officer.

This difference of approach is difficult for house officers to accept. They feel that missing an important psychological fact is the equivalent of not hearing a significant cardiac murmur or of not feeling a spleen. They have trouble becoming accustomed to the psychiatrist's patient acceptance of the fact that in a brief interview one can catch a glimpse of only a fraction of a patient's personality. To be sure, the psychiatrist hopes and tries to see quickly all the outstanding characteristics of a patient's personality, but often that is impossible. It may be necessary to interview a patient repeatedly until the situation becomes clear.

Mr. M.'s case affords an opportunity of assessing the effectiveness of the methods used at the Beth Israel Hospital to teach psychiatry to nonpsychiatric physicians. As mentioned above, the psychiatrist, in dealing with the psychological problems of medical patients, bases his approach on concepts formulated by Edward and Grete Bibring. Briefly summarized, this approach consists of making an evaluation of the patient's fundamental personality structure, paying special attention to the characteristic behavior patterns and defenses used by the patient. In dealing with the patient, the attempt is then to support these defenses and to avoid challenging them. The approach followed by both the house officer and the psychiatrist illustrates the use of this technique in a clinical situation. This approach is the basic blueprint for determining the best method of handling the psychological difficulties of medical patients.

How useful is this blueprint for teaching these methods to nonpsychiatric physicians? As a teaching method, the approach was brilliantly successful in involving the house officer in an attempt to deal with Mr. M's psychological problems. From the history and the patient's behavior, she quickly spotted the major trends in his personality and knew how to help him with his difficulties. This landed her right in the middle of a complicated situation. The significance of her experience will be evident to anyone who has tried this kind of teaching. Students have a strong tendency to remain aloof from situations like these, either ignoring them or philosophizing about them from a safe distance; this house officer, however, was really involved in trying to understand and help this troubled man. To my mind, this is one of the great strengths of this method of teaching. The conceptual system evolved by the Bibrings is sufficiently simplified so that it can readily be grasped by people who are unfamiliar with psychodynamic theory. It has immediate and convincing impact on those who may never have the opportunity to explore psychiatric theory and understand fully its complicated concepts. Even though simplified, however, this approach focuses attention on aspects of personality which are central to the problems encountered in the medical management of patients. In many cases, knowledge of the patient's defensive structure will by itself suffice to indicate to the physician the most effective way to deal with the patient. Even in the case of Mr. M. which was selected to illustrate a failure of this method of teaching, we can see that the house doctor was on the right track; with a little more background, she might have achieved a real gain in understanding. Even as it was, her management of the case in line with the psychiatrist's suggestions was effective, although she could not understand why.

Nevertheless, this approach has the defects of its virtues; it presents the problems which inevitably arise when an attempt is made to use a simplified or abbreviated version of a complex conceptual scheme. If complications arise for which the simplified scheme makes no provision, the person who knows only the simplified scheme is helpless to deal with the complications. He is like a person who has a set of instructions telling him how to get to the City Hall. Assuming he knows nothing about the topography of the city except what is in his instructions, he is lost if he makes one wrong turn or encounters one detour. If he has a good general knowledge of the city, however, he will know when he is headed in the wrong direction and will be able to make appropriate corrections.

This is clearly what happened in Mr. M.'s case. A transference problem arose, and the house officer found herself in an area which was entirely unfamiliar to her. Such complications arise fairly frequently when house officers attempt to use this approach in dealing with troubled patients. To help them meet these complications, it is essential that the psychiatric teacher remain in close contact as they attempt to apply the technique. If he does not, they will encounter too many frustrating failures and will become convinced that attempts to understand the patient's personality are a waste of time. In order to establish a continuing contact between the house officer and the psychiatrist, the training of house officers ought to evolve in the direction of setting aside a certain period of time each week to be used for psychiatric supervision.

From the discussion so far, the reader may feel that an important element in this case has been overlooked, that is, the problem of countertransference between the house officer and the patient. The problem was obviously present and did contribute to the initial difficulties that were encountered. However, in teaching nonpsychiatrists there is often a tendency to put too much emphasis on problems of countertransference, and the discussion of this first case has purposely focused on conceptual problems. Still, problems of countertransference certainly cannot be ignored, and the second case to be presented illustrates some of these problems.

A word should be said about these first two cases. Both are rather dramatic. For that reason they are useful for presentation not only because they are interesting, but also because they highlight certain aspects of the kind of teaching under discussion. By themselves, however, the more striking cases give a misleading picture of how this teaching proceeds. The day-by-day teaching is routine and rather uneventful, and the cases presented here stand out just because they are exceptionally vivid illustrations of certain principles.

The house officer involved in the second case replied in a surprising manner when the psychiatrist first introduced himself and explained his activities on the ward. The house officer said flatly that he did not want to learn anything about the patient's feelings. At the time the psychiatrist had no idea why the house officer adopted that attitude, so he contented himself with accepting these remarks in an affable manner. It soon became apparent that the house officer's attitude proceeded not from deep hostility to psychiatry, but rather from the fact that he felt quite unsure of himself. To others, it was clear that he was a bright and talented person, but he had difficulty accepting that view of himself. He liked to clown and poke fun at himself. If anyone challenged his professional judgment he was apt to "shoot from the hip," to come back at the person with the first thought that crossed his mind rather than to wait and give a well considered answer. Such responses sometimes had the effect of making it appear that he was in the wrong even when his judgment was right. But it was apparent to most of his coworkers that if one waited him out, he would recover fairly quickly and behave in a reasonable way. In the course of a conversation, a second house officer mentioned that an important male member of the first house officer's family was an eminent professor who had the reputation of possessing truly encyclopedic knowledge of his field as well as a flair for displaying that knowledge prominently.

The psychiatrist assumed that the first house officer really wanted to learn about the feelings of his patients in spite of his disclaimer and looked about for a good teaching case. One soon presented itself in the person of Mr. A., a bearded, 68-year-old Jewish patriarch who was convalescing from a stroke. He had recovered in large part the use of his paralyzed arm and leg, but he was refusing to eat and in spite of intravenous feedings was steadily losing weight. He was bitter and depressed, but after some conversation he was able to express his anger at his children and at the hospital personnel, who, he said, considered him "as good as dead" and consequently neglected him. He described himself as a man of learning whose opinions and prerogatives had been respected in former times by his friends and family, a situation which he contrasted bitterly with his present state, lying in bed, ill and used up. He was hurt most by the fact that his children visited him infrequently. With strong feeling in his voice, he said, "What is the sense of living if nobody cares any more?"

When Mr. A.'s case was discussed with the house officer, it was apparent that he was carrying a crushing burden of guilt over the patient. He felt he was responsible for Mr. A.'s failure to improve, and as a consequence he felt acutely uncomfortable in the patient's presence and tried to make his visits as brief and infrequent as possible. The psychiatrist and the house officer discussed in a general way the extent of a physician's responsibility, and it was suggested to the house officer that he try to understand the patient's feelings with the same objective but sympathetic attitude he displayed when he investigated the patient's organic illness. This, the house officer said, was impossible for him to do. He said that if Mr. A. died of another stroke, he would not feel guilty because that lay beyond his responsibility, but while Mr. A. continued to waste away he felt guilty because it was his duty to persuade his patient to eat. During his rounds, the patient would criticize him and then he in turn would get angry and scold the patient. The patient would refuse to eat and the doctor would feel helpless and frustrated.

The psychiatrist asked the house officer if he thought it possible that the patient, without being aware of it, *wanted* doctors to feel helpless and guilty, and that the reasons for this desire arose primarily from Mr. A.'s previous experiences. As they reviewed the patient's attitude toward his family and his illness, the house officer was able to formulate for himself the cause of Mr. A.'s refusal to eat. He saw that the patient was angry at his family because he felt neglected and carried his anger over to the doctors and other hospital personnel. He saw that the patient's refusal to eat was partly the result of his depression and partly an attempt to get back at his family and the doctors in a peevish, self-punitive way. As the discussion continued, the house officer was able to formulate an effective way to deal with this problem. He decided that Mr. A.'s family should be encouraged to visit the patient more frequently and that the medical staff should make a special effort to show their respect for Mr. A. and their desire to help him recover.

An interview was arranged with two of Mr. A.'s sons, who had been mildly tyrannized by him for many years. Mixed with their fondness for their father they felt a certain resentment toward him for his irascible ways. They said that since his stroke he had become impossible to deal with. He had accused his family of neglecting him and told them that if they were so ungrateful they shouldn't bother to visit him at all. They had responded by making their visits less frequent. This response apparently was based in part on angry retaliation and in part on the feeling that their visits only seemed to make their father worse, so that it seemed to them just as well to visit less often. It was explained to the sons that their father's behavior was caused by his feeling that he was a used-up invalid whom no one could respect. The suggestion was made that now was the time to redouble the amount of affection and respect they showed him. The sons agreed with this analysis, and one of them remarked that such behavior was just like their father. In the past, when anyone in the family crossed him, he would have an outburst of temper and sulkiness. Oftentimes the family had had to consult with one another to see who had offended him, so that the culprit could go and make proper apologies.

The patient's family were conscientious about increasing the number of their visits. They divided the day up into shifts, and since the family was large, the patient had visitors for the greater part of the day.

The house officer made a practice of visiting the patient for ten minutes each morning and each afternoon. During this time he endured the patient's criticisms, encouraged him to eat, and praised his efforts at eating and at using his paralyzed side. He also listened to the patient's stories and found to his surprise that the patient was a learned and interesting old man, whose bitterness was an ineffectual response to the hurt of feeling himself abandoned. The patient responded rapidly to these measures, and in a short time the problem of his not eating disappeared.

This result was very satisfying, but the most striking outcome of the case was a remark made by the house officer several weeks later, when he was approaching the end of his rotation on the ward. Looking back on this case, he commented that his part in it had been the most important experience he had had during his training. Clearly, that is saying too much; it is perhaps another example of his tendency to state things in the most dramatic way; but at the same time there is some truth in his remark. As a result of this experience, the house officer handled his patients with more confidence, and at least the possibility opened up that in his new position as a doctor he might be stimulated to evolve new methods of handling situations rather than automatically falling back on the old methods which had serious disadvantages for him.

The case of Mr. A. illustrates the collapse and re-establishment of an emotional relationship between the doctor and his patient. The patient, frightened by the illness which had struck him down, feared that his family and his doctors might desert him. This anticipation led him to attack the very people on whom he depended for love and care. The doctor, recoiling under this barrage of anger, which touched on certain sensitivities of his own, found it too painful to maintain an emotional contact with the patient and began to withdraw from him. This withdrawal had dire consequences, since it seemed to the patient that it confirmed his fear of desertion. He then began to destroy himself in order to punish the doctor for faithlessness. The situation had reached the point where the patient's successful recovery depended on the doctor's ability to re-establish an emotional relationship with him. The doctor had to come back into contact with the patient's hatred and self-destructive feelings. He could neither flee from those feelings nor respond to them with counter-aggression.

In the event, the house officer solved his problem, with the excellent results which have been described, using the classical psychiatric approach to such a situation. He took the first step toward a solution when he was able to describe his relationship with the patient. Actually, the simple act of describing his relationship had the effect of changing it. When the ego is pointedly called in to observe certain feelings, one's attitude toward these feelings is altered in profound and subtle ways. Once the house officer had described his difficulties with Mr. A., it became much more difficult for him to relapse into his familiar, automatic response of angrily avoiding Mr. A. as an impossible old crank. By discussing the situation, he acquired a greater degree of detachment and a greater readiness to see the patient's behavior as a problem which should be examined and understood.

Aided by this understanding and detachment, he began as the next step to re-establish his emotional relationship with the patient. As he did so, it became clearer that the patient's rage had little connection with him as a person, but rather was directed toward persons and situations in the patient's past. His increased awareness made it easier for the doctor to establish an attitude of tolerant neutrality and sympathetic understanding, which in turn reassured the patient that his anger would not drive the doctor away nor injure him. Having tested out the situation and found that it was safe, the patient became much less frightened. As a consequence, he did not need to be so angry and he became a more tractable patient.

The learning experience was important for both patient and doctor. The patient learned that he need not automatically assume his habitual stance of defensive aggression. He found that he could risk exposing some of his underlying feelings for he could count on the doctor to understand his needs and to respond to them in an appropriate and helpful manner.

The doctor learned the value of a sympathetic and emotionally neutral attitude in approaching a patient. Taking such an attitude permitted him to circumvent Mr. A.'s defensive hostility and come face to face with the underlying fear of being abandoned which provoked it. He had the new experience of following Freud's method and thus being able to catch a direct glimpse of the unconscious forces hidden behind the manifest behavior. He was personally involved in dramatic demonstration of the fundamental psychiatric premise that behavior is the end product of a complex process in which unconscious impulses play a major role. To the extent that he could apprehend the unconscious impulses at work in this particular patient, he could realize that his own response of guilt and anger made no sense whatsoever. Understanding that, he could perceive the correct way to deal with the patient: it became easy and natural to respond by enduring the patient's scoldings while acting in a manner that reassured him that his fears were groundless. Simultaneously, the patient began to sense that his physicians understood some of the deeper meanings of the painful interactions in which he found himself embroiled. Even though the patient himself could not understand these interactions, his feeling that his physicians understood gave him confidence in them and enabled him to tolerate tactful intervention on their part. The importance of this reciprocal learning experience that can go on between the doctor and his patient has not received the emphasis it deserves. For any medical patient, whatever the state of his emotional health, it is the most reassuring experience that the doctor can provide.

In everyday practice, the doctor and the patient are, to a greater or lesser extent, deprived of the benefits of this learning experience. Illness, in addition to creating reality problems, usually puts heavy pressure on the patient's unresolved unconscious conflicts. In Mr. A.'s case, for example, illness heightened the patient's fear of being unworthy of love and of being abandoned. Under pressure, a patient will often be compelled to utilize his customary defenses in ways less flexible and frequently less successful than usual. When he turns to his physician for medical help, he anticipates that he will also be helped with his emotional problems. In order to help, the physician must create an atmosphere of sympathetic understanding and tolerant neutrality which will encourage the patient to expose his unconscious conflicts and defenses. Ordinarily, the physician will not clarify these conflicts and defenses for the patient, but he must have a clear understanding of them in his own mind. This understanding will enable the physician to respond appropriately and to give the patient the feeling that the physician has understood what is disturbing him.

All too often, however, the sympathetic atmosphere is not set up and the understanding is not achieved. As a result, many a patient feels that his doctor doesn't understand him, doesn't listen to him, doesn't answer his questions, doesn't allay his concern, doesn't explain what's going on, or is unavailable when a crisis arises. If a careful poll were taken, most conscientious physicians would be astounded to find how many of their patients had the feeling that their doctor just wasn't available when they needed him. In most cases, these feelings are not based on fact. They are based on the patient's dimly recognized perception that somehow, between his own reluctance to talk and the doctor's unwillingness to listen, he has been prevented from airing certain nameless worries which are troubling him. Of course, most patients have enough emotional health to endure this extra burden without excessive difficulty. Only an unusual patient, like Mr. A., will break down under this strain. But it is clear that if the physician fails to establish the atmosphere that will encourage the patient to reveal pressing unconscious feelings, he misses a golden opportunity to reassure the patient, to increase the patient's confidence in the physician, and to have the satisfaction of helping the patient through a difficult period.

From this point of view, Mr. A.'s case represents one of a series of minor crises that recur frequently during a physician's development. The doctor in this case had to decide whether he would encourage the patient to reveal his unconscious conflicts and defenses so that the doctor could help him find a way to deal with them, or, on the other hand, whether he would decline to recognize the patient's feelings and force him to cope with them as best he could without outside help. Every young physician faces this choice every day of his career. The cumulative weight of his responses to this choice will push him in one direction or the other: he may find himself becoming increasingly at ease in perceiving patients' unconscious thoughts and feelings, or he may find himself adopting one of the stereotyped bedside manners that are designed to spare the physician anxiety by limiting communication between the patient and the doctor.

It is interesting to observe that if the physician cuts himself off from the patient's feelings, the loss to the physician is far greater than the loss to the patient. In the case of Mr. A., we can see that a doctor who did not develop a method of encouraging Mr. A. to express his deeper feelings might easily dismiss him as an unpleasant old man who had decided to be impossible. But, as we have seen, behind this patient's behavior was concealed a fascinating scientific problem. There are standard methods of elucidating this problem, and there are lessons to be learned that are applicable to many other cases. If the physician dismisses this patient as a crock, it means that in order to spare himself discomfort he has decided to cease making meaningful observations of the patient's feelings. It means that in a difficult area of medical science he has chosen to abandon rational methods and to permit himself to be guided by habit and prejudice. Unfortunately, as medicine is being taught today, many house officers fall into this erroneous position without realizing its implications.

As the foregoing discussion has stressed, the ideal attitude for the physician to take is to encourage the patient to reveal his deeper feelings by conveying the impression that the doctor will respond in an understanding and helpful manner. The technique cannot be learned in the same way that one learns to hear a cardiac murmur. To establish a constructive relationship with a patient, a doctor must make use of certain basic elements in his own personality. Since these elements are more or less fixed, teaching is unlikely to change or influence them directly; but although this limitation must be borne in mind, there is a great deal about the technique that can be taught to house officers. In fact, it was surprising to find during this study that in general it is easier to influence a house officer's attitude toward his patients than it is to teach him psychiatric concepts. One explanation may be that when a psychiatrist interviews a patient in order to demonstrate the establishment of this sort of relationship, the complex and subtle components of the relationship materialize in a manner which promotes sudden recognition and comprehension. Apparently, there is no comparable method by which psychiatric concepts can readily be made manifest. These underlying concepts, which are the bones of our understanding, are difficult to demonstrate. We have no X ray which will permit us to see them through the overlying mass of data in a flash of understanding. The concepts and their interrelations can be understood only after countless laborious dissections, only after one has observed and thought through many clinical events.

There is, of course, considerable experience in supervising psychiatric residents in the technique of forming a relationship that encourages the patient to reveal his unconscious thoughts. It is not clear, however, how appropriate the methods which have been useful in this area of teaching will be in the task of teaching house officers in the setting of a medical ward. Since there is as yet no consensus on this point, it may be well to review in detail the teaching methods which were employed in the case of Mr. A. While this case is special in certain ways, it is important to see if any general principles are discernible.

The main point to be emphasized is that an extended period of preparation was necessary before the teaching could become effective. When the house officer first came on the ward, he and the psychiatrist had many friendly, informal chats together. These chats permitted them to get to know and trust one another. They also allowed the psychiatrist to begin to understand the house officer. It was immediately apparent that his saying he "had no interest in learning about patients' feelings" was an outrageous bit of humbug; it was more nearly true that he was excessively concerned about patients' feelings. The psychiatrist was also able to observe the conditions under which the house officer learned most readily: since he had a habit of doubting his own judgment, it was important to encourage him to evolve an idea on his own, with the teacher's contribution limited to suggestion and guidance. When he had reached a worthwhile conclusion, he needed support to keep him from disparaging and discarding it.

Another important part of the preparatory process was that the house officer had had an opportunity of observing the contribution that psychiatric knowledge can make to the management of medical patients. From day to day, as various problems arose on the ward, he was able to see that psychiatry is not irrelevant to the practice of internal medicine but rather that it has many practical and useful suggestions to offer the internist.

He had also had an opportunity to observe at first hand the attitude that a psychiatrist takes toward a patient's feelings. He had seen that, in an atmosphere of tolerance and sympathetic understanding, the patient can be comfortable while discussing his feelings and revealing what sort of person he really is. The house officer had had a chance to observe the variety of ways in which this relationship is useful to the patient and to the doctor in their combined effort to help the patient deal with his illness.

With these experiences in the background, the psychiatrist was gradually able to introduce the idea that physicians have varied feelings toward their patients. It was pointed out, in a general way, that these feelings affect the way a doctor treats a patient. By degrees, the psychiatrist was able to make the discussion more specific and to show the house officer that *he* had certain feelings about certain patients which affected the way *he* treated these patients. As matters went along, the psychiatrist tried hard not to push the house officer, but to give him the feeling that the services of a psychiatric consultant were at his disposal. The house officer might use them as much or as little as he chose. The psychiatrist also encouraged the house officer to feel that he could talk freely about his feelings toward patients with confidence that he would meet with a tolerant and helpful response. The fulfillment of this careful preparatory work came when he was able to tell the psychiatrist about his anger and guilt and his need to avoid this particular patient. Here was a decisive moment in this case, a step which made the later successful treatment possible. It represented an unusual exposure of feelings that are ordinarily well guarded, and would not have been possible unless the preparatory process had been successful.

This preparatory process will be familiar to all psychotherapists. It resembles the establishment of a therapeutic alliance. In the case under discussion, however, it was an alliance in a much attenuated form. It appears that the most effective teaching of medical psychology to house officers will require the development of this kind of attenuated therapeutic alliance between the psychiatric teacher and the house officer, especially when the teaching involves the house officer's countertransference feelings.

In spite of his disclaimer, this particular house officer clearly wanted help in dealing with his patients and welcomed the help that was offered. Most house officers would be more chary of accepting help from a psychiatrist and few would be ready to accept so much help. In teaching these other house officers, it is just as necessary to develop a therapeutic alliance, but it is technically a far more difficult problem.

An important source of the difficulty apparently lies in certain attitudes which are characteristic of young house officers. It is illuminating to compare students at different stages of their medical training and to note how they react to psychiatric teaching. Speaking generally, second-year students respond most eagerly and derive the most profit from psychiatric teaching. Third-year students are less accessible to psychiatric teaching and fourth-year students still less, while the nadir of responsiveness is reached during internship. After that period, recovery sets in, and most (but certainly not all) house officers and young physicians seem progressively easier to teach as they advance in their training. But a shocking change occurs between the beginning of medical school and internship. The medical students who have been relatively ready to use psychiatric insights in their dealings with their patients become transformed into interns who seem rigid and far less concerned about their patients' feelings. The question that inevitably arises as to how they have managed to forget so much in a few years may be answered in the following way.

The medical student allows himself to make a tentative identification with the psychiatric teacher. He assumes easily, perhaps even glibly, the vocabulary, techniques, and modes of thought peculiar to psychiatry. At the same time, he is not in a position to assume responsibility for their effectiveness. The educational process requires that he make many of these tentative identifications with his various teachers, and at some point integrate them into a professional identity of his own. The house officer sees himself in quite a different position. To a certain extent, he feels that what has gone before is make-believe, but that now he faces a test which will reveal whether or not he has the inner qualities which will enable him to become a good physician. He feels that responsibility for his patients rests heavily on himself. It becomes increasingly difficult to act like a student and passively accept substantial amounts of help from his teachers. It is important for him to demonstrate (mostly to himself) that, on his own, he will be able to treat his patients correctly. As a result, he sharply narrows the focus of his interest to the central ideas of making sure that he misses no important diagnosis and omits no life-saving treatment. He recoils from ideas which seem in any way irrelevant to these goals, or which seem unproved to him or which are not sufficiently concrete. In the course of this process, most of psychiatry is dismissed as nebulous, speculative stuff which is not fit intellectual fare for a practical man who wants action and not just talk.

While it is true that the house officer exaggerates the amount of responsibility that he actually has, still this change in attitude represents, at least in part, a healthy, forward step in his growth as a physician. That the more practical, skeptical attitude which the house officer assumes is better suited for dealing with the prickly, unyielding facts of clinical practice should not, however, obscure the fact that his reaction against psychological teaching is far too extreme. While it is clear that the bath water must be thrown out, is there no way to avoid discarding the baby?

These observations should warn us that there is a serious flaw in the process of educating physicians. We can hardly remain content with an educational system which demands that students in the course of their progress should abandon some of the most valuable parts of their learning experience. It is important to emphasize that the problem lies in the system and not in the individual personalities of the students, a fact that is apparent to anyone who has seen perceptive, psychologically attuned students who become dismally unresponsive as interns but who can successfully retrieve their perceptiveness as they go on to become physicians or even sometimes to become psychiatrists.

The first two cases dwelled most heavily on the problems of understanding psychological concepts and on the technique of establishing a therapeutic alliance. While these considerations are always of fundamental importance, the psychiatric teacher ordinarily does not present them to the house officers as explicit issues. Instead, as the third case will illustrate, the emphasis is placed on a rather more elementary concern of psychiatric teaching, the relationship between psychological factors and physical illness.

The patient, Mr. B., is an insurance adjuster, single and in his 30's, who was admitted to the hospital because of a second episode of bleeding from a peptic ulcer. The psychiatrist was asked to see him because he had been ignoring his diet and medications while at home. There had been some discussion of surgery for this patient, but it was decided that he should have one more try on a medical regimen. The feeling was that eventually he would come to surgery. When the psychiatrist saw him, Mr. B. was sitting in bed with his pajama top unbuttoned to reveal a hairy chest. His manner was one of studied nonchalance, and there was nothing spontaneous about either his gestures or his posture. He seemed to be continually striking poses which could have come directly from the pages of a physical culture magazine. When he adjusted his body carefully from one pose to the next, the psychiatrist half expected to hear his muscles ripple. From time to time, he would rub a part of his body with a gesture that was almost a caress. He had a handsome tan, and it was not surprising to learn that he was an L Street Brownie[1] and an amateur weight-lifter. While Mr. B. was talking about these activities, the psychiatrist commented that Mr. B. was a man who was very proud of his physicial condition. This remark established rapport between them and Mr. B. continued at some length to describe his body-building activities. Later in the interview, the psychiatrist asked him why he found it so difficult to stick to the medical regimen. He said that he palled around with two or three good buddies. They went to sporting events and stock car races. They had a favorite bar where they hung out. At all these places they'd drink beer and eat pizza. He didn't want to spoil everybody else's fun by not going along with the crowd.

When he was asked if his buddies knew that he had an ulcer, he said he'd never bothered to tell them. It seemed silly for a big strong guy like him to be having stomach trouble. Besides he wouldn't want anyone to think he was a complainer. His mother had indigestion. Every night after supper she would lie down on the sofa with a bellyache. The family was disgusted because they thought she was putting on.

The psychiatrist said that Mr. B. had done such a fine job of getting himself into good condition that it was a shame he neglected something as important as his stomach. He went on to say that the doctors' job is to help people to get into good physicial condition. They admire anybody who can do that, although there aren't many who ever get into really excellent condition. The psychiatrist said that here Mr. B. had done unusually well, but it was disappointing that he was ignoring his stomach, since that might undermine all the rest. Mr. B. seemed to be listening carefully, so the psychiatrist went on to ask if his buddies were weightlifters too. He said, "Oh, yes, they'd go down to the gym to work out or go over to one another's houses and fool around with the weights." The

---

[1] For readers unfamiliar with local Boston customs, the Public Bath House is located on L Street. The Brownies are so called because they pride themselves on bathing throughout the year and thus have a glowing tan even during the frigid Boston winter. In passing, it is interesting to note that since they bathe nude, this tan covers their entire body and has misled more than one physician into believing that he had discovered a case of Addison's disease.

psychiatrist commented that his buddies probably paid a lot of attention to keeping in shape and were careful to protect their health. They probably would feel badly if they found out that they had caused him to harm his health. This suggestion was too much for Mr. B. to accept at that moment; he looked at the psychiatrist in surprise.

The discussion turned to what he might eat when he went out with his buddies. He considered the possibility that he might eat a Swiss cheese sandwich, or just eat nothing instead of pizza, and that he might drink coffee with a lot of milk rather than beer, but he looked doubtful about these ideas. When he was asked about dates, he said that he had broken up with a girl several years before. He had gone with her for five or six years but she had started to get bossy so they had a fight. He was sorry to break up with her. He was kind of lonesome and if he happened to meet the right girl he would like to get married. At present, he was only dating once in a while. After his last disappointment, he didn't want to get too involved with a girl.

Since the psychiatrist thought that the patient would eventually come to surgery in spite of efforts to avoid it, he decided to introduce gently the idea of a possible operation. The psychiatrist said that doctors certainly preferred that people did not have operations if they could be avoided. The doctors would do everything they could to help him stay in good health so that he wouldn't need an operation, and they hoped he would co-operate. Mr. B. became visibly anxious when the possibility of an operation was mentioned. He began to ask many questions about it. The discussion was kept brief, and the emphasis was on the point that for the present they would concentrate on making sure that he received the best possible medical care. If further difficulties arose in the future, they would review the situation with the patient, and together they could decide what treatment would be best for him.

When the interview was over, the house officers had a lively discussion about the patient, and it was clear that they had a good understanding of his personality. From his poses, his self-caresses, and his comments about himself, they saw that he had an enormous emotional investment in his own body. They understood that his life was dedicated to developing a perfect body. He and his buddies formed a little society devoted to body-building and to such masculine pursuits as stock car races and sporting events. It was essential to him to have the admiration and esteem of these buddies. The house officers could understand that in this masculine Garden of Eden women were troublesome creatures. He had broken up with his girl after a long, drawn out engagement and had dated infrequently since then. More significantly, he described his mother as weak, complaining, malingering, despicable and sick. Unhappily, the patient suffered from stomach trouble, the same sickness that his mother had. The house officers realized that it would probably be impossible for Mr. B. to admit to his buddies that he had this feminine disease. They understood what the psychiatrist had attempted to do during the interview and saw that he had appealed to this man's great pride in his physique to motivate him to take proper care of his ulcer. It was explained to them that this maneuver is what Grete and Edward Bibring refer to as manipulation— that is, an attempt to help a patient meet a crisis by bolstering his customary methods of dealing with situations (E. Bibring, 1954; G. L. Bibring, 1956). They discussed whether the doctors' admiration for him for following the medical regimen might possibly restore some of the self-esteem he feared to lose by confessing that he had an ulcer. They recognized the unsuccessful attempt to open up the idea that his buddies might share his fear of being imperfect and might view his illness with sympathy rather than contempt. The house officers were encouraged to keep working on these issues while the patient was in the hospital. They discussed the point that if he came to surgery, as seemed likely, he would have considerable anxiety about the operation. It would place a severe burden on this man to have his body's integrity violated, to sacrifice part of a vital organ, and to be left with a disfiguring scar. They ended with a discussion of latent homosexuality which was linked to the patient's low opinion of women. The psychiatrist was pleased when an intern made the insightful comment that this patient would do poorly with a woman physician, and that they should be prepared for that problem if he were readmitted.

A revealing episode occurred when the group returned to the ward after their discussion. The assistant resident had missed both the interview and the discussion, but when he returned, the psychiatrist began to relate to him the interview with the patient as it had occurred. The rest of the group, who were still carrying on their discussion of the case, broke in with animated remarks to amplify what the psychiatrist was saying. As time went on, the assistant resident became more and more distressed. He could understand the words that were being said, but they conveyed no meaning to him. Here again is a vivid illustration of the difficulties caused by the conceptual gap between psychiatry and medicine. The assistant resident, on his side, was struggling to understand, and the psychiatrist, on the other side, was struggling to explain, but they were totally unable to communicate. If the assistant resident had been a psychiatrist, a few comments about the patient's body narcissism and past history would have given him a firm grasp of the situation. This incident underlines the importance of the medium which is used to convey psychological information to nonpsychiatrists. It suggests that practically no information can be transmitted by a written consultation or verbal communication between the psychiatrist and the medical doctor. Information can only be conveyed by interviewing the patient in the presence of the medical doctor.

To examine this premise in greater detail, we may ask why it was that the group that participated in the interview acquired a vivid appreciation of the patient's personality, while the assistant resident understood nothing. With both, the same words were used to describe the patient. In talking to the assistant resident, the psychiatrist tried to reproduce almost word for word the discussion which had just finished. It is clear that the interview had provided a background which permitted these words to acquire meaning. To someone who had missed the interview, the words were meaningless.

When we examine the interview, several facets are worthy of attention. The first is that in the interview the psychiatrist's first few steps were a process of establishing an atmosphere in which the patient would feel comfortable while talking about his intimate feelings. The patient began to see that the interviewer would not criticize or laugh at his feelings but would treat them with the utmost tact and respect. He began to accept the idea that the interviewer needed to understand his feelings so that he could help the patient to deal with the difficulties arising from his illness. The effect of this procedure was to forestall the patient's developing pernicious defensive attitudes directed toward his physician. In the cases discussed earlier of Mr. M. and Mr. A., we saw that each of these patients quickly began to involve the physician in his emotional problems. Both patients saw their physicians as antagonists in the psychological conflict which was harassing them. As a result, the physician was unable to establish himself as a neutral figure and was blocked in his attempt to help the patient deal with his difficulties. With the third patient, Mr. B., however, the initial interview set up an atmosphere in which the patient and the doctor could work together in their attempt to find a solution to the patient's problems, undisturbed by transference reactions. This atmosphere is unfamiliar to house officers. Those who observed the interview could see it evolve and could sense the new opportunities which it opened up. To them, it made sense to say such things as "Praise this patient for sticking to the medical regimen and perhaps it will compensate him for the humiliation of admitting he has an ulcer." They had seen the psychiatrist use this approach with the patient and, in the setting of the limited therapeutic alliance which had been established, they had seen it have some effect. To someone who had not observed the interview, on the other hand, it might well seem doubtful that such an approach could have any effect whatsoever.

The second point to observe about this interview is the clear way in which the patient displayed his inner feelings. He posed, flexed his muscles, caressed himself, and talked with great feeling about body building. It was apparent to everyone present that this man had an enormous investment in his own body and that this was indisputably the strongest emotional force in his life. To comprehend it, one did not require an understanding of psychiatric theory, one needed only a sound pair of eyes and ears. To those who observed the interview, it immediately made sense that this man would rather endanger his health than humiliate himself by admitting to his buddies that his body had a defect, especially one that he saw as womanish. To someone who had not seen the interview and who was unfamiliar with dynamic psychiatry, this proposition might seem incredible. The interview thus bridged the conceptual gap between the house officers and the psychiatrist. The patient revealed his inner feelings so clearly that they were apparent even to those who were unfamiliar with psychiatric concepts.

Third, the interview established a clear connection between the patient's psychological make-up and his medical illness. Those who sensed the strength of this man's body narcissism realized that it was not merely a peripheral oddity that might be of interest to a psychiatrist. They saw that it was a compelling emotional force that would probably defeat any attempt at a cure.

In summary, the interview with Mr. B. demonstrated the effectiveness of a therapeutic alliance, it spelled out the dynamic forces in the patient's personality with unmistakable clarity, and it showed how those forces were relevant to the medical situation. The earlier discussions of Mr. M. and Mr. A. have dealt with the first two points; let us now turn our attention to the third point.

In Mr. B.'s case, the assistant resident had great difficulty in understanding that this patient's intense narcissism had important implications for his medical treatment. In the interview, it was easy to demonstrate these implications, but having missed this convincing demonstration, the assistant resident remained skeptical that the patient's narcissistic feelings could have an important effect on his treatment. His attitude is one which is widespread among house officers and among medical doctors in general.

They have great difficulty in understanding in what way a patient's psychological make-up is relevant to his medical illness.

Unfortunately, it is not always recognized that this problem of understanding exists. For a number of years, many of the most thoughtful and
progressive physicians in both medicine and psychiatry have emphasized
the importance of integrating the two fields. So strong has been the feeling that integration would be worthwhile that we may have convinced
ourselves that we have made much more progress in that direction than
has actually occurred. The physicist Percy Bridgman made the comment
that in order to understand what a concept means to a scientist, one must
ignore what he *says* about it and observe how he *uses* it. If we examine
the patients' medical charts, we can reach some understanding of how
medical doctors use psychological concepts and thus, by inference, what
these concepts mean to them.

Medical charts are the raw material and basic stuff of which clinical
medicine is composed. They are the equivalent of the scientific protocols
or the experimenter's notebooks in other branches of science. If a patient
enters the hospital with cardiac failure, certain observations are recorded
which establish that diagnosis. Then digitalis and other forms of treatment are given, and certain observations are recorded to indicate that
the cardiac failure is cured. The medical chart thus becomes the keystone
of the scientific method as it is utilized in clinical medicine. By referring
to this record of observations and procedures, medicine checks and con-
firms its hypotheses, students observe and become convinced of the correctness of medical precepts, and research workers perceive the direction in
which further advances must be made. The startling fact is that medical
doctors seldom record on a chart any observations of psychological events.
In the three cases discussed in this chapter, the most important events
that occurred were psychological events. The medical problems and the
psychological problems were so intertwined that neither could be solved
without the others; yet in the charts, the house officers typically described
the medical events fully but made no mention of the psychological events.

Surely no science can progress if it systematically excludes from its basic
record one half of the relevant data. The medical chart of today offers
convincing evidence that the tradition of medicine is strongly antagonistic
to treating psychological data in the systematic, scientific manner that
is accorded to physiological data. The ideal of contemporary medicine
should be to eliminate this illogical distinction. The rational, critical
method used by medical doctors to deal with physiological data should be
extended to include psychological data. At the present moment, un-

fortunately, this goal is completely out of sight. Medical doctors lack a conceptual system that would enable them to observe and appreciate psychological events. In most cases they lack the skill to set up a therapeutic alliance which would permit them to obtain information from their patients and then to use that information to influence their patients in a psychologically effective manner. And last, the tradition of medicine operates to preserve an arbitrary and obstructive distinction between psychological and physiological events.

These are three of the important problems encountered when teaching medical house officers about the psychological aspects of illness. At present, the psychiatrist's teaching efforts are concentrated mainly on dealing with the third of these problems: the emphasis is on demonstrating that the patient's feelings play an important part in his illness. The first two problems are not dealt with directly, but are avoided and rendered inoperative, as the case of Mr. B. clearly illustrates. Here the psychiatrist set up a therapeutic alliance with the patient which in part could be successfully transferred to the house officer in charge of the case. The psychiatrist was fortunate to find a patient who described his feelings so clearly that they could be understood by observers who were unfamiliar with psychiatric concepts. Having established an alliance and elicited those feelings, he could then demonstrate to the other physicians that the feelings were highly relevant to the patient's medical problem.

Physicians need to have demonstrated to them repeatedly that a patient's emotional state is always relevant to the rest of the medical situation. Unfortunately, demonstration by itself is insufficient for genuine understanding. In fact, interviews such as the one betweten the psychiatrist and Mr. B. can even be deceptive to the observer. It looks so easy. Two people sit down together and, before long, they are talking about the patient's intimate feelings and the patient is placidly accepting suggestions that touch him in sensitive areas. That can happen only, of course, because the interviewer has set up a therapeutic alliance and has understood the deeper psychological implications of what the patient is saying, but an observer is apt to overlook these prerequisites. Such an interview is useful for demonstrating that psychiatry is a relevant part of medicine, but as a learning experience, it lacks roots. Before a house officer could conduct a similar interview, he would need to know how to set up a therapeutic alliance and he would need to understand thoroughly the basic psychological concepts.

Providing house officers with competence in both these areas should be the long-range goal of psychiatric teaching in general hospitals. House

officers should become proficient interviewers who are able to set up therapeutic alliances with their patients. They should also have sufficient
comprehension of basic psychiatric principles so that they are able to
understand the unconscious forces at work within their patients. Experience to date makes it appear that considerable progress can be made in
teaching techniques of interviewing to house officers. On the other hand,
teaching them the conceptual framework which underlies psychiatry remains a formidable problem for which our present methods of teaching
offer no adequate solution.

# Teaching Dynamic - Psychological Principles and Their Application to General Medical Care

CECIL MUSHATT, M.D.

RICHARD E. CUTLER, M.D.

HENRY G. ALTMAN, M.D.

THIS CONTRIBUTION IS intended as a report on the teaching of psychoanalytic principles and their application to general medical care in three areas of the overall psychiatric teaching program for nonpsychiatric medical staff at the Beth Israel Hospital. Courses were given to (1) allergists in the Allergy Clinic, (2) general practitioners working in the General Medical Outpatient Clinic, and (3) house officers in the General Medical Outpatient Clinic. The course for allergists was conducted from 1950-1953, and that for the house officers has been conducted continuously since 1956. The course for general practitioners began in 1959, and has been maintained to date. Impressions and conclusions to be reported here have also been derived from observations made in the course of less intensive teaching of staff in the Endocrine and Prenatal Clinics.

The aims of these courses have been (1) to study the value and effects of efforts to help nonpsychiatric medical staff to incorporate the use of

We are greatly indebted to Dr. Grete Bibring, Dr. Herrman L. Blumgart, Dr. Harry Derow and the United States Public Health Service for encouragement and help in pursuing these studies. We are particularly grateful to the Commonwealth Fund for interest and support in undertaking this work in its early phases. We appreciate the cooperation of all the physicians who participated in the courses. Acknowledgment is also due to Miss Dorothy Bernstein, R. N., Nursing Supervisor of Ambulatory Services, and to Miss Evelyn Rosen, R. N., formerly Nursing Supervisor of the Outpatient Department for facilitating our work in the various clinics at the Beth Israel Hospital.

psychological principles into their over-all study and treatment of their patients, (2) to test out a particular method of teaching, and (3) to study the problems involved both for student and teacher in pressing for such integration of psychological principles into the practice of medicine. In this last respect, we were especially concerned with the study of the determinants of the universally experienced negative, and often highly emotional, attitude of a large segment of medical, surgical, and obstetrical staff in general hospitals toward the use of psychological concepts as an additional significant and rational approach to medical care. Consideration of this phenomenon of resistance, as well as the method of teaching chosen in order to overcome it, will receive special emphasis here.

### General Orientation and Theoretical Approach

As in the rest of the program at the Beth Israel Hospital, our aim in teaching has been to try to help nonpsychiatrists to acquire sufficient knowledge which would enable them to provide psychological management of a limited nature in their routine practice. The goals of treatment are to bring about remission of physical or psychiatric symptoms, to speed up convalescence, to help patients tolerate medical and surgical procedures more easily, to make medical and surgical management more effective, and to make symptoms more tolerable. Essentially, the aim in such treatment is to reduce the intensity of conflict or to facilitate repression of it and to remove, temporarily at least, the necessity for symptoms so that the patient can function more effectively, though within the relative limitations of his personality. It has been found that such results can be achieved very frequently with only limited knowledge and psychological procedures, both in the case of physical illness with emotional components and in emotional illness. Often improvement has been maintained for prolonged periods. Ambitious goals, such as aiming at cure in the sense of reorganizing the individual emotionally with the undoing, for instance, of his susceptibility to reaction in physical terms, in the majority of cases are either not necessary or are impractical as far as routine practice by nonpsychiatric physicians is concerned.

Our orientation in regard to the subject matter and principles to be taught was determined by early exploratory discussions with the allergists. The latter objected strenuously to an approach which they would consider to be a presentation of general psychiatry. They were afraid that by a course with such an orientation, they would feel too much pressure to be responsible for all forms of psychiatric illness. Such responsibility, they felt, could be undertaken only by specialization in psychiatry. It is pertinent to remark here on the fact that this is a source of fear in many physicians who undertake limited training in psychiatry under the program of assistance to general practitioners offered by the United States Public Health Service. Such a fear may be responsible in part for the fact that increasing numbers of such physicians are abandoning general practice to undertake the long-term training for specialization in psychiatry. In this way, the purposes of the program are being defeated.

The allergists made it clear that it would be much more acceptable to them to be addressed primarily in terms of a psychological approach to people with physical illness. As a result, the initial focus in our courses has been on the psychosomatic concept. For this reason, the ensuing description of our general orientation toward principles which are taught will emphasize the psychosomatic viewpoint, in particular the psychosomatic theory of F. Deutsch (1940, 1953, 1955, 1959).

We present Deutsch's broad view that every case of physical illness can be regarded as having psychological components, whether in the form of reactions to illness per se which aggravate symptoms, or in the form of reactions of the environment to the illness which affect the patient adversely, or whether they are determinants in the precipitation, maintenance, or causation of the illness. The relative importance of the psychological elements needs to be evaluated. For successful treatment of many cases of physical illness, attention to the psychological needs of the patient is essential, whether it is given consciously and by design or unconsciously and intuitively. This does not mean that the development of a specialized branch of medicine is advocated under which are to be grouped specific physical disorders. The concern is with a special approach, namely that of psychological considerations in the study of all forms of physical illness. Questions about whether somatic or psychic factors are primary or secondary become academic when it comes to the matter of application of psychological principles to medicine. Furthermore, the need for recognition of psychological elements in physical illness does not imply that psychological management should supersede or displace the utilization of medical methods which have been developed on the basis of knowledge of physical processes considered in physical terms. There is required an integration of all available resources.

According to Deutsch, from the beginning of life, bodily processes become fused and amalgamated with emotional processes by symbolization. This fusion is a process which is part of and essential to normal as well as pathological development. Bodily functions, through their symbolic representations, become a bodily language expressing the individual's relationship to himself and his environment. Physical dysfunction with emotional significance essentially symbolizes disruption of relationships or disharmony between the individual and the present and past significant persons in his environment. This in turn can become a representation of disharmony between the individual and himself in the various parts of his personality. Good function, from a psychological viewpoint, can be considered to depend on resolution of conflict between the individual and key persons in his past and present life. The resolution of such conflict has the effect of loosening the entanglement of emotional processes and physical functions.

This broad theoretical framework helps to bridge the gap between psyche and soma and helps to make understandable the interrelationships of the two modes of human functioning and expression. Through it one can present in psychological terms a unified concept of mental and physical functioning. It provides an acceptable rationale for the introduction of material on all aspects of emotional and personality development, normal and pathological, and for discussion, for instance, of the nature of emotional experiences in life from birth onward, which maintain psychological health as well as disrupt it.

This viewpoint also lends itself to examination of the significance of depressive elements which underlie many physical disorders with strong psychological components, and to discussion of the views of many authors (Daniels, 1940; Deutsch, 1959; Knapp, 1960; Lindemann, 1945; Ludwig, 1954; Mushatt, 1954, 1959; Sperling, 1946) regarding the central role of reaction to loss and separation, actual and symbolic, in the precipitation, maintenance, or aggravation of physical and psychiatric illness. An understanding of depression and its protean manifestations and of its determinants provides the means of being of significant help, through limited psychological management, to a great majority of patients with physical illness.

In these courses, from the point of view of approach to limited treatment, focus thus tends to be on the study of the interaction of the individual with his past and present environment, largely in terms of ego psychology. In regard to instinctual life, there has been more emphasis on understanding of aggressive components than on sexual aspects. There is no special stress on the need to study the sexual life of patients, even though psychosexual development holds such a central position in the evolution of the personality. This de-emphasis of sexual life derives in part from the application of our theoretical viewpoint (Mushatt, 1954,

1959) in regard to etiology in psychosomatic, borderline, and psychotic states, namely that the basic difficulty arises from impairment in ego development and in development of object relations. Mastery and transformation of sexual and aggressive impulses are certainly usually impaired as a result of disturbed ego function, and this in turn hinders ego development. In the limited management that can be provided by nonpsychiatric personnel with restricted training, detailed study of sexual life usually is not necessary nor does it belong there, just as exploration of unconscious fantasy life is inappropriate to such work. Even in hysteria and obsessive-compulsive neuroses, where the symptoms arise from inability to master sexual (and aggressive) drives, in limited work one should approach the sexual conflicts via the ego derivatives and representations. In such cases this can be done with hope of some measure of success. Our avoidance of emphasis on this special area also stems from our belief that the intense sexualized transference which ordinarily develops with extensive exploration of a patient's instinctual life would make it difficult for both the physician and patient to proceed with ease and objectivity in regard to total management. However, some knowledge of unconscious processes and of instinctual life is necessary for the physician to be able to understand and utilize effectively his patient's conscious and preconscious communications. It is necessary, too, for understanding of the doctor-patient relationship.

## Approach to Teaching

The general approach to teaching has been clinical and the format in all courses essentially the same. One of us (C.M.) was originally impressed with the clinical approach both in the form of the conferences and of the individual contacts with the physicians as described in the report on the Commonwealth Fund's experimental course on psychotherapy in general practice given at the University of Minnesota in 1946 (Witmer, 1947). The major shortcoming of this experiment lay in the brevity and intensity of the course. It was felt that such a model was likely to be most effective and more consistent with the realities involved in teaching and learning if it were used over an extended period with any one group of students. All learning involves a slow process of assimilation which is dependent not only on intellectual understanding, but also on emotional processes (American Psychiatric Association, 1952). This is true for all aspects of medical education where the influence of unconscious reactions is very pronounced. It is especially true for psychiatry.

In all areas of medical training other than psychiatry, not only is teaching done through the didactic or abstract intellectual method, but emphasis is placed on the active participation and association of the student with the medical and surgical instructors in the direct study and management of the patient. Through the latter procedure, highly complex emotional or psychological processes are brought into play which facilitate learning. One major process, for instance, is that of identification. One cannot expect to teach all that has to be taught in medicine. Exploiting the process of identification mobilizes and enhances the individual's capacity for learning on his own through experience and study. The opportunity for identification with the instructor is also of help to the student in facilitating mastery over unconscious reactions to confrontation with illness in people, and with the procedures required in examination and treatment. This in turn aids learning. In psychiatric teaching, both of psychiatric as well as of nonpsychiatric trainees, the tendency is for the clinical application of theory to be taught in the abstract. Clinical experience, when offered, is mostly provided, in contrast with other areas of medicine, without the apprenticeship experience of direct witnessing of the instructor in action by the student, and without the instructor directly assisting the student in his immediate contact with the patient. As a result, an already slow process of learning is made even more difficult.

In addition, in medicine and surgery, abstractions are more readily translated into concrete conceptualizations for use in application to the study and treatment of the patient. Psychological principles, by contrast, are probably among the most difficult to teach and learn. Aside from the greater emotional impact which they have on the students, which burdens both teaching and learning, they do not lend themselves to the same clear, dogmatic, and organized presentation of knowledge as, for instance, medicine or surgery. Moreover, abstract knowledge of dynamic psychology is not easily utilizable in the service of clinical skills. For instance, in the first clinical procedures in contact with the patient, namely history-taking and physical examination, it is relatively easier, after a period of instruction, by following a prescribed outline, to learn to take a medical and surgical history and to do a physical examination which would provide a reasonably adequate guide to physical diagnosis and medical management. A psychological-medical history, taken according to a comparable outline, most often would result in the collection of a vast amount of material concerning a patient's life in a form which may be of little value for diagnosis and for decision in regard to treatment. It is a much more difficult matter to use one's theoretical knowledge of the kind of information needed and of the difficulties that may be encountered in trying to obtain not only facts but those facts which in the light of the psychoanalytic concept of genetic relationships may throw light on the nature of the illness and the relation of the patient's problems to it (Deutsch, 1940). The physician, in order to gain a reasonably useful knowledge of the patient's life, has to have some awareness of these difficulties and of methods of overcoming or reducing them. The latter involve what are to be regarded as therapeutic maneuvers which have to be used from the beginning in order to gather significant and diagnostic information.

Again, in regard to the investigation of the patient beyond the anamnestic stage and in regard to therapeutic procedures, it is easier in other areas of medicine for a student to grasp both from theoretical knowledge and from clinical demonstrations why certain procedures may or may not be done. Psychological study tends to be more subtle and indirect, and the relation of cause and effect is less dramatic and much less obvious. Predictions or evaluations regarding cause and effect cannot easily be accepted by skeptical students. One major reason for this lies in the fact that, in psychological study, some knowledge of the unconscious is necessary for the understanding of a patient's communications. One cannot devise therapeutic measures satisfactorily if the patient's communications are approached wholly in terms of conscious or overt content. The skepticism of students in regard to the validity of the theory of the unconscious is most likely to be overcome in the clinical setting.

### Organization and Procedure in Teaching

The courses for the allergists and general practitioners were each set up by invitation to all participants. In the initial planning, Dr. Herrman L. Blumgart, former Chief of the Medical Service, Dr. Grete L. Bibring, Chief of the Psychiatric Service, and Dr. Harry Derow, former Head of the Medical Outpatient Clinic, took an active personal part. We have found that such personal involvement of the chiefs of service has been very important and helpful.

In the allergy group, there were five members originally. They attended the clinic regularly throughout the year. Two members withdrew from the course after a considerable time; the others continued for three years. In the general practitioner group, there were seven members in the first year. In the second year another member of the clinic staff joined the course at his own request. All members have remained through the four years of the course. In the case of the medical house officers in the Outpatient

Clinic, at any one period there were one or two assistant residents and two interns on a ten- and twelve-week rotation respectively.

The course for the general practitioners was the most intensive, and will therefore be described in some detail. It was organized as follows: (1) A conference lasting one hour and three quarters was held every week throughout each year. It was attended by all members of the group and was conducted by the senior instructor (C.M.) assisted by the two other instructors. The latter attended for the purpose of maintaining continuity of teaching and relationships between conference and clinic setting. In the second year, each instructor in turn presided at conference, with all three attending. In intense and prolonged courses, strong student-teacher transference relationships develop which are important for the learning process. We found it desirable to have all instructors present at conferences for the first two years so as to avoid too much of a split in transference. In the third year the senior instructor attended regularly, while each of the others was present for two sessions per month. (2) The group was divided into two sections, each attending the clinic on a different day in each week throughout the year. Each member was expected to spend one and one half hours weekly in the clinic. Two instructors attended the clinic on both days during the first two years of the course. In the third year only one instructor was present at each clinic session. Each instructor attended on the same day every week. (3) All three instructors met weekly to review experiences during the first year, and less frequently after that.

The programs for the allergists and house officers were conducted along the same lines. In both, a psychiatric instructor was present in the clinic throughout the year once weekly for two hours and this was followed by a conference with all members of each course lasting one to one and one half hours. In the case of the allergists, one instructor (C.M.) conducted the entire course. With the house officers, for part of the time two instructors (C.M. and R.E.C.) participated, but subsequently one instructor (R.E.C.) was responsible for all the teaching.

With all groups, teaching was not restricted to these formal meetings, but informal discussions were held at every possible opportunity outside as well as within the clinic. Informal contacts were found to be especially valuable.

Teaching in the group conference was done as follows. In the initial meetings, an informal lecture was given on our views of the part played by psychological factors in physical illness and on the psychoanalytic concept of the genetic relationships in personality development. This was fol-

lowed by talks on the concept of the unconscious and of the mental mechanisms of defense, both intended to lay the groundwork for instruction in
interviewing and evaluation of interviews. After that, the main approach
was through case presentations. The physicians would present cases from
the clinic or their private practice and, as much as possible, the patients
would be interviewed by the instructor in the presence of the group. The
interviews would last about forty-five minutes. Frequently, one instructor
would see the same patient at a number of successive conferences and in
several instances for as many as five to six sessions. In their second year,
the physicians in the General Medical Clinic were encouraged to conduct
the interviews before the group with the help of the instructor. This undertaking, a difficult one for the physicians, created a powerful stimulus
for interest and involvement on the part of all members of the group.
The case material would be used to discuss interviewing techniques, but
primarily it would be used as a starting point for an extemporaneous talk,
with discussion by the group of topics considered significant for the understanding of normal as well as pathological personality development. We
tried to avoid limiting the case discussion to evaluation and suggestions
for management of the particular patient. At first, there was very little
emphasis on treatment. An effort was made to lift out material from successive cases in such a way as to maintain and develop central themes
over a number of weeks. Subjects previously discussed would be approached repeatedly from different aspects and for further elaboration.
This was especially useful when it was observed that certain topics had
had an emotional impact on members of the group and had been marked
by defensive responses. In this way one could not only allay the physician's concerns, but undo or circumvent the resistance to assimilation of
the concept in question.

When there would not be any specific case presented or patient interviewed, questions would be brought up for discussion by members of the
group. Often, for instance, ideas expressed in the course of casual social
conversation preceding the start of the formal conference would be used
as a starting point for an extemporaneous talk and discussion. In instances
where a theme had been dealt with repeatedly but in a diffuse manner,
an organized lecture on the topic would be given.

It can be seen that we did not give a systematized series of lectures on
psychiatry or psychiatric syndromes. We rigorously avoided this in spite
of repeated pressure from the doctors. Only in the case of the general
practitioner group was a brief systematic course of didactic lectures given,
but this was done only in the third year. A reading list was offered in

the second year at the request of the general practitioners and it was left to the members to choose and expand their own reading from this. Primarily, we felt that systematized didactic lectures on psychiatric syndromes, if given early, would structure the teaching too much in the form of traditional medical teaching and would not lend itself to the major task of teaching both normal and pathological personality development. It would not permit the kind of emotional response and involvement which we feel helps the physician to gain a greater inner freedom in dealing with the day-to-day problems in his contacts with patients. We would like to add that, when we have had the opportunity to participate as leaders of small discussion groups for students after class didactic lectures, it has become clear how much need there has been for such mutual exchange through free and lengthy discussion between students and instructors. It was also observed how good didactic lectures inevitably aroused considerable inner personal concerns in students.

We have been impressed too with the frequency with which psychiatric instructors take it for granted that students and fellow physicians can grasp the emotional significance and impact of everyday experiences on the individual. Often they do not show appreciation of the complex emotional mechanisms which prevent the student or doctor from affective understanding of the effect of even the most commonplace experiences on the life of an individual. Often the expectations for psychological awareness are too high. Primarily didactic teaching does not permit this problem to be dealt with successfully, nor does it give the instructor the opportunity to become aware of any shortcomings in respect to it.

The purpose of the instructors' attendance in the clinic was exclusively for teaching through individual contact and supervision of the physicians. Case consultation and treatment were not provided by the instructors except indirectly as the result of the use of cases for teaching. On occasions when it was found that patients needed specialized psychiatric treatment, they were referred to the psychiatric clinic. Such instances offered an opportunity to demonstrate the manner in which one could bring about in the patient a readiness that would make such a referral acceptable and useful. Too often patients are frightened and antagonized by the manner of referral even by the best-intentioned physician.

The instructors, as far as possible, have avoided interviewing patients alone without the presence of the patient's physician. It is very easy for the psychiatric instructor to find himself pushed exclusively into the role of a consultant and therapist to whom cases are referred for psychological evaluation, management, and disposition. Under such circumstances, the psychiatrist frequently finds himself isolated in his clinic office, so that other members of the clinic, beyond receiving reports on their cases, have little opportunity to learn to use the psychological information in their own management of their cases. Nor do they feel the pressure to assume responsibility for the psychological management of their patients.

The teaching in the clinic setting with the individual physicians reinforced that done in the group conference and vice versa. We feel that for the teaching to be done more effectively, it is desirable to maintain contact concurrently for a considerable time with the doctors individually in the clinic and as a group in conference. It is not at all easy to get physicians to become involved emotionally in the study of dynamic psychology. By this kind of intensive contact their inner resistance can be more easily overcome even though only gradually, and the learning process facilitated. In the clinic setting, it has been our practice for the instructor to sit with the individual doctors in turn while they interview and examine their patients. The instructor participates in the interview for periods of varying length to help the physician keep the interview moving or to demonstrate techniques of interviewing. As far as possible, the instructor avoids taking over the interview completely. The instructor discusses the patient with the physician after the patient has departed. Where possible, the other doctors are invited to join in the discussion. Often the instructor will see the same patient with the doctor over a number of follow-up visits. Long-term follow-up with supervision has been encouraged, but we have not met with much success in developing this.

Consideration has had to be given to the pressure of caseloads in the clinic. On very busy days there often has been very little activity on the part of the psychiatric instructor. The physicians have been encouraged to limit the number of patients seen for lengthy interviews, and in the remainder of cases to limit themselves to ten to fifteen minutes. Under the pressure of clinic and private practice, physicians cannot realistically be expected to spend a great deal of time with all patients. In this sense, of necessity, they must be selective. Ordinarily most doctors appear unconsciously to feel guilty at not being able to do enough for their patients. To press them to do more than is feasible under the conditions and the realities of clinic and office practice burdens them even more with a sense of failing their patients. This antagonizes them and impedes their work. We feel also that limited management depends for its effectiveness primarily on the development of a strong positive transference reaction. Only this can explain the striking remission and control over symptoms, even though most often only very modest in duration, which we have observed repeatedly following ten- to fifteen-minute sessions with patients in general medical and specialty clinics. Stress is placed on the value of setting out to develop a good working relationship with the patient and upon the methods by which this can be done in brief interviews.

Some comments on interviewing by instructors at conferences and in the clinic may be of interest. Essentially, the interviewing technique has been associative in character, encouraging questions about physical symptoms and about personal relationships in an associative context (Deutsch, 1939). In this way, affective relationships can be readily recognized, and the significant relationships in an individual's life, especially those that bear on the illness, can be found and focused upon most easily. This method also helps to impart to students the value of listening not only to content but, for instance, to themes of communications, and through this to teach how to use material from patients, what to say to patients, and how to observe the manner in which an individual unconsciously works over a problem. Communications, otherwise seemingly trivial or irrelevant, can be seen more readily in a significant light.

The presence of the doctors in the interview conducted by the instructor seems to be more advantageous than that of having them listen to interviews on a tape recording or through a one-way screen. The physicians are drawn into participating in the emotional climate of the interview and, as a result, they can relate more empathically with the patient, thereby appreciating the interview more effectively. At the same time, identification with the instructor is fostered. Our impression, too, is that once the patient has been put at ease in the conference—usually there is some discomfort—the interview can be made to proceed just as effectively as a one-to-one interview from the point of view of the kind of material that needs to be elicited for limited management.

For the instructor, interviewing before the group is certainly not identical with interviewing in isolation but, with experience and care, it can approximate it. One difficulty to be overcome, for instance, is the tendency to try too vigorously to do something for the student by way of bringing out material suitable for teaching purposes, just as the physicians, and especially medical students and house officers, often seem in a great hurry to bring about results in their patients. This often provokes greater defensiveness or the mobilization and expression of excessive emotions on the part of patients. The latter, particularly, has been found to disturb medical students and house officers. This tendency serves only to distort the interviewing and therapeutic process and to reinforce the physician's own attitude of impatience with the psychological approach.

When we have been aware of disturbing the interview by such activity, we have discussed it freely with the group, taking the opportunity to discuss, for instance, the theory of defense mechanisms and their manifestations and bringing in symptom formation as one of these defenses.

### Reactions of Physicians

Some reactions of the physicians which bear on the problem of resistance and on sources of difficulty in teaching will be described and discussed.

In the case of the allergists, at the outset a great deal of concern was expressed about the attitude of psychiatry toward their specialty. There was considerable feeling from their reading and attendance at lectures that psychiatrists believed that emotional factors were the sole or primary etiological agents in allergic states. As a result, the allergists felt that in approaching them, the psychiatrists would devaluate their specialty as such and would shake their confidence in their work. An associated concern was a suspicion that the psychiatric instructor's real aim was that the group should become psychiatrists and abandon their own specialty. This sense of threat to their organic orientation and interests presented obstacles repeatedly in spite of the pains we took to prevent such misconceptions of our viewpoint. In defense, the allergists reacted with rejection and devaluation of the role of the emotions in physical illness, with devaluation of psychiatry in general and with attacks on psychiatrists. Strikingly, among the general practitioners in our group, this problem was not at all prominent. There was ample skepticism at first about the value of the psychological approach, but no evidence of fear of devaluation of the general practitioner's position. The interval between the course given for the allergists and for the general practitioners was six to seven years. During this period all three instructors were aware that they had acquired greater skill and sensitivity in regard to the presentation of their subjects. With greater awareness of the kind of knowledge needed for limited management, there has been a gradual change in focus and points of emphasis. This factor may account in part for the striking difference between the allergists and the general practitioners in regard to this problem.

In part, however, the insecurity of the allergists appeared to stem from their uncertainties about their own special area of interest. There is often a wide discrepancy between the vast body of knowledge about immunological and allergic processes in the body and the application and efficacy of treatment based on this knowledge. Another explanation for the contrasting reaction of the allergists and the general practitioners has to do with the difference for the individual between specialization and general practice in the sense that on the part of the general practitioner there is greater emotional readiness to extend his interests into a new and unknown and even provocative field, especially with the probability of acquiring only a very limited knowledge of the latter and of having to function with only limited skills. All individuals, when faced with new situations and undertakings with which they have little affective familiarity, react with special concerns and self-questioning. This was evident in all groups, but seemed much more pronounced in the allergists. One allergist described his dilemma eloquently during one conference. He had become very argumentative on this occasion, and when he was asked what was making it so difficult for him to accept what was being presented, he replied, "The whole situation is like this to me. It is as if I had already completed a painting and it is framed. Then someone like you comes along, takes off the frame, puts a dab here and a dab there and I am faced with a large canvas and I don't know what to do with it or how it will end." The general practitioners, by contrast, quickly showed evidence of increasing self-confidence and self-esteem in their work. In addition, the general practitioner, as seen in our small and relatively select group, seemed to have a greater tolerance for psychological closeness to his patients.

In all groups there was evidence of considerable anxiety about the use of psychological investigation and treatment. They often expressed the fear that a little knowledge was dangerous. In early conferences, this was expressed by one physician as follows: "You know, I am scared to death by the whole business. I am more scared for the others than for myself because I have had some training in psychiatry. They may begin to think they know something and then begin to interpret things to patients and make them worse . . . . It takes years for a psychiatrist to know what to say to a patient, but you want us fellows to do this in eight to ten lectures." The unconscious distortion of the actual plan for the course expressed in "eight to ten lectures" only emphasizes the anxiety expressed. The intense concern over insufficient knowledge and the dangers felt to be inherent in this for the patient and the doctor is by no means restricted to psychology. We have seen ample evidence of it on all levels, from medical students and house officers, in whom it is especially pronounced, to senior staff instructors in regard to their medical and surgical work with patients. It seems to us that the physician's overidentification with the patient forces upon him an unconscious striving to meet the patient's unconscious demands for omniscience and omnipotence. This creates an overdetermined sense of personal responsibility for human life. Failure to meet these demands arouses feelings of inadequacy and of guilt toward patients. The actual limitations in our total medical and surgical knowledge and skills enhance this sense of inadequacy and guilt. In medical students and house officers the problem is expressed in the form of impatience with their supervisors or instructors, in impatience with the task of gaining experience, in excessive studies of patients and in urgency and overtreatment of patients. In relation to the psychological approach, it is difficult for them to accept the subtleties and relative slowness of therapeutic procedures, and especially the concept of limited goals in treatment. The latter implies for them a failure to do everything possible for the patient. We have the impression that one psychological determinant for specialization derives from these sources. The acquisition of extensive knowledge of one organ system, and, as a result, the legitimate relative restriction of one's interest to a specific area of the body and person serve as a defense against feelings of inadequacy and unconscious guilt, though they do not always provide a successful protective maneuver.

While the confrontation with physical illness unconsciously mobilizes in the physician personal concerns regarding his physical condition, the exposure to dynamic psychological concepts tends to be even more provocative for him and to threaten his defenses against self-awareness even more. One physician commented, "You cannot talk about such things as personal problems and personality development without stepping on someone's toes. We all tend to think in terms of ourselves and we all have problems." This remark seemed to explain further the uneasiness with psychological concepts that has been apparent in all groups. In all groups, every member went through a period of introspection and concern about himself or about members of his family. On occasion, some members consulted the instructors privately, or had a member of their family evaluated. Only in rare instances was treatment recommended. In these cases, we do not feel that this need resulted from provocation by the courses, but, on the contrary, participation in the courses had enabled these men to recognize emotional problems in themselves and to come to terms with the need for treatment.

Most often inner personal concerns in regard to teaching material were not expressed directly as such, but were manifested in various ways such as by devaluating and rejecting attitudes toward the concepts, hostile and aggressive behavior toward the psychiatrist, irritable argumentativeness, sleepiness, irregular attendance, etc. A striking example was seen in one instance: After considerable preparation through the discussion of a male patient's difficulty in marital adjustment, the concept of the childhood oedipal phase in boys was discussed, together with the manner in which the carry-over of childhood unconscious guilt over sexual interests and activities derived from this phase may impede adjustment in marriage. At one point, one of the group heatedly questioned the usefulness of such information for the practice of his specialty. At the time, the question was answered in very simple but inadequate terms. Over the ensuing few weeks the topic was approached repeatedly in various ways. Finally, when the instructor led into a discussion of the problems of adaptation confronting the medical student in regard to the abandonment of ordinary social taboos in the interests of study of the patient, the same physician casually told of his inhibition as a medical student in regard to certain aspects of physical examination, and of the conscious struggle within himself to overcome this, as he did successfully when he graduated. These remarks were not explored further, but we felt that they explained the doctor's earlier resistance to certain aspects of the discussion of the oedipal phase. We felt that we had successfully achieved in him a tolerance toward the subject which made it possible for him to discuss his earlier inhibitions without self-consciousness and which made it possible for him to utilize the information presented to him. It is inevitable for the doctor-student to show reactions and to go through periods of introspection. It is the task of the psychiatric instructor to bring into the teaching situation the same kind of skills which he uses to establish a working relationship with his patients, but in this situation not in terms of treating the doctors as patients, but in terms of recognizing the problems presented to the doctors by his presence and the concepts he teaches, and in terms of attempting by his manner of approach to present his subject in such a way as to arouse least anxiety and to allay anxiety or depressive reactions when aroused.

We do not believe, as some do (Balint, 1961; Berman, 1950a; Walters, 1961) that, because of such phenomena, nonpsychiatrists should be taught psychological concepts through the medium of group psychotherapy, that is, that they should enter into group therapy so as to gain knowledge of individual psychology through study of themselves. It would be pertinent to add here that we do not agree with European writers (Baerwolf, 1961; Balint, 1961) who state that "partial knowledge is always more dangerous than utter ignorance particularly for the patient" and that "for the use of psychotherapeutic measures in any form full psychoanalytic and psychiatric training is necessary." We feel that such ideas arise from the lack of appreciation of the value that limited goals and relatively superficial study of the patient may have not only in regard to medical psychology or psychoanalytic medicine, but also in the management of individuals with overt psychiatric illness.

Very frequently growth and maturation in relation to the emotional aspects of the tasks of his profession can be effected in the doctor through a system of teaching conducted over an extended period, without having recourse to a formal procedure overtly and primarily designed as a therapeutic situation. Because psychotherapy frees the individual for further maturation, it should not be confused with education. Education and psychotherapy are not synonymous, nor are they substitutes one for the other. Nor is formal psychotherapy always necessary to bring about maturational changes in an individual. When teaching is done with respect and awareness for the impact of the subject on the students and for other difficulties involved in learning it, not only can a large body of knowledge and information about the psychology of the individual be passed on and assimilated, but inner changes can be brought about unconsciously in the students which give them a greater tolerance for themselves and for their patients. In this way, the learning process can be facilitated. Such inner changes not only help the learning of psychology, but we believe that they also affect in a very positive way the capacity to learn medicine and surgery as well as the capacity for objectivity in these areas. An example of this was seen in the second year of the course for general practitioners. An elderly woman had been interviewed at length. She was extremely depressed, and presented a painful story of a succession of deaths in her family with particularly trying circumstances associated with them for the patient. After the interview, one physician laughingly remarked, "I was bushed by the end of the interview, but not like I would have been a year ago listening to this kind of interview. I was listening all the time."

Frequently, general questions brought by the physicians for discussion before the group and in private discussion with the instructors have been raised out of concern by the physicians about themselves. In our courses, where we have tried to keep the discussion of the personal lives of the doctors at a minimum, we usually have been on the alert for the personal implication of the doctors' questions, and we have tried to deal with them with great care and circumspection. Most often the personal element has been involved only unconsciously by the physician. This was seen most strikingly in the observation of the kinds of patients presented by the individual doctors. For instance, there were instances in which the same physician presented cases repeatedly which turned out to be almost identical in the nature of the presenting problem. Often this has been an expression of difficulty which the doctor has had in dealing with this particular problem in his patients. In one instance it became apparent that the physician's interest in a special kind of case and his excessive concern for these patients were determined by problems with which the physician was beset in his own personal life. The patients he presented were invariably late middle-aged widows in conflict with their children over the latter's efforts to develop independent lives for themselves. In recognizing the general nature of the physician's problem, we tried to approach the individual cases by discussion of the tasks normally involved in maturation, of the interplay between parents and children, of the inevitable reactions as the developing son or daughter tries to move in the direction of independence. There was no direct reference to nor questioning of the physician in regard to his personal life. In this oblique fashion, we hoped to lend support to the physician and to offer some measure of insight. It became apparent that his work with these patients became less emotional and more objective. The impression of sustaining this physician through a difficult period was confirmed by the fact that, after some time, he came to conference early and before the others had arrived, and told of his own specific problem and of how he had been trying to deal with it in the preceding weeks.

A lesser, though important, determinant for the fear already referred to that pressure is being put on the physician to become a psychiatrist and that the organic point of view is being challenged is to be found in the fact that, in discussing cases, for the purpose of teaching there tends to be almost complete preoccupation with psychological factors. It is highly desirable for the instructors to see to it that the physicians be encouraged to discuss the organic point of view in cases. This not only helps the physician to maintain perspective, but it is of advantage to the instructor who on his part usually has a great deal to learn about the organic side of medicine, and who through such discussions can obtain a better appreciation of the realities of medical practice. One other valuable effect of such discussion derives from the fact that in all teaching situations, irrespective of the age, experience or status of the student, a strong transference relationship is built up between the student and teacher with the mobilization of elements of child-parent reactions. By encouraging discussion of their medical knowledge, an unconscious reaction is aroused in which the doctor-student feels that the instructor respects his knowledge and skill. This in turn enhances the student's own self-respect and confidence and enhances the relationship to the instructor, which in itself facilitates learning.

A continually perplexing situation for the doctor-student has been the fact that so often psychiatrists and nonpsychiatrists think in such different terms about their patients' communications that often it seems as if they speak a different language. We are not referring here to the use of technical language. The latter has been avoided as much as possible in our courses. The psychoanalytic psychiatrist certainly does think in a different manner. He not only thinks about the actual content of the patient's communications, but is constantly and busily trying to think on another level, namely, on the level of what the patient is trying to express unconsciously. It is extremely difficult and frustrating for the nonpsychiatrist to see how the psychiatrist finds so much in so little. It is difficult for him to appreciate why so much attention is paid to experiences ordinarily regarded as commonplace or normal, and especially why he pays so much attention to commonplace expressions.

There is a great deal of difficulty for the doctors in coming to grasp the full significance of the concept of the unconscious in a way that would lend itself to application to everyday study of their patients. This has been exemplified by their difficulty in understanding the concept of the unconscious mental mechanisms of defense and, for instance, in learning to appreciate the psychological significance of a symptom as a defense against psychic awareness and preoccupation. They find it hard to understand that people for whom physical symptoms serve this purpose cannot tell directly of their emotional difficulties. One extreme example of this was seen in the case of a middle-aged lady who had been attending the Allergy Clinic for a considerable time because of asthma and recurrent bouts of coughing. When she was interviewed in the presence of her physician, at first it was only with difficulty that a clear and detailed description of her recent individual asthmatic attacks could be obtained. Very gradually she began to elaborate on her symptoms and, in doing so, she began to introduce events and circumstances surrounding each bout. Finally, she spoke of events in her life which occurred about one year after her marriage, and she expressed her belief that these events had precipitated her bouts of coughing and wheezing. These events related to her moving away from her hometown to that of her husband and to her disagreeable reception by her husband's family. She then remarked that she had always felt that her symptoms were emotional. After she had left, her physician, in discussing her, became angry at the patient and expressed the naïve view that she had deliberately and maliciously withheld information from him. It is only by a gradual process that an untrained person can become able to think in terms of psychological meaning and language. As already described, this requires certain inner changes in the physician.

These experiences and observations have led us to some conclusions in regard to unconscious motivations for the rejection by such large segments of the medical profession of the validity of the findings of psychoanalytic psychology and of the need for integration of the latter into medical and surgical care. This rejection, as well as the overemotionality displayed by many physicians and surgeons in regard to this subject, is a never-ending source of difficulty and discouragement for psychiatric staff working in the milieu of general hospitals. Some authors, such as Alexander (1939) ascribe this difficulty to the historical change that took place in the nineteenth century with the development of the scientific era not only in the natural sciences, but also in medicine. The discoveries by Virchow marked the change in medicine and advanced medical knowledge immeasurably. At the same time Virchow's views that all functional change was preceded by structural change, that there were in effect only diseases of organs and cells, led to the exclusion of consideration of the influence of emotional life on bodily function. We feel that the exclusive assertion of the organic point of view following Virchow's contributions arose from the need for a powerful defense against the psychological stress involved for physicians in confrontation with the physically and emotionally ill, just as preoccupation with the logicality of the natural sciences may be used as a defense against the irrational in man. The attitude that dynamic psychology threatens the objectivity of scientific medicine and therefore has no place in the latter, has complex sources in the very nature of human personality development and especially in the nature of the psychological adjustments required of every physician. The understanding of this process is important for medical education as a whole. For stimulation in consideration of this point of view we are indebted to Murray (1950). Some aspects of the problem may be described as follows.

The experience of the medical student throughout his training and even afterward can be regarded as unique. At a time when he has barely come through a trying and harassing developmental period in life, namely adolescence, the medical student is confronted relentlessly with realities of life that are highly charged, such as birth, aging and death, disability, injury to the integrity of the human body and mind, injury to the integrity of human relationships by illness, and separation through illness and death of people who have played vital roles in the lives of individuals. Psychologically, because of the symbolic meaning of various parts of the body, the disruption of the integrity of the human body through physical illness is intimately connected with the problem of disharmony in personal relationships. Unconsciously, physical illness is a reminder of such problems.

In addition, the student is expected to be able to see, hear, touch, and smell in both a physical and psychological sense without compunction or reserve. He is faced with the resolution and mastery of conflict in regard to the conscious and unconscious taboos which he has acquired in the course of his emotional development against the fullest use of all sensory modalities. He is expected to use the latter in a way that demands de-emotionalization or dehumanization of the emotional aspects of all sensory perceptions. For instance, he is expected to look at, touch, examine, and explore the naked human body, male and female, in a manner detached from all the emotional and sexual, heterosexual and homosexual, implications that such activities have in nonmedical experience. The psychological counterpart is the need to be able to look into the most intimate experiences and feelings of the individual without feelings of guilt, and, in addition, to feel, smell, and taste in the sense of empathic experience all that an individual patient has gone through without reaction in personal terms. In addition, aggressive acts against the human body which under other social circumstances are regarded as destructive and even criminal are now to be undertaken in the constructive service of the individual, as for instance, the cutting and excision of parts of the body in surgical procedures. This requires a reorientation of previously strongly developed attitudes. All this carries with it the implication that the doctor is expected to be omniscient and omnipotent and in full control of his subjective experience, an expectation which not only the patient has of the doctor but, unfortunately, the doctor often has of himself. It is worth noting that the patient is usually expected by the doctor and auxiliary medical personnel to respond with the same equanimity and detachment to exposing himself physically and psychically and to respond with the acceptance of procedures that, in other circumstances, would be considered aggressive acts on the human body and human dignity (A. Freud, 1952).

One can easily visualize how formidable a task of adjustment is required of the student and physician. The process, to a large extent, goes on unconsciously. How the adjustment takes place varies from individual to individual, depending on his personality structure when he enters upon the study of medicine. There is no doubt that everyone is changed as a result of the experience. To a great extent, the change represents growth or maturation as a result of the unconscious mastery over so much that ordinarily presents sources of conflict and stress for all individuals. Such mastery can be expected to take place only gradually and laboriously. However, as part of the price of adjustment, there frequently occurs a denial or repression of the awareness of and of responsivity to human emotions. The confrontation with the need for incorporation of psychological understanding of the individual into medical practice reawakens the whole range of responses to the emotional problems of adjusting to dealing with the sick, and this in turn awakens preoccupation with one's own emotional development and attitudes toward one's own self. In large part, the reactions are unconscious or only close to consciousness but they manifest themselves in various ways. Gross examples are seen in every medical student in his periodic concern about the health and integrity of his body and even of his mind when he first encounters illness in patients. Physicians in their late forties, when confronted, for instance, with the frequency of coronary disease and cancer in this age group, often become very concerned about themselves. Most frequently reactions appear in the form of impatience with the patient's questions and concerns, whether they be reasonable or illogical, excessive fatigue, and irritability with patients when they talk of intimate personal experiences and when they show excessive emotionality over their life situations. When confronted with aspects of emotional development and with the nature of interpersonal family relationships which affect a patient's life adversely, physicians, no less than anyone else, become preoccupied and concerned about themselves consciously and especially unconsciously. It can be expected that this interferes with objectivity in the study of patients. It is a provocatively imposing task for the physician who wants to work effectively with his patient to accept the necessity of trying to appreciate the experience of the patient through empathy. The latter requires identification with the patient which must be kept tightly encapsulated, as it were, and separate from his own personal life. When one considers all that is involved, one cannot expect too much from the physician, and one can expect that the capacity for achievement of an appropriate attitude toward the patient and toward himself can take place only gradually and slowly like all maturational processes.

### Results

We would like to summarize our impression of the results of our teaching in regard to its influence on the physicians and their work. In the case of the house officers, it is hard to estimate the effect of this part of the teaching program. A serious defect lay in the short period of contact with them and in the erratic nature of their service in the Outpatient Clinic. In the context of the year-round contact of the house officers with psychiatric staff, we felt that we supplemented the teaching that was maintained on all services, and the total beneficial influence of this teaching is abundantly evident throughout the hospital. There was significant value in this particular setting in helping the house officers to adjust to the very special experience associated for them with work in a general outpatient clinic, especially in helping them to overcome their feelings of hopelessness and helplessness in regard to the chronic patients, especially the elderly. We could help them to see how often chronicity, even in the elderly, could be broken up, though frequently only temporarily, by the addition of relatively simple psychological procedures to their medical management.

In the case of the allergists and the general practitioners, there is no question that they acquired a great deal of psychological knowledge about patients over the course of the three to four years of continuous teaching. Even as early as at the end of six months, changes were observed. These are expressed in the following remarks of one general physician. "Since taking this course, the fog has lifted. Now I feel I can keep patients going on a day-to-day basis and I feel better about it. I no longer feel a charlatan and I can get patients to talk about themselves without fear of causing mental trauma. I feel I do things as I have always done, but I have more insight about what I do." Shortly after this remark, the same physician reported that formerly, when he received a night call from a patient who was emotionally disturbed, he would get irritated and give the patient the name of a psychiatrist to contact. He now no longer reacted this way, but offered the patient an appointment at the earliest possible time, preferably the next day, and tried to arrange the session so as to have ample time to explore the patient's situation, such as before or after regular office hours.

We observed in the Allergy Clinic how, when patients were referred there from other clinics for study, they often were returned to the referring clinic not only with reports on allergic sensitivities, but with recommendations for exploration of certain areas of the patients' emotional lives, which might have a possible bearing on the illness.

The newly acquired skills were not limited to the management of patients with physical illness, but the doctors found themselves able to be of significant, even though restricted, help to patients with almost every variety of psychopathological state, including ambulatory psychosis, alcoholism, reactive depressions, hysteria, and obsessive-compulsive states. "We are no longer afraid of the diagnosis," was a comment illustrating this change.

Significant was the fact that the acquisition of new knowledge was not only on an intellectual and abstract level, but the successful utilization of it was determined by an affective appreciation of psychological concepts. There has been considerable evidence of emotional change in the doctors not only in regard to patients, but also in regard to themselves. This finding is of particular interest for the elucidation of the phenomenon of resistance or hostility of the medical profession to the utilization of psychological concepts. In a questionnaire submitted to the general practitioners at the end of two years, all remarked on their greater tolerance and patience with individuals with emotional problems, and on their greater tolerance of themselves and of their own emotional conflicts into which they had acquired some insight. These changes became evident through observations of their approach to their patients and of the change in the manner in which various recurrent topics were discussed. The staff seemed easier to work with in the clinic and there was less tension for auxiliary staff in dealing with them in regard to patients. Even in a busy clinic and private office where time is realistically severely restricted, the doctors are now able to give the patient a feeling of leisurely interest, and this is reflected in the manner of history-taking. The stereotyped mechanical fashion of history-taking so frequent in medical practice, and which so often causes patients to react negatively to the doctor because it evokes the feeling of being "just a case record," has changed. Histories and follow-up examinations are now done in a manner more conducive to the facilitation of the patient's efforts to establish a psychological relationship with the doctor. In addition, this has made for greater accuracy in the gathering of information from patients in regard to symptoms.

One aspect of the changed attitude in regard to history-taking stems from the value that affective insight into psychological development has in helping the physicians to be less afraid of a psychological closeness to their patients. Some of the doctors have remarked on their awareness of having become less involved with patients through identification, so that they feel that they can be more objective. From very early in the courses, we became aware of the doctors' strong unconscious fears of their patients' dependency on them, even though such dependency is a prerequisite for successful medical treatment. An interesting example of this was that of one physician who had a very obvious difficulty in interviewing patients, namely, he would ask questions and with scarcely any time given to the patient to reply in any detail, he himself would begin making comments.

Much thought was given to the question of how to approach this matter with the physician tactfully, but he himself courageously solved it. After witnessing the instructors interviewing patients, and after he had raised many critical questions about the interviews, this physician decided to make a tape recording of one of his interviews with a private patient. He played the recording for himself, and to his consternation, according to his own account, he mostly heard only himself talking. He volunteered the opinion that this was due to his anxiety and discomfort with patients and with their demands upon him.

Devaluation and scorn for patients with emotional problems which were seen in the early period of all groups for the most part disappeared later. Expressions such as "constitutional inadequacy," "cerebral stenosis," and "mental degeneration," etc., which were often used, especially by the allergists, disappeared completely from discussions. One physician commented that "the personal effect of the course was considerable in that some entrenched prejudices have been removed and more objective reasoning has replaced it."

This change in the physicians was dramatized by their change in attitude towards the discussion of sexual topics. The general practitioners in particular are consulted for advice on sexual matters frequently and they were concerned about their lack of knowledge regarding sexual development. In the early phase of the course the physicians brought, in a repetitive way, cases of patients who had come to them with sexual difficulties. When a number of such cases had been presented, an effort was made to present in a systematic way the psychoanalytic theory of sexual development, starting out with an attempt to show how the various cases presented could be seen to have symptoms derived from a hierarchy of developmental phases in normal sexual organization and showing the significance of these phases for total personality development. The lecture created a great deal of uneasiness in all the physicians. They discussed it quite emotionally both in the conferences and in the clinic with the individual instructors. There was a desire expressed generally by the physicians that sexual topics should not be introduced by members of the group as frequently as had been done. The subject of sexual development was introduced subsequently by the instructors from time to time without any special emphasis and in a limited way, usually in terms of its significance in relation to the total development and in terms of expression of ego strivings. By contrast with this early responsivity, at the end of the second year in the course for the general practitioners a case which was presented lent itself to a detailed discussion of homosexuality, a topic into which it is invariably difficult to enter freely. This was received by the members of the group with notable equanimity and readiness for exchange of views. The freedom which the instructor felt in taking up this topic in detail at this time derived from his impression of the inner tolerance that had been developed in the physicians toward all aspects of personality development.

Most of the doctors reported that they felt that they now worked with patients with much greater ease. This was especially appreciated with chronic cases with previously intractable symptoms. In addition, the general practitioners expressed the feeling that in some way their sense of status as physicians had increased, and they felt more confident about their work.

There is little question but that the courses have been of considerable benefit to all participating. The results demonstrate that nonpsychiatric medical personnel can be helped to acquire a working knowledge of dynamic psychological principles and enabled to integrate it into their over-all management of their patients, whether the latter have physical or psychological disorders. The method of teaching and the orientation chosen are effective in achieving this end. Moreover, the results provide confirmation of our conclusions regarding the sources of resistance on the part of the medical profession to psychological concepts, and regarding the difficulties in teaching the latter.

We feel that courses such as those described here can be of great help in medical education, not only in regard to the utilization of psychological concepts, but also for facilitation of the learning process in medicine and surgery and for the development of a healthier and more effective adaptation to life as a physician and surgeon. We feel, too, that short didactic courses alone or short periods of exposure to psychological concepts often evoke disappointment and hostility rather than stimulate interest. Extended courses not only permit the acquisition of knowledge to take place solidly by helping the physician to go through the experience of testing himself out gradually, but they make it possible for the student and physician unconsciously to make the kind of inner emotional changes necessary to enable them to assimilate and utilize the concepts easily. After completion of courses, it is desirable to maintain contact with the physicians, even in very limited form, in order to sustain interest and to support the physicians in work that in itself is very trying. It is rarely recognized that regular medical and surgical conferences which are regarded as absolute necessities serve a purpose beyond their instructive and informative value, namely that of sustaining the physicians and surgeons in their demanding endeavors.

# Integration Clinic: An Approach to the Teaching and Practice of Medical Psychology in an Outpatient Setting

DON R. LIPSITT, M.D.

SINCE GRETE L. BIBRING (1951) introduced the teaching of medical psychology into the training program of Beth Israel Hospital, the indispensability of integrated medical practice and psychological thought in the general hospital has been amply demonstrated (G. L. Bibring, 1949; 1956). The special needs and problems of developing such a program are extensively noted in other chapters. It is clear that the successful integration of medicine and psychiatry in the general hospital will, in part, depend upon the ability of the training program to assist the hospital in meeting the needs of the community it serves. The history of the training and teaching program at Beth Israel Hospital demonstrates the effectiveness of its alliance with a variety of services within the hospital through Consultation Service (Kahana, 1959). Teaching Rounds (Dwyer & Zinberg, 1957), Home Care Program, Obstetrical Clinic, Tumor Clinic, General Practitioner Training Program, and others. Through constant reassessment of the general hospital's evolution (Solon, 1958, 1960; Lee, 1958) and newer developments in the field of psychiatry, it is possible to extend both service and training to keep pace with the needs of patients, hospital, and staff. One of the more recent extensions of the psychiatric teaching program has been the establishment of the Integration Clinic, a clinic intended to further co-ordinate Medicine and Psychiatry through its focus on the practice of medical psychology in the hospital's outpatient clinic service. This paper will describe the indications for such a clinic, as well as its scope and purpose. Inasmuch as clinical experience varies with the setting in which it occurs, some of the special problems encountered in Integration Clinic will be discussed.

## Indications for the Clinic

The need for the Integration Clinic was indicated by several evolutionary changes in the hospital:

### Expanding Usefulness and Applicability of the Medical Psychological Approach

The Beth Israel Psychiatric Service, although essentially an outpatient facility, has had as its objectives the study, treatment, and teaching of emotional problems of patients in a general hospital. It has therefore distributed its service over the existing wards and clinics of the hospital without segregating patients in a separate psychiatric ward. In this way, it was possible to bring to the physician's other specialties a psychotherapeutic approach which could be applied within the framework of his medical function. Over the years, there has been, in addition to the increasing demand for outpatient psychotherapy, a greater demand by other hospital services, both inpatient and outpatient, for psychiatric opinion. Such demand has resulted in a greater burden upon the Psychiatric Service and, at the same time, the widening applicability of the medical psychological approach led to a certain degree of diffuseness of psychiatric participation in all medical management. This demand and widening applicability invited a more focused, centralized approach to the use of medical psychology in the outpatient department.

### Changes in the Referral Patterns of House Officers and Attending Physicians in Outpatient Clinics

Although one aim of the teaching program is to prepare nonpsychiatric physicians to recognize and treat appropriate psychological problems in general medical practice, a concomitant result of successful training is a sharpened awareness of psychiatric problems which the physician feels untrained to treat. This has resulted in certain changes in the referral patterns of house staff and attending physicians. There has also been some indication that these physicians consider more and more patients suitable candidates for psychotherapy and refer them for this service. However, it seemed that referring house officer and evaluating psychiatrist often had disparate opinions regarding such suitability. Perhaps the house officer, briefly trained in psychological medicine, has a higher expectation for psychiatric treatment than his psychiatrist colleague. If this is so, it suggests that some familiarity with screening and evaluation techniques would be an important addition to the training program of medical personnel, although the final assessment of suitability for psychotherapy is more appropriately the special task of the trained psychiatrist. Over the years, it appeared that many patients referred from outpatient clinics for psychiatric evaluation were found to be candidates, not for the more structured types of regularized insight psychotherapy, but rather for a variety of supportive and perhaps manipulative types of therapeutic measures which were individually "tailored," to meet the special needs of these patients. It was felt that patients for whom the treatment of choice was long-term or brief psychoanalytically oriented therapy, required an extensive evaluation in order to define goals, character structure, and predominant conflict areas. But patients for whom other types of therapy were preferable seemed adequately assessed with more abbreviated evaluation methods. To test the accuracy of these impressions, a survey was made of representative series of patients referred from outpatient clinics for psychiatric evaluation.

A preliminary review of two series of consecutive referrals to Psychiatric Service, each of 11 patients, was carried out in 1960-1961. Of the 22 patients, 9 were referred from outpatient clinics of Beth Israel Hospital. Of these 9, only 2 patients completed the psychiatric evaluation and neither of these was recommended for intensive psychotherapy. Those not completing evaluation came for only one interview or refused to come at all (Table 1).

TABLE 1

| Referral source | Cases | Completed Evaluation | Accepted for Intensive Therapy |
|---|---|---|---|
| Outpatient clinics (BIH) | 9 | 2 | 0 |
| Self-referred | 7 | 6 | 4 |
| Community sources | 6 | 5 | 2 |

A survey of these data indicated that about one third of the patients in these series were from outpatient clinics and that a majority of incomplete evaluations was in this group, rather than in either the self-referred or community-source-referred groups. Furthermore, it seemed possible that these OPD patients were less likely to be accepted for intensive psychotherapy. This suggested, besides possible differences in patient motivation (perhaps self-referred patients are predominantly psychoneurotics without major medical or physical complaints), the possibility of inappropriate referrals, as well as wasteful use of clinic resources.

To pursue these issues further, a consecutive tabulation was made of all referrals for psychiatric evaluation in a two-month period. This showed that, of a total of 125 referrals, 54 per cent came from outside the hospital and 46 per cent came from intramural sources. The latter consisted of 4 major sources: Out-Patient Department, hospital wards, Emergency Ward, and Health Service. Forty-one per cent of all intramural referrals were from OPD, indicating this as the major source of psychiatric referrals within the hospital itself (Table 2).

TABLE 2

Consecutive Referrals to Psychiatry
(Two-month sample)

|                        | N      | per cent     |
|------------------------|--------|--------------|
| Extramural Referrals   | (67)   | (54)         |
| Intramural Referrals   |        |              |
|    OPD  | 24     |              |
|    Wards | 18    |              |
|    E. W. | 8     |              |
|    Health Service | 8 |          |
|                        | (58)   | (46)         |
| Total                  | 125    | 100 per cent |

A majority of OPD referrals was from Medical and Surgical Clinics. These data confirmed the general pattern observed in the smaller series.

The records of ten successive patients referred from outpatient clinics and completing psychiatric evaluation were then selected for a detailed review, which revealed certain common characteristics: (a) All had had extensive contact with a variety of outpatient clinics. (b) Nine were women over 58. (c) Chief complaints were often vague and nonspecific, e.g. dizziness, headache, insomnia, fatigue, stomach distress, etc., and were very often refractory to symptomatic treatment. (d) The diagnosis of depression, possibly chronic, was usually entertained and entered into the record only late in the patient's clinic course. (e) These patients were thought to be very dependent by interviewing psychiatrists. (f) Many exhibited a strong, anti-psychiatry bias. (g) In the psychiatric evaluation, chronic depression emerged as the most common diagnosis; masochistic features were often prominent. (h) None of these 10 patients was accepted for psychoanalytically oriented interview psychotherapy, although most were felt to be in need of some psychiatric assistance. (i) Prescription of treatment comprised a wide range of dispositions, including referral back to the OPD clinic, with recommendations for management and treatment with psychoactive drugs; referral to social service and family agencies; situational and environmental manipulations; referral to family physician for "total" treatment; supervised supportive care by a medical student; referral to General Practitioner Medical Clinic for management with psychiatric consultation.

These findings and observations seem to confirm a number of impressions: that outpatient services represent a significant user of the Psychiatric Service; that patients referred from OPD are usually not suitable candidates for intensive psychoanalytically oriented therapy and seem to represent a special group of patients for whom the medical psychological approach is most aptly suited; that these patients possess in common a number of characteristics which present special problems for the physician; that specialized screening and evaluation techniques would probably be helpful, economical, and expedient for both Psychiatry and other services. A special clinic designed to address itself to these issues seemed indicated.

### Antipsychiatry Bias of Patients Referred for Psychiatric Evaluation

As indicated above, many patients referred for evaluation appeared strongly opposed to psychiatric assessment. In spite of the increased public education and sophisticated enlightenment of patients and physicians, it is clear that the tendency to look upon psychiatry as "different" from other medical specialties persists. In part, this may be realistically based on the fact that psychiatry *is* different from other medical specialties in its conceptual framework, its terminology, and its techniques. But since orthopedics, for example, is different from obstetrics in similar ways, perhaps a greater part of the attitudes toward psychiatry may be attributable to certain more or less obsolete beliefs (or even superstitions), as well as a kind of mystical aura that psychiatry still holds for some, especially in the average or lower intelligence groups. Many older patients, who seem to comprise a large part of the population that frequents outpatient clinics, still believe that psychiatry is for the insane only; these people are more comfortable in a setting more typically medical in its accoutrements. Other less tangible factors come from the realm of attitudes, emotions, and misconceptions which are the accretions of individual experience, of both patient and physician. Referral of a patient for psychiatric evaluation is often an outgrowth of a unique interaction between a specific patient with a specific doctor, each with particular special needs and attitudes. Some patients may be reluctant to accept referral to a psychiatrist; others may comply with their physician's recommendation but demonstrate apprehension, fear, or negativism in the evaluation. Others may completely ignore a referral.

Experience in the application of psychological concepts to a variety of medical problems has taught that psychiatric evaluation may be of considerable benefit to both patient and referring physician, although referrals may not always be suitable for the traditional forms of insight psychotherapy. But it is the psychiatrist's challenging task to bring to the patient with an antipsychiatry bias a form of medical treatment which the patient requires, but basically opposes. The extensive experience with psychiatric consultation to the major hospital services has demonstrated repeatedly that patients who are otherwise not receptive to psychiatric treatment or referral usually accept willingly (and often gratefully) a psychiatric assessment which is proferred in the more familiar traditional medical or surgical ward setting. It is recognition of this phenomenon which suggested that psychiatric evaluations of certain outpatients might be performed more effectively in a clinical setting which minimizes the inherent differences between medical specialties; such a clinical setting could potentially facilitate the referral process itself as well as the psychiatric assessment of a patient's total medical situation.

### Increasing Awareness that Depression and Anxiety often Appear in Disguised Forms as Somatic Complaints, and that Depression Itself Is a Broad-Spectrum Illness, which Often Calls for Psychiatric Evaluation or Treatment

A majority of patients referred from outpatient clinics give the impression that depression is a significant part of their illness. Often the house officer or attending physician is interested in an assessment of the depth of depression, as well as recommendations for treatment. Many physicians feel competent to treat certain forms of depression but prefer to do so with the security of knowing the patient has been cleared by a psychiatrist. Others are fearful of the suicidal potential of depressives and will refer anyone who appears depressed to any degree. Many such patients can be managed by a psychiatrically knowledgeable physician, perhaps with adjunctive drug treatment, and do not necessarily require the specialized services of a psychiatrist beyond the initial screening evaluation. A clinic which can provide this kind of consultative back-stop, as well as teaching and service, seemed an important need in total medical management.

### The Expanding Use of Psychopharmacologic Agents

It is quite likely that antidepressants and tranquilizers are used more extensively by medical specialists other than dynamically oriented psychiatrists. Although the physician often turns to the psychiatrist for a clearer understanding of the uses and abuses of such drugs, he is sometimes disappointed to find that his own experience and knowledge of these agents far exceeds that of the psychiatrist. The use of all drugs, including placebos, has a critical role in the doctor-patient relationship and is therefore an important part of medical psychology. The introduction of drugs which have demonstrated their efficacy in certain specific psychiatric conditions provides the psychiatrist with an excellent teaching aid, since the doctor-drug-patient model of interaction is the more familiar medical framework of all physicians than is the psychiatrist's more purified doctor-patient relationship. It is in the matrix of the former framework that the beginning physician is more readily able to assimilate psychological concepts. A clinic which functioned within such a framework would serve an important teaching function in a general hospital.

### "Problem" Patients with Histories of Prolonged Contact with Outpatient Clinics

Every general hospital has recognized a category of patients that presents special diagnostic and therapeutic challenges. They are sometimes referred to contemptuously as "crocks" or as "thick chart patients," or as hypochondriacs, "hysterics," or "neurotics," terms more often than not diagnostically inappropriate. They usually have been to most of the specialty clinics in the outpatient department, over a period of years, yet seldom seem to obtain relief from their persistent complaints. They are usually well known to all hospital personnel and frequently look upon the hospital as a kind of "second home" (Reider, 1955). For some it represents a social as well as a medical resource, and it is not uncommon to hear of marriages between patients who have attended the same clinics for years. They evoke a variety of responses in physicians, from intense annoyance to friendly sympathy and even overprotectiveness. Some become "clinic orphans" in that they are unable to find a stable relationship with any single physician, while others form strong bonds with a single doctor for as long as he remains with the hospital. It would appear, therefore, that the character of their interaction with physicians has a great deal to do with the number of clinic referrals they experience and the length of time they continue their affiliation with the hospital (Lipsitt, 1961, 1962). Some of these patients are ultimately referred for psychiatric evaluation, perhaps as often out of desperation and frustration as out of need for psychiatric attention. Many of them exhibit unusually intense conflicts over dependency, difficulties in the expression of angry feelings, or poor object relations. It appears that they frequently try to utilize their clinic experiences, often futilely, to work out certain of these paramedical problems. The Integration Clinic, by placing itself in the path of "clinic rotators" or "clinic orphans," could more carefully observe and try to understand their unique problems and needs. A better understanding of the psychological make-up of these patients could be used to teach other physicians more appropriate ways to treat this very significant group of clinic patients. All of these considerations strongly supported the establishment of the Integration Clinic.

### The Clinic: Its Setting, Structure, and Function

Integration Clinic meets three afternoons a week in part of the Medical Clinic on the first floor of the Out-Patient Building, where the majority of outpatient clinics meet. The major Psychiatric Service is located on the third floor of this building and utilizes special appointment-making techniques, waiting areas, and interview rooms, some of which are equipped with couches. Interview rooms in the Medical Clinic have the bare essentials of a desk and two chairs, medical examining table, wash basin, and a wall-attached blood pressure apparatus. In order to appear as much like other specialty clinics as possible, Integration Clinic uses the same appointment-making, billing, and cancellation methods as these other clinics. Unlike Psychiatric Clinic, where the referred patient deals directly with the psychiatrist in setting up an appointment, patients referred to Integration Clinic deal with secretaries or nurses rather than the physician. This practice seems to minimize manipulativeness in some patients and to lessen their tendency to see appointment-giving by the doctor as an indicator of interest, concern, or affection.

Initially, during the exploratory phase of the clinic, staff consisted only of one psychiatrist and an on-call social worker; however, psychiatric residents now rotate through the clinic as part of their training experience. Patients are referred to Integration Clinic primarily from other outpatient clinics whenever a psychiatric opinion is desired by the clinic physician. Before the establishment of Integration Clinic, the thirty-five outpatient specialty clinics could refer any patient to the Psychiatric Service for evaluation. The evaluation procedure consisted of usually one to three one-hour interviews by a resident psychiatrist, psychological testing when indicated, staff presentation for formulation, recommendations, diagnosis, and disposition. Depending upon the vagaries of scheduling, as well as the number of patients on the waiting list, the total time duration from referral to disposition might be a matter of months. The evaluative procedure in Integration Clinic consists of thirty to forty-minute interviews, intended to force an early tentative diagnosis and formulation, in an attempt to make as expedient a recommendation and disposition as possible. This avoids long delays between referral and initiation of treatment and manages to eliminate most waiting-list problems by seeing the patient within two to three days of referral. Disposition is often immediate, especially when social service or family agency appear to be the more suitable referral. In some cases, additional appointments are arranged for either further evaluation or supportive medical psychological treatment which seems most suitably carried out by a psychiatrist.

Although most patients seen in Integration Clinic are referred from other outpatient clinics, some are also referred by ward physicians. These are usually patients who have had an emotional reaction to surgical or medical treatment which has required a psychiatric consultation. These patients are more receptive to an Integration Clinic visit rather than psychiatric referral for follow-up after hospital discharge. Occasionally, patients who are seen on the Emergency Ward by a psychiatric resident are referred after the resident assesses or alleviates the acuteness of the situation. Also, patients who are seen in casework occasionally require interim psychiatric evaluation to determine mental status, level of employability or disability, depth of depression or suicidal tendency, or perhaps merely to help the social worker in management of the case. An additional type of referral is the patient who has undergone brief psychotherapy with a supervised medical student who has left the hospital; such a patient sometimes requires only periodic follow-ups, supportive treatment, or further disposition.

Brief evaluation and screening of all referrals is not intended to be a total intensive depth investigation, but rather concerns itself with the predominant aspects of a patient's total medical situation. For example, the approach is a medical psychological one which focuses the patient's chief complaint, his major conflict areas as they have been mobilized by his medical condition, his physical status, drug treatment, and the patient's understanding of his medical situation. It also assesses the nature of the doctor-patient interaction as revealed in the patient's previous experiences in various clinics as well as through direct observation in Integration Clinic. Some assessment of personality structure, based on the principles of personality diagnosis as taught in the Psychiatric Service, is felt to be essential for adequate disposition and treatment. On the basis of this assessment, an impression is gained of the patient's suitability for insight psychotherapy. If there are sufficient indications that the patient might benefit from such treatment, he is referred to the Psychiatric Service for a more intensive depth evaluation. Otherwise, the patient is recommended for adjunctive drug treatment, supportive psychotherapy, referral to social service or family agency, referral to another treatment facility (e.g., psychiatric hospitalization), or referral back to the referring physician with consultative aid in the patient's total treatment. A note is entered in the chronologically correct place on the patient's chart in every instance, recording as succinctly as possible relevant history, diagnostic impressions, recommendations, and suggestions for psychological management based on personality diagnosis. If the use of drugs is recommended, method of administration as well as dosage schedule and possible side effects are clearly spelled out. Whenever possible, a personal conference is held with the referring physician or social worker, in order maximally to use the referral for its multiple teaching potentials.

**Results**

Use of the Clinic

In a six-month period, 197 appointments for psychiatric assessment were made in Integration Clinic by other specialty clinics. The total number of appointments were made for 108 individual patients; 90 patients followed through and 18 failed to appear at all. Fifty-nine appointments were missed by a total of 18 patients, since each patient missing an appointment is offered at least 3 rescheduled appointments and may also be re-referred by another clinic. In the six-month period, no patient was seen more than 6 times, and the great majority attended only one or two times prior to definitive disposition (Table 3).

When Integration Clinic was first established, there was some concern that the ease with which referrals could be made might precipitate a flood of referrals, especially of problem patients. However, a comparison of data for the first and second three-month periods indicates that the rate of referral has been fairly stable.

TABLE 3

| Number of times seen | First 3 months | | Second 3 months | | Combined 6 months * | |
|---|---|---|---|---|---|---|
| | Pts. | Visits | Pts. | Visits | Pts. | Visits |
| 1 | 29 | 29 | 39 | 39 | 63 | 63 |
| 2 | 13 | 26 | 6 | 12 | 14 | 28 |
| 3 | 3 | 9 | 3 | 9 | 8 | 24 |
| 4 | 0 | 0 | 2 | 8 | 3 | 12 |
| 5 | 0 | 0 | 0 | 0 | 1 | 5 |
| 6 | 0 | 0 | 1 | 6 | 1 | 6 |
| Totals | 45 | 64 | 51 | 74 | 90 | 138 |

* Figures in this column do not represent a sum of figures in the other columns, since some of patients seen second 3 months were the same ones seen the first 3 months.

It is difficult to assess the significance of missed appointments on the basis of available data, but some patients seem reassured by the knowledge that if they miss an appointment, they may call in to re-schedule another. Some patients seem to find as much security in knowing the hospital is always available to them in time of need as do patients who must spend many hours sitting in the waiting rooms. For example, one very masochistic woman, who was seen three times in a six-month period, felt that she would like to see how long she could "manage on my own" after she was assured she could come in any time. In her third visit, she explained that she was feeling quite well, had taken a part-time job for the first time in eighteen years, looked less depressed, and explained her visit as a "way to prevent myself from slipping back." Several times after this, she would make an appointment, only to call and cancel the day before, explaining to the secretary that she was "feeling OK for now." Some patients are wary of Integration Clinic, expressing curiosity as to its function and purpose; but, for the most part, patients take their referral as a matter of course, talk freely and volubly about their problems, and do not seem concerned about the particular orientation of the physician. Some patients demonstrate a certain degree of naïveté as to whether psychiatrists are truly doctors or not, yet seem very reassured when they are told that the doctor in Integration Clinic is a medical doctor with psychiatric training. One patient who, during her hospitalization, refused to talk to an identified psychiatrist on the ward, was referred to Integration Clinic on discharge and, after asking something about the clinic, interrupted explanatory comments by insisting that it was Medical Clinic she was being seen in, since she had been there before. Some patients become highly inflamed at the suggestion that they require psychiatric treatment, yet seem readily able to accept help with "their nerves," which seems to convey the preferred impression of organicity, often reinforced by the giving of drugs.

Many patients who have, in the past, rejected psychiatric referral, have been able to accept referral to Integration Clinic. This was clearly indicated in the author's experience when a patient had been contacted two years previously by the author as a resident, at which time the patient irately complained that she should not have been sent to Psychiatry by the outpatient doctor since she was not crazy; however, two years later, she came willingly, although somewhat timidly, to Integration Clinic, where she announced that she did not believe in "talking treatment" and then talked volubly about her problems for the entire interview.

Although adjunctive drug treatment seems to support the preference of some patients to see themselves with physical rather than emotional disease, there are some patients who seem pleased to find a change in the pattern of their clinic experience when they are simply given a repeat appointment instead of more and more medication. It appears that, for many, the giving of pills has become something of a trademark of their transactions with physicians, and it is difficult for them to dispense with it. Yet many smile and agree that perhaps medicine does not help them, or that they have the strength, self-knowledge, and ability to get along without drugs.

### Types of Dispositions Made

Of the 90 patients seen in Integration Clinic in a six-month period, only 7 patients were further referred to Psychiatric Service for intensive evaluation for psychotherapy; 6 of these were accepted for insight psychoanalytically oriented psychotherapy. By far the largest number of patients were returned to the referring clinics, with recommendations for management, including drug treatment when indicated. About one third of the patients seen have been treated with psychopharmacological agents, either in Integration Clinic or the clinic which ultimately carries responsibility for the patient. Three or four borderline or psychotic patients were referred directly to psychiatric hospitals for admission, an occasional patient was transferred to a family agency, and several were referred in their first visit to Social Service, sometimes starting casework evaluation that very day. A number of patients were told to return on a PRN basis, either to Integration Clinic or the referring clinic. A few patients were recommended for one month of supervised supportive and exploratory treatment with a fourth-year medical student.

## Types of Patients Seen

As was expected, a large percentage of patients seemed to be hospital "orphans," that is, it was seldom certain which was the most appropriate facility for these patients; they often become "rotators" with multiple visits to many of the specialty clinics. Some of these patients have on occasion been referred to Psychiatry, but such a referral often appears to be a gesture of desperation or finality rather than a hope for definitive treatment. It may very well have been a mutual recognition of this by both patient and referring physician which accounts for the failure to complete psychiatric referral, as noted earlier. Although the "rotators" seem to travel in the same circles, they are by no means a homogeneous group. Referral for psychiatric opinion is usually based on recognition by the referring physician of the element of depression but the depression is of various types and degrees. Usually, somatic symptoms are prominent and often demonstrate a remarkable constancy over a period of many years. A variety of drugs, orthopedic devices, diets, and such, have frequently been recommended, often without symptomatic improvement, in which case the patient either moves on (or is moved on) to the next specialty clinic. Very rarely is a referral made for psychiatric opinion after a single Medical Clinic visit, unless the patient is overtly psychotic or has a history of previous psychiatric illness. One new patient, with a well-documented, fairly classical agitated depression, was referred after a month of extensive work-up in Medical and Surgical Clinics, including GI series, barium enema, sigmoidoscopy, gall-bladder series, laboratory studies, and examinations. He was ultimately referred to Integration Clinic where the nature of his depressive illness was explained to him. He was treated with medication (Tofranil and Librium) and showed a marked response within two weeks. It seems very likely that many of the "rotators" have had just such a beginning in their outpatient "clinic careers." The patient mentioned here was passive enough to comply with recommended procedures in hopes of finding help, but the annoyance and anger over what seemed to him like endless tests was not yet deeply submerged, and it was possible to discuss this with him. With the more chronic patients, angry feelings toward the clinics and doctors are almost always a prominent, although often deeply hidden, part of the clinical picture, and are usually acted out in the context of their ambivalent interactions with doctors, nurses, secretaries, elevator operators, cashiers, and other personnel, rather than verbalized in their clinic visits. It appears that when some opportunity is allowed for ventilation of this anger, there is some decrease in the frequency of clinic visits, suggesting that one use of clinic facilities is the repetitive attempt to resolve conflicts engendered in part by the vicissitudes of the doctor-patient relationship.

Among patients referred to Integration Clinic, a variety of depressed types seem definable, although there is, of course, considerable overlap. Table 4 categorizes the major types of patients.

## TABLE 4

1. Masochistic Depressive Group
2. Agitated Depressive Group
   a. Mid-life (involutional) depressions
   b. Stress or loss reactions of the aged
   c. Severe reactive depressions
3. Chronic (nonagitated) Depressives
4. Miscellaneous
   a. Borderline and Psychotic Group
   b. Hysterical Conversions
   c. Severe Phobics

The masochistic depressives usually have a long history of apparent misfortune and suffering, some appearing more accidental than others. These patients may, for example, often bemoan the real loss of loved ones, but may also complain of the sacrifices they have made in a lifelong marriage of misery which they have chosen to preserve. They sometimes verbalize the dynamic meaning of their illness when they complain that "this is what comes of always being self-sacrificing and trying to help others—you end up with some incurable illness that medical science has no answer for." They frequently have a single severe symptom, such as lifelong headaches or generalized pruritus, which is refractory to the usual treatment methods. These patients seem to arouse guilt in physicians more quickly than any other type and new house officers are often quick to suggest a new treatment method on first meeting. In a sense, these patients invite, or even challenge the doctor to cure them, only to achieve their satisfaction by pointing out the doctor's failure. They insist that "the doctor knows best," but repeatedly demonstrate that he doesn't. The result is very often referral to another clinic for some other treatment.

In this manner, a string of hostile-dependent relationships is established with a variety of doctors without actually ever resolving the difficulty. In their continual search for acceptance, they repeatedly provoke rejection, often with a heightening of anger and hostility in both patient and doctor. As long as this anger remains at the core of the transaction, patients seem to have a need to return to clinics in an attempt to work this out. Management of these patients seems more effective when it adopts a pessimistic rather than an optimistic approach, when it supports the strong and independent part of the character. One can often see an immediate lifting of depressive demeanor in these patients when they are told it is extraordinary that they have managed so well in the face of their terrible life experiences. The doctor-patient interaction seems to lose some of its hostile-dependent overtones when patients are told that perhaps the doctor does not always know best, that perhaps patients themselves have good judgment about themselves in certain situations, and perhaps even know what medicines help them most. Unless these patients are acutely agitated or depressed, it seems more appropriate and beneficial to withhold medication and to encourage them to utilize their natural resources to solve their problems. If drugs must be given, they seem more effective when the patient is told that they may not help at all, and when the patient is allowed some latitude to experiment with drug dosage on his own. If a strict regimen is set up, these patients almost always come in complaining of unbearable side effects or discontinue medication without giving it an adequate trial.

The next largest category of patients is the agitated depressive group. This group encompasses a variety of conditions, including the involutional depressions of mid-life, acute depressive illness in the elderly, and severe reactive depressions to physical illness or severe trauma. The age range in this group is wide and patients may present single or multiple symptoms. They are often treated for anxiety in Medical Clinic with sedatives, hypnotics, and tranquilizers, because anxiety frequently masks their underlying depression. Very often, treatment of the anxiety component alone allows depression to break through in extreme forms and many of these patients often report worsening of their condition after initial early improvement. In one such case, a fifty-year-old housewife was seen in Medical Clinic for a check-up because she was worried about a pain on her left side of two months' duration. A thorough work-up recorded the impression of "no disease," and she was advised to return in one month. This time she was limping because of intensified pain in her left hip, and she was complaining of menstrual flow changes. A diagnostic impression of "sciatica" was recorded, X rays were ordered, and a referral was made to Orthopedic Clinic where examination revealed "no significant findings" and a diagnostic impression of "static strain" was made; treatment consisted of new shoes, back-strapping, and a bed-board. She failed to keep her next Orthopedic Clinic appointment and was not heard from again for over a year, until she finally returned to Medical Clinic to explain that she had been hospitalized in a state hospital with acute involutional depression. She continued to be depressed and was referred to Integration Clinic, where Tofranil 25 mg. TID and Librium 10 mg. TID were prescribed, and the patient was returned to Medical Clinic for continued care. Notes on the patient's chart indicate that she has been happy and calm for several months and has, for the first time in many years, returned to work as a restaurant hostess. The patients in the agitated depressed group are more capable than the masochistic group of minimizing their contact with outpatient clinics when their illness is in remission. Furthermore, they seem to respond best to adjunctive drug treatment with psychopharmacological agents.

A third group of patients seen with some frequency are the chronic depressives, with a host of vague, mild complaints, but no significant agitation or anxiety. They are usually older people, who have been isolated to a large degree from outside contacts and who seem to use the clinics for support, ventilation, and a source of supplies. Sometimes their only request is to have their blood pressure taken or to be given a bottle of laxative, or to be weighed. They respond very well to being given things, even if only vitamins or aspirin; and they often look upon their clinic visits as a kind of social event, an opportunity to meet their patient colleagues, to chat with nurses, secretaries, and elevator operators, to learn the latest medical news of their friends. These patients attribute magical powers to the clinics and the doctors; although their relationships are often ambivalent, they seem predominantly to manifest affection for them. They seem to have developed a way of life which is surrounded with an aura of depression and, quite often, attempts to treat them with antidepressant drugs result in a worsening of their condition, perhaps through some disruption of their lifelong adjustment. Unfortunately, these patients do not represent a medical challenge for many hospital physicians, and they are therefore sometimes discharged without follow-up. But it is possible that the treatment for such patients is the very type of dependent relationship upon the hospital which they have established for themselves. The medical challenge here may very well be the deliberate planning of a treatment program which, until now, has been allowed to develop casually and haphazardly. Unlike the masochistic group, these oral-dependent patients cannot be expected to return readily to clinics on a PRN basis and must be *given* additional appointments to avoid further regression and to maintain them in some marginal adjustment.

Other splinter groups of depressives include a small number each of borderline and psychotic patients, a few patients with chronic brain syndrome, a few hysterical conversions with deeply masked depression, and a few severe phobics who become depressed over the "senselessness" of their fears. This group seems to benefit from appropriate drug treatment and noninterpretive but clarifying and educative, support.

## Teaching

The ultimate objective of teaching nonpsychiatrist physicians the principles of medical psychology is partially met in Integration Clinic in a variety of ways. By working in the same setting as other clinic physicians, the psychiatrist in Integration Clinic is able to decrease the gap between medical specialties, to affiliate more closely with other physicians in an attempt to understand and treat common problems, and to participate in vis-à-vis informal discussions centered around medical problems met with in all outpatient clinics. A succinct note in the patient's record instead of a lengthy separate psychiatric consultation also seems to improve the clinic physician's attitude toward the psychiatrist. Furthermore, a note by the psychiatrist reassures the clinic physician that he may proceed attentively with his medical or surgical procedure without being assailed by doubts and fears which interfere with his clinical function. The ready access of psychiatric opinion also seems to lessen the anxiety in some physicians that arises when they are concerned that they may not be able to obtain psychiatric assistance when their patients need it most. Another boon to the teaching of medical psychology has been the use of psychopharmacological agents in Integration Clinic. Whereas it is often extremely difficult to convey the concepts of medical psychology and personality diagnosis to new house officers in a relatively pure form, it does seem to be more acceptable or palatable to them when the use of medication is part of the doctor-patient interaction.

## Miscellaneous Results

In the brief time that Integration Clinic has existed, there has been a noticeable decrease in the number of referrals to the Psychiatric Service from intrahospital sources. This has permitted a more effective use of psychiatric facilities for evaluation and treatment without being hampered by overloading. There has also been a noticeable decrease in the number of emergency psychiatric consultations requested. It has been observed in the past that physicians often request emergency psychiatric consultations even in nonemergency situations, and it has been presumed that this is at least partly explainable as the physician's concern that consultation will not be available when it is needed or that waiting lists militate against *any* psychiatric evaluation *except* on an emergency basis. Besides advancing the physician's knowledge of psychiatric principles, there is some concomitant education of the lay public through Integration Clinic contacts. Some patients with antipsychiatric attitudes seem to modify their bias and even become receptive to psychiatric assistance when they belatedly discover that they have been seen (and perhaps even helped) by a psychiatrist in their visits to Integration Clinic.

**Discussion and Summary**

The chronic clinic-goer represents a difficult management, treatment, and rehabilitation problem in most general hospitals. In addition to seeking solutions to medical problems, such patients try to solve emotional problems through their relationships with doctors, clinics, hospital, and a variety of personnel. The satisfaction of these emotional needs by the OPD appears to be highly fortuitous, resulting sometimes in distress to the patients and leading to a costly use of hospital and community resources. Clearly, before significant changes will come about in this situation, it is the task of the physician to understand more about this group of patients. If chronic depression is a major illness in this group and data suggest that it is, then this must be recognized, and depression must be treated early in the patient's contact with clinics, rather than as a complex of independent somatic symptoms treated over a long period of time in a variety of specialty clinics. Or, patients whose major goal in various clinics is seeking satisfaction of dependency needs should be treated in ways which provide more direct and less complicated means of satisfaction. A clarification of the ways in which patients use clinic facilities, the nature of the transactions which result in multiple clinic referral (often spoken of as "unloading" or "dumping"), and the influence of such practices on the course and duration of illness, may permit earlier interruption of processes which can lead to chronic invalidism. It will allow treatment and course to be influenced by plan rather than, for example, by the chance reactions of a specific doctor to a specific patient. There is clearly a need for better matching of treatment to the patient's needs and personality structure.

The doctor-patient relationship is the building block of all medical practice, and the course of the patient's illness is as greatly influenced by the vagaries of this relationship as it is by the skill of a surgical procedure or the efficacy of a drug (Balint, 1957).

Integration Clinic evolved as a logical extension of the prominent emphasis placed on the teaching of medical psychology at Beth Israel Hospital. Its orientation, in keeping with that of the Psychiatric Service, is one which stresses that treatment of any kind for any patient or group of patients is best prescribed on the basis of personality diagnosis. In addition to providing specialized treatment, evaluation, and screening, it is the clinic's objective to bring psychiatric help to reluctant or apprehensive patients, to facilitate further research into and understanding of a variety of special problems encountered in outpatient settings, and to teach the general principles of medical psychology as well as the specific characteristics of these special patients to nonpsychiatric physicians who constitute the first line of medical defense. It is apparent that certain affective disorders, such as depression, are manifested in a wide spectrum of symptoms and have a variety of meanings to the individual patients experiencing them. Furthermore, patients exhibiting similar illnesses use the doctor and the hospital in a variety of ways to work out their conflicts; they therefore require differential treatment. Integration Clinic is in a position to study intensively patients' needs, to clarify some of the complexities of the utilization of outpatient facilities, and to explore the relationship of such utilization to chronicity.

# The Psychiatric Service and the Community

# Mental Hygiene for Educators: Report on an Experiment Using a Combined Seminar and Group Psychotherapy Approach

LEO BERMAN, M.D.

ANNOUNCEMENTS WERE MAILED to educators in the Boston area who were thought to be actively interested in what modern psychology could contribute to education. It was stated that the seminar was to consist of twelve weekly sessions of two hours each and that the fee for attendance was twenty-five dollars. It was decided to draw up the application blank in a rather conventional manner and only information about professional training, experience, and present position was requested. This was done with the thought that it may help minimize the stirring up of undue misconceptions and anxieties about the course. There was no screening of the ten individuals who applied, and they were all admitted to the group.

### Report On the Group

The group consisted of nine members and the leader. A tenth member was present in the first two sessions and then dropped out with the explanation that she could not attend because of illness in the family. A secretarial employee of the Massachusetts Society for Mental Hygiene was present from the fifth session on and took verbatim notes. There were seven women and two men. Four women were unmarried. The age range was from the middle twenties to the early fifties with seven of the members thirty-five or older. There were two psychological counselors, a director of guidance with an academic background in education, a supervisor of

---

Reprinted in abridged form from *The Psychoanalytic Review*, 40:319-332, 1953.

This experiment was conducted under the aegis of the Massachusetts Society for Mental Hygiene.

teachers of religion, a teacher supervisor in a public school system, an assistant principal, two principals, and Dr. Bower, the Consultant in School Projects for the Society. Dr. Bower came to occupy an interesting position in the group: she was a member of the group and at the same time she was regarded by the others as assistant to the leader. In some respects she actually functioned as such, as for example when she was asked to take notes during the meetings. (This practice was discontinued after the fourth session as it was not altogether satisfactory.) In all, individuals from four different public school systems from the Boston area attended. Two of the group members worked in close collaboration at the same school, and two others had known each other prior to the group meetings. Three members were veterans of another experimental group learning situation, the Bethel workshop sponsored by The Research Center for Group Dynamics and The National Education Association.

The group met evenings in a large room used by the Society. All were seated around a table. The atmosphere before and after the meetings was informal and typically the buzz of conversation could be heard. However, with the start of a session there was a definite increase in tension. There was some verbalization about this tension in the very first session: various members said they felt that they didn't know much about dynamic psychology and thought that perhaps others in the group knew more. It gradually became clear to the group that it was an escape on to "safe ground" for them to engage in "shop talk." The group also soon learned that silent periods were a result of resistance to talking about themselves or one another.

Despite the tension clearly present in the first session, the leader was impressed with the liveliness and eagerness of the members to talk of their technical problems and of themselves. For example, B. in a somewhat self-enhancing fashion was talking of her achievement at school, when C. interrupted to bring up an entirely new subject. The leader called attention to this sequence and made some remarks about feelings of insecurity. B. saw the point and commented in rather friendly fashion: "We give and take. We slap down and get slapped down.'" Because of the evidently high "group morale" the leader discarded his original plan of giving some introductory lectures on dynamic psychology. Upon his suggestion it was agreed that the group decide for itself when it would discuss a more formal presentation of a school problem by one of the members and when there would be a session devoted to a freer discussion of their own feelings in the handling of school problems. The latter was characterized by a member as a situation of "being under fire."

During the twelve sessions, a total of five reports were given. These were presented at the second, fourth, sixth, seventh, and ninth sessions. Difficult problems were presented involving children, parents, and teachers and there was much useful discussion which developed. These reports also provided an opportunity for the leader to talk in a more didactic way about the psychology of adolescence, the rejected child, the compulsive personality, etc. However, it became increasingly clear to the group that such sessions were also in the service of resistance. It was interesting to observe how the group wavered back and forth between the need for the safe haven of a discussion "outside" of themselves and their wish to face the evidence accumulating during the sessions that irrational feelings in them impaired some of their functioning as educators.

For example, the third session was a very active one in which member D., who had reported on a problem in the second session, was the chief subject of discussion. As the group investigated D.'s reasons for feeling very hostile toward a teacher who, she felt, was not sufficiently understanding of a dull boy of an underprivileged background, D. brought illuminating personal material from her past. This stimulated various other members to tell of their overaggressive and "bristling" reactions to certain school situations they encountered. With the help of occasional comments and questions by the leader, the discussion then proceeded to the subject of their resentful feelings against their parents when they were younger. Another aspect of the discussion of exaggerated and irrational hostile feelings was that it resulted in a "spilling over" of aggression into the group itself which led to one or two rather pointed attacks by a member upon another. A certain self-regulatory functioning of the group then became evident when some of the members tried to divert these aggressive feelings into more peaceful and potentially useful channels.

In the fourth session there was a report by member E. It was clear to E. and to the group that the report, although technically interesting, was presented in a somewhat detached and impersonal way, and that E. had difficulty in speaking about herself. However, the leader felt that the impersonal nature of the discussion that followed the report was probably also a reaction to the more personal and open quality of the previous session. Such sequence is a familiar phenomenon from individual psychoanalytic treatment and from group psychotherapy. There was no report in the fifth session which was characterized by considerable openness by many of the members. Despite the fact that almost all the members expressed a preference for sessions without a formal report because "that's where we get most help," the sixth and seventh sessions were both largely taken up by reports and a technical discussion of them. These two sessions had the lowest attendance (Grotjahn, 1950) of the entire course. The group then seemed to gain in security so that by the end of the ninth session they reached a decision not to have any reports in the remaining three. As one of the members put it: "A presentation is not our greatest value here. It serves as a jumping-off point."

Out of the abundance of data and impressions that can arise out of twelve sessions, I should like to illustrate the vitality and constructive movement that was evident in the group with a more detailed example. In this example attention is focussed primarily on the effects of the interaction of a particular group member with the group. Some of the pertinent material and its evaluation have been altered or omitted out of consideration for the privacy of the individuals involved.

W. was one of the senior members of the group in terms of his age, experience, and the responsibility of his position. His membership in the group was but one expression of his varied interests in raising the level of functioning of the school which he headed. He had, for example, gone ahead despite opposition in instituting progressive changes at his school. In the first sessions he showed himself to be well informed on things psychological and readily engaged in some of the technical discussions that came up. At the same time he maintained a cool reserve in talking about himself at a time when several of the members had already described and discussed various of their problems. This tendency was further re-enforced by the careful, somewhat overrespectful way in which the group generally handled him. Matters were undoubtedly complicated by the fact that in some ways he was the actual superior of two or three other members in the work situation outside of the group. The only more direct evidence of a problem area that was apparent to the leader in the early sessions was a certain sharpness and edginess in W.'s exchanges with a younger male member of the group. At this time W. was circumspect in his relation to the leader.

The leader began to feel that it would be a major gain both for W. and the others if W. could more genuinely become part of the group. W. was actually a person of importance in the group, but in addition he probably represented, especially to the younger members, a friendly, but also somewhat fearsome father figure. The leader visualized the possibility of W.'s being helped through attaining a better awareness of some traits which he would certainly want to master were he more cognizant of them. Such improved awareness could then perhaps lead to some work on the origins of such traits in his earlier life in order to provide him with a more effective lever in helping himself. In the course of such development, other members of the group would have occasion to go through a learning experience in delineating a person more objectively by correcting the more distorted conceptions of him resulting from unconscious transference processes.

In the fifth session there was some evidence to show that W. was participating more as a member of the group rather than remaining the detached and cautious observer outside of it. He had been sitting by in almost complete silence for about one hour listening intently to an active discussion going on among various members. This discussion centered around the problem of finding oneself pushed by strong feelings, against one's better judgement, into strict and harsh attitudes toward others. Some school and personal material had been brought up which led to a comment by the leader to the effect that even though we may consciously reject certain ideas of our parents we may unconsciously feel just as they do. This comment was followed by corresponding personal material by several previously silent members. After a while W. suddenly remarked with some enthusiasm that this was very helpful. He then went on to report on a certain situation at school which troubled him as he did not know whether he was being too self-assertive. In the course of the brief discussion of what W. reported, S. raised a question as to whether W. appeared as "a figure of authority, an army sergeant, a father figure" to the involved person at the school. No one in the group picked up this comment and the leader felt it would be premature to focus on it at the time. However, some minutes later the leader found occasion to touch on it in a less direct fashion. A member had commented on her difficulty in talking in the group and the leader raised the question whether the age or status of the members in the group played any part in her difficulty. Shortly after, at S.'s suggestion, all the members, including the leader, gave their ages. At several points in the course of the remainder of the session, W. talked in a more personal way of some problems in his work. One of the points he brought up dealt with a problem which has so often sorely tried not only the educator: his emotional reactions to children who were disobedient and provocative. At the end of the session, during a discussion of plans for the next meetings W. volunteered to bring a report.

W. was not present at the sixth session. (He had also missed the third session.) In the seventh session he reported on a difficult problem he had been contending with for several years. An adolescent boy had been acting up in such ways as to be quite disturbing to all who dealt with him at school. W. wanted to do everything possible to avoid the last resort of expelling him. Various teachers, guidance counselors and psychiatrists had not been able to help very much. Some of the students were complaining about what seemed to them to be favored treatment being accorded the boy by the school. The mother of the boy seemed weak and ineffectual in dealing with him, and the father, who for years had been remote and indifferent, was, in more recent years, alternatingly harsh or overindulgent. When the school attempted to deal with the father, he was most uncooperative, defensive, and at times explosive. W.'s report was sensitive and comprehensive, and his mixed feelings toward the boy, of frustration and anger together with a need to suppress such feelings and show extraordinary forbearance and patience, came out clearly. This was commented upon by the leader who also indicated that one could, in such case, consider having the boy removed from the school. At the end of the session, the leader asked what the group would like to plan for next week: another report or a discussion of why this boy got under W.'s skin. (The pattern had already developed in the group of having a more open and personal discussion of a reporter in the session following a given report.) A member of about the same seniority as W. quickly remarked that she would like an open discussion very much. The others maintained a tense silence which was finally broken by E.'s remark that W. should have two votes in deciding what should be scheduled for next week. W. then said he did not know how he would be feeling next week but he was willing to have the personal discussion.

The first half of the eighth session was again characterized by the group's gingerly handling of W. The leader commented on this and asked if it was because of W.'s rank. This question was followed by more direct questions and comments by two older members. One of them expressed a feeling that W. sometimes tends to stand on authority, and again somewhat later asked W. directly, "Why do you put on a cloak of authority with the youngsters?" A younger member, S., expressed a similar feeling. These comments obviously made an impression on W. In the latter half of the session, with further prodding by other members and the leader, W., for the first time, began to bring personal material from his earlier life, which was closely related to more immediate problems under discussion. He also commented at one point that more recently he found that he was not reacting so emotionally to the boy he had reported on to the group. At the end of the session there was a rather friendly, relaxed feeling in the group. When the leader asked about the program for next week, S. thought there should be more discussion of W. W. suggested that another member bring a report in which W. played an important part. A younger member laughingly commented that was a good idea. A member who had known W. for some time commented on the favorable changes W. had undergone in the last years.

Important parts of the ninth and tenth sessions were characterized by material similar to what had come up in the latter part of the eighth session. At one point W. spontaneously returned to the earlier remark by a member of a need to cloak himself in authority and linked it up to certain feelings of insecurity he had had some years ago and which in more recent years were diminishing.

The latter half of the eleventh session and the twelfth and last session were strongly influenced by a tapering off process. This process was touched off when a member inquired about different group approaches. The leader went along with the interest the group manifested in this subject for two reasons: (1) After the personal nature of the sessions, he felt it would facilitate a return to a more ordinary kind of interpersonal relationship among the members to discuss a particular subject rather objectively. (2) The subject of groups provided an opening to the leader to ask how the members felt about this group and the functioning of its leader. In the course of these discussions it was of interest to note W.'s remarks on the learning process in the group. He defended the technique of presenting reports because, "you have to have a real situation before you can get anywhere." He stressed the importance of feelings in learning and added that one goes from emotional experience to learning from interpretation rather than from intellectual understanding. He said that twelve sessions was a very short time and wished there were more. He rather approved of the leader's approach in "bringing a person out" so that the person was not too uncomfortable, but he rather disapproved of the extent of the leader's silence and suggested that it frustrated the person involved.

### Discussion

The experiment yielded some positive results and also raised many problems. To varying degrees, all the members seemed to feel it was a valuable experience for them in which they had deepened their psychological understanding of others and learned helpful things about themselves. There was a unanimous feeling that the group should meet further with the primary purpose of learning more about themselves. Those members who had attended the Bethel workshop stated that the approach used in the present experiment complemented the Lewinian approach in that some of the personal factors making for a loss in effective functioning were exposed and worked on constructively. The writer came away with the feeling that the experiment was promising and that further explorations of the approach were worthy of study. It appeared to indicate that in a group one could successfully enter into the seeming shadowland in which education and psychotherapy, as ordinarily understood, merge into one another. The experiment was also a demonstration that the theoretical criticism by psychoanalysts that there was a relative neglect of genetic considerations in Lewin's work could have some practical significance (Hartmann & Kris, 1946).

There are broader implications in the effective development of a combined seminar and group psychotherapy approach from the mental hygiene point of view. Such approach could provide a means through which many people fulfilling important functions in the community could be reached. Most of these people would never think of consulting a psychiatrist, quite apart from considerations of time and money, because of the minor nature of their neurotic difficulties and/or an unawareness of how these difficulties affected their work. In an attempt to clarify somewhat some of the problems confronting us in developing such techniques, the remainder of this discussion will take up briefly some points highlighted by this experiment and by other work in group psychotherapy.

### Some Theoretical Psychoanalytic Considerations

When a group meets for a definitely limited number of sessions, it is important for the leader to try and see to it that by the final session there be no *excessive* amount of activated conflicts and anxieties present which then leave the members uncomfortably suspended in mid-air. It is self-evident that the more limited in number the sessions are, the more important it becomes to avoid more highly charged conflict areas. In the group here described the leader deliberately avoided the sexual area although various openings presented themselves in the course of the sessions to enter into it. There were two or three brief, quite intense exchanges in the ideological area, involving religion and labor unions which the leader felt would be too "group-disruptive" to deal with in a group of this type. In addition to the helpful effects of various transferences, partial identifications, suggestion, and catharsis, the help derived from discussion of personal problems in this group is better referred to as a process of "clarification" rather than as one leading to "true insight" (E. Bibring,

1953). By that it is meant that the insight gained refers to preconscious material rather than to strongly repressed unconscious material. There is some reason to believe that other more intensive psychoanalytic group therapy approaches do result in a gain in true insight.

## The Group

This group was a very mixed one from various aspects, and no attempt was made to screen the applicants. Except for Dr. Bower, the writer had never seen any of the other members before the first session, and the only information about them available to him derived from the application blanks. This lack of information was a point of some concern to the leader, but he hoped that his clinical experience in both individual and group psychotherapy would guide him through this difficulty. It is not possible to say from this single experiment whether there was a significant chance factor present which made for this group's effective functioning, or whether the generalization can be made that a well-trained and experienced leader should be able to contend with practically any group similarly organized. This important point will have to await further study.

Some data are available from this experiment on the problem of the psychologically vulnerable member who participates in such a group. A member who was quite active in the first six sessions had a flare-up of an old psychosomatic condition for which she had been and still was in psychiatric treatment. She missed the next four sessions because of this illness. It was of interest that when she became ill she phoned Dr. Bower and, for the first time, told of the details of her illness and suggested that Dr. Bower keep the leader informed. When she felt better, she phoned the leader and asked if she could rejoin the group. Upon her return to the group she described some aspects of her illness. This led to an interesting discussion of the guilt feelings of some of the members, including the leader, who felt that perhaps some of their remarks had contributed to her relapse. She recalled instances of transient somatic symptoms after two sessions when certain material was brought up by herself and by the leader. She did not think the sessions had any direct bearing on the recurrence of her illness, but on further questioning thought it might be a possibility. Without further information the writer does not see how one can go beyond this evaluation. However, this incident does suggest that a tactful way should be sought to obtain more background information on prospective group members.

As regards the somewhat delicate matter of the participation in the same group of individuals of varying status from the same school or school system, it seemed from this experiment that the advantages outweighed the disadvantages. Here, too, a final answer will have to await further experience with the method. The possibility has also to be kept in mind that a psychopath may be inclined to use the personal material of the members that comes up in the group against these members on the outside. There was no such development in this group although one of the members complained that several others had made some remarks of her behavior in the group to mutual acquaintances outside. This point was taken up in the group and it seemed that the members then saw more clearly how important the matter of strict keeping of confidences, which had been agreed upon in the first session, was.

In closing this brief discussion of the group some additional impressions are noted which may be worthy of further investigation: (1) Some of the material from this experiment centering around Dr. Bower and certain experiences from psychoanalytic group therapy suggest the possible value, especially for certain personality types in the group, of the presence of a semi-official mother figure to work with the leader (father figure). (2) The optimum size of the type of group discussed here is probably ten to fifteen members. (3) It may be of value to increase the number of sessions in a single course to fifteen and also to consider a plan of additional courses annually for the same group.

### The Leader

It is quite evident from the above that a leader of such a group should be a well-trained and experienced person. This is of particular importance in the present experimental phase of this method with its various possibilities of undesirable side-effects. More concretely, it seems to me that the leader should be psychoanalytically trained with clinical experience in individual and group psychotherapy, and also in the problems reported on by the members in the seminar part of the course.

The nature of the leader's functioning in the group deserves some comment. There are some analysts who believe that the analyst actually participates, to a certain degree, in a personal and emotional way in the individual psychoanalytic treatment situation and that such participation is a significant factor in the therapeutic process (Berman, 1949). The degree of such participation by the leader of a group seems to be greater. For example, the leader in the course of the group work described here felt it to be appropriate to refer to his age and guilt feelings when these points came up for discussion among the members in regard to themselves. Apart from these infrequent instances, when the leader, as it were, verbally demonstrated that he was a member of the group, he was also aware at different times that the impact of the group on him aroused certain anxieties, and he found himself working on these anxieties both during and after sessions like the other group members do. One may say that the leader is also a member of the group in the sense that he, to a certain extent, participates emotionally in the group process and benefits from some of its educational and therapeutic effects (Grotjahn, 1950).

To summarize: a group approach to enhance self-understanding and the understanding of others with the chief purpose of improving the group members' functioning level on the job has been described and illustrated. This approach is so oriented as to encourage the active participation of individuals fulfilling important functions in the community. Some of the problems posed by this method were noted and discussed.

# Psychoanalysis and Group Psychotherapy

## LEO BERMAN, M.D.

PSYCHOANALYTIC PSYCHOTHERAPY is showing a wholesome tendency toward more experimentation in an effort to deal with the old problem of extending substantial help to the many who need it. For example, some analysts are experimenting with variables like the technical handling of the interview itself, or the length and frequency of interviews. Others are exploring further the potentialities of working dynamically with the patient after his ego state has been altered through drugs or hypnosis. The various types of group psychotherapy in use at present represent another avenue of approach. Whatever the future may decide about the value or lack of value of these efforts, there is no question but that interesting clinical data are being brought to light.

After some brief introductory notes on group psychotherapy it is the purpose of this paper to examine the analytic situation in its group aspects, and to comment on some unconscious and ego psychological aspects of group psychotherapy. It is hoped thereby to somewhat further our understanding of both these forms of therapy. In connection with these considerations some suggestions will then be made in regard to certain possible lines of additional investigation in group psychotherapy.

As there are different types of group psychotherapy, the writer would like to specify that for the purposes of this paper those group psychotherapies are under consideration which are based more or less on analytic thinking, and are carried out with smaller sized groups, not exceeding ap-

Reprinted from *The Psychoanalytic Review*, 37:156-163, 1950.

proximately eight or ten patients. Thus the work of representative writers like Ackerman, Lowrey, Redl, Schilder, Slavson and Wender come under consideration.

There are, of course, a number of obvious differences between psychoanalytic treatment and group psychotherapy. These can be illustrated with a few selected examples. The fact that more than two individuals are present in the therapeutic situation allows for an increase in transference possibilities, both as regards the transferences between patients and therapist, and among the patients themselves. Because of the identification mechanisms in play, it develops that there are not only a group of patients and one therapist, but several therapists, or perhaps to put it more precisely, an hierarchy of therapists, with the actual therapist at the apex. Instead of a resemblance to a parent-child situation as in psychoanalysis, one deals more with what corresponds to a family situation of a parent with a number of children.

For the analyst who is a beginner in group psychotherapy, these and other complications may be rather taxing. The therapist has constantly to keep a triple orientation in mind; he must note the behavior and verbal material of the individual patient as in analysis; he must try to be aware of the specific effects any given behavior or material of an individual patient may have on the other individual patients, and he has to consider the group as a whole, the direction it is taking, and whether the "group climate" (Redl 1944, 1944a) is favorable toward therapeutic aims. However, I found that beginning work in group psychotherapy was approximately as difficult as beginning work in analysis. After a while one feels more at home in it and seems to develop what Redl has referred to as a "group action memory."

It is important to note that it is not easy to draw the line between the concept of individual psychology and that of group or social psychology. Freud (1922) noted that, in a certain extended sense, "Individual psychology is at the same time social psychology as well." Redl (1944, 1944a) and Erikson (1945) illustrate the opposing points of view on this subject. Whereas Redl speaks of a deep-seated difference between individual motivation and group psychology, Erikson questions the existence of any really different psychological laws which apply to the individual in a group, as opposed to the isolated individual.

To pose an unfamiliar-sounding question, can psychoanalytic treatment be viewed as a kind of group therapy? Although in practice we refer to a situation of patient-therapist as an individual psychotherapy, and patients-therapist as group psychotherapy, we are faced with the fact that the former situation is one consisting of two individuals. Whether we care to refer to such situation of two individuals as a "group" or not is a matter of semantics. Freud (1922), for example, cautiously referred to the hypnotic relation as a "group formation with two members." The important thing to note is that the psychological field in both situations of individual and group psychotherapy includes an entity "individual patient" and an entity "therapist." Such viewpoint, of course, highlights the similarities of both types of therapy, as opposed to some of the contrasts noted above. Slavson's (1947) conception of group psychotherapy as treatment of the individual in the group rather than through the group seems closely related to this viewpoint.

Apart from the fact that objectively it is a situation *à deux*, certain rather familiar observations in analysis show that subjectively the patient frequently experiences the walls of the analyst's office as being semipermeable. There are chance meetings with other patients, real or imagined, perception of a warmed-up couch from the preceding patient, cigarette stubs in waiting-room ashtrays, the analyst's secretary, etc. Some of these experiences remain uncathected in the analysis, while others may become important parts of the analytic situation. For example, significant infantile rivalry constellations both as regards oedipal and sibling jealousies may be activated by these real experiences continuous to the therapeutic situation. Thus, although in group psychotherapy a number of individuals are spacially and temporally contiguous during the actual therapeutic session, it may be seen that in psychoanalysis, in connection with the patient's experience of the unsharp boundaries of the analyst's office and the timelessness of the unconscious, the patient may react to the analytic situation as if there were more than two individuals present. It may also be noted that some experiences like hearing the analyst talk on the telephone, or seeing him talk to his secretary are important in that they help the patient in his anxious, searching and indispensable evaluation of the analyst as a real person.

In contrast to the above instances in which the representations of contiguous real persons were, so to speak, thrust upon the patient to become vectors in the analytic situation, there is another set of familiar phenomena occurring during analytic treatment in which the patient takes a more active role. I refer to acting-out phenomena outside of the analysis. From the point of view of the analytic situation as constituting a group of two, the patient can be impelled, for various reasons, to enlarge this group. Psychologically considered, the added real person or persons then become integral parts of the analytic situation for a period. Occurring typically in connection with the transference situation, the acting out may consist, for example, of sexual behavior, or, in cases of psychologically determined physical symptoms, a seeking of medical attention. From the way the patient refers to such behavior during a session, it is almost as if the person with whom the acting out occurs were actually present at the patient's side, with both pitted against the analyst. One gains the impression in some cases that without this psychological enlargement by the patient of the therapeutic group of two, the pronounced anxieties of the patient in connection with the transference could lead to the patient's flight from the analysis.

There are, of course, other evidences pointing to the intrapsychic experience of the analytic situation by the patient as consisting of more than two individuals. In the transference the analyst can represent a number of persons, at times even simultaneously, as for example, when he represents both parents. In cases in which strong pregenital tendencies are present, and in which the unity of the body ego is impaired, partial objects are experienced as independent entities, and furthermore, various inanimate things like furniture, etc. come alive. However, these instances do not come under consideration in this paper, as we are concerned only with examples of rather real, whole objects who become a part of the analytic situation, and who continue to retain a large degree of their individuality in the patient's mind. Only such examples show a correspondence to what obtains in group psychotherapy.

The above considerations suggest that there is no sharp line between individual and social psychology, and that individual psychoanalytic treatment can in a sense be considered a group psychotherapy. From the point of view of these considerations, it is not surprising that some descriptions of unconscious and ego-psychological factors in group psychotherapy, and of differences between psychoanalytic treatment and group psychotherapy impress one at times as somewhat misleading. This is in part a result of an insufficient appreciation by some authors of the fact that many of Freud's illuminating statements on group psychology are based on descriptions of mobs, and do not, without modification, apply to the ordinary therapeutic group.

A recent paper (Pederson-Krag, 1946) on unconscious factors in group therapy appeared to me as representative of the thoughts of some analysts about group psychotherapy. After noting Freud's observation that when an individual becomes part of a group his unconscious mental processes tend to dominate his conscious processes, the author suggested a classification of the various group therapies based on the "preconscious fantasies they best exemplify." One gained the impression from this paper that the author felt that the gratification of various preconscious fantasies was the chief element in the deeper therapeutic effect of the treatment. The concluding sentence in the paper likened the group therapy situation to certain religious ceremonies used by the priests to control and lessen the anxiety of the congregation.

There is no doubt that various unconscious factors weigh heavily in the so-called "repressive inspirational" types (Thomas, 1943) of group psychotherapy. Although of theoretical and practical importance, these are in some ways of lesser interest to the analyst. It is questionable, however, how justified Pederson-Krag was in assigning the same importance to such factors in the analytically oriented type of group psychotherapy. She did not distinguish between those group therapies in which the therapist gratifies various infantile wishes, either naïvely or planfully, or analyzes them to further insight. Therapy groups, like the analytic situation, favor the activation of various regressive phenomena. However, the crux of the matter in both situations lies in the use of his knowledge of the dynamic situation by the therapist for the specific goals he has set for the treatment.

As opposed to the one-sided consideration of group psychotherapy as a process which offers primarily a gratification of infantile wishes, there is also another tendency to view it either primarily or in considerable part as a kind of educational experience, as a "more real experience than individual therapy," which is "less bound to the irrationalities of the unconscious and is weighted on the side of allegiance to social reality," (Ackerman, 1945). Activity group therapy has been described by its originator, Slavson (1947), as "predominantly an ego therapy" in which "ego strengthening" is the counterpart to insight gaining which occurs in individual psychotherapy and in interview group psychotherapy. Slavson also described the therapeutic process in activity group therapy as being based upon acting out and leading to "derivative insight; namely derived from the patient's own growth rather than from interpretation by other members of the group or the therapist."[1]

In attempting to evaluate the above-quoted and other formulations, the problem is not that they do not carry a certain ring of truth in them as being representative of the clinical data. Rather, they impress me as occasionally tending toward exaggerated emphasis of the differences between individual and group psychotherapy. It seems to me, for example,

[1] It should be noted, however, that Slavson (1947) believes individual and group psychotherapy are based fundamentally on the same psychodynamics.

that no psychoanalytic treatment can be successful unless it becomes a "real experience," and the analyst becomes a "real" person. All psychotherapy, including psychoanalysis, works only with and through the ego, and achieves its results by increasingly strengthening the ego. As the ego, during psychoanalysis, grows in strength, it is likely that much "derivative insight" occurs, as was described in activity group therapy. It can also be stated that psychoanalysis, like various group psychotherapies, indirectly helps the ego achieve some successful repressions of a more stable sort, through increasing the strength of the ego. A reading of the "Symposium on the Theory of the Therapeutic Results of Psychoanalysis" (Glover et al., 1937), while keeping in mind the observations and formulations described by various group psychotherapists, will offer much stimulation to the interested analyst. It may be noted here that closer consideration of the commonly used terms "education" and "treatment" leads to difficulty in determining where the one ends and the other begins. A sampling from psychoanalytical writings reveals a wide range of opinion in regard to this point, and emphasizes the need for more precise formulation.

If it is true that group psychotherapy can be approximately as effective in attaining the limited goals which any sound psychoanalytic psychotherapy (apart from regular psychoanalysis) strives for, then it is deserving of systematic investigation. This is particularly the case when we consider that larger numbers of patients can be treated, and, from the qualitative point of view, that certain patients who experience the single interview situation as an insurmountable barrier, become accessible in the group. There are two variables of paramount importance which are inherent in the group psychotherapy situation, and which lend themselves readily to experimental manipulation. These variables are the size of the group, and the individual make-up of the group.

The goal in manipulating these two variables is to help attain optimum transference and anxiety levels in the individual patient to facilitate the flow and the handling of conflictual material. This material comes up not only in the form familiar to us from psychoanalysis, but also in the transference reactions of the patients to one another. The pitfalls to be avoided are groupings which offer too much gratification, and those which are too anxiety-provoking. It is very striking, for example, to observe how the addition or removal of a single patient in a small group can affect the capacity of the other group members to use the treatment situation effectively.

We need clinical data based on careful study of groups of increasing size, beginning with the smallest, a group of two patients and the therapist. What are the advantages and disadvantages for patients with specific problems and backgrounds to be placed in a group of a specific size and composition? Is it advantageous or disadvantageous to construct a resemblance in the group to the actual size, age, and sex distribution of the patients' families? It can readily be seen that it is possible in this way to achieve in a more natural manner what Moreno arranges through his psychodramatic technique. How homo- or heterogeneous should the group be as regards the psychodynamic diagnosis, symptomatic picture, present life situation, prognostic outlook, etc.? Any hunches or impressions one may have should be tested clinically.

There is also the problem of concomitant individual psychotherapy. How regular a feature should it be during group psychotherapy? It would be of much interest to study different groups whose individuals receive varying amounts of individual psychotherapy, including psychoanalysis. Which is preferable in a given patient; to have him seen individually by his group therapist or by another therapist? It is clear that a well organized research project will require a team of workers to investigate these and other questions.

In conclusion, I should like to draw attention to the following. It perhaps has not been sufficiently realized that the development of group psychotherapy as a therapeutic tool provides a favorable opportunity for the analyst to further his contribution to the study of social psychology. He is now in a position to apply his special skills to the direct study of groups. Such work may help to extend the interrelationships of psychiatry and other allied fields. Although much important work in group psychotherapy has developed along psychoanalytic lines, it is noteworthy that relatively few psychoanalysts have actually engaged in such work. Psychoanalysts have tended to delegate the actual work with groups to social workers or psychologists under their supervision. It is hoped that this paper may stimulate some psychoanalysts to work more actively in this field.

### Summary

Considerations have been advanced which underline certain similarities between psychoanalysis and group psychotherapy. It was suggested that in a sense, psychoanalysis can be viewed as a group psychotherapy, and that group psychotherapy is neither uncontrollably dominated by unconscious forces nor simply educational in a superficial sense. Some suggestions were made about further research in group psychotherapy, with particular emphasis on problems of grouping in relation to the attainment of optimum anxiety levels and transference reactions.

# A Group Approach in the Contexts of
# Therapy and Education

NORMAN E. ZINBERG, M.D.

DAVID SHAPIRO, PH.D.

IN THIS PAPER WE describe a psychoanalytic group approach with nurses, psychiatrists, educators and college students. The group work was conducted primarily within an educational setting, and in the main, the participants accepted the groups as professional training requiring the expression of personal ideas and feelings that might bear on their professional status.

The groups were conducted for two purposes: (1) to learn about individual problems of professional identity and development, emphasizing how individuals respond differently in similar professional environments and how, with increased understanding of this interaction, more flexibility in these situations is possible—the groups might enable participants to state consciously the values that define for them a concept of competence in their work; (2) to learn about group dynamics and process through group observation and self-study in order to increase understanding of daily professional meetings and conferences where so much of what goes on remains unspoken—group participants would hope to learn more about, and avoid, the irrational personal reactions in themselves and in others that interfere with the stated purposes of the groups and with the goals of their daily work.

In the group approach, selected elements of psychoanalytically-oriented individual and group psychotherapy are utilized in combination with an "objective" kind of discussion, as in conventional teaching.

Typically, the groups are set up in the following manner: Each group

Reprinted from *Mental Hygiene*, 47:108-116, 1963.

meets with a group leader for fifteen weekly sessions of one and one-half hours each. Group members are asked to describe situations and incidents from their daily work which occasioned their undue or untoward reactions.

These accounts are then discussed, with the goal of clarifying some of the subjective and objective components which helped bring about such reactions. Inquiries may then lead to a limited and selected exploration of pertinent adolescent or childhood situations.

As the development of the group proceeds, increasing attention is paid to the emotional reactions of group members to one another and to the group leader. An effort is made to relate these reactions to psychological factors which interfere with professional growth and development of the participants themselves. At selected points during such work, the group leader utilizes some of the interactions which have occurred during the meetings as concrete illustrations of various psychological phenomena which are otherwise difficult to grasp in a meaningful way, as in lecture or written material.

The arrangement for fifteen sessions allows the groups to follow a traditional educational period (semester). The limitation of time keeps the situation to a restricted number of goals and helps put a ceiling on the amount of personal material brought into discussion. Although the groups are offered as part of regular teaching programs, it is made clear at the beginning that membership and continuing attendance is voluntary. Experience has shown that group memberships up to fifteen can work effectively. The size of the groups may be limited by the particular requirements of the institution or situation. It is important that the group leader be well trained and experienced in individual and group therapy, and also conversant with the particular professional problems of the participants.

The basic rationale of this group approach was stated by Dr. Leo Berman (1953a).

> The group leader (the writer) saw in the experiment a potential usefulness from the practical and research points of view. The seminar approach with an experienced clinician offered an opportunity to deepen the educator's psychological understanding of these students and colleagues in a way which could be more meaningful than other more academic approaches, as in some college courses and lectures for example. At the same time, it offered the possibility of dealing constructively with some of the minor subjective anxieties and conflicts of "normal" individuals fulfilling important functions in the community.

It is well-known to psychoanalysts, from teaching experiences with social workers, psychiatrists, and others, that difficulties may arise during the learning of psychological material because of the specific subjective meanings of this material to the individual concerned.

The individual may be consciously aware of such difficulty, as for example, when he becomes anxious and preoccupied when subject matter dealing with masturbation or intense rivalry comes up. He may also be unaware of the difficulty because the conflictual area may have been more or less repressed. In such instances the individual may feel bored and conclude that this or that subject is unimportant or he may manifest hostility, insisting that the material is absurd, etc.

Although, of course, there are individual differences, it is not yet entirely clear as a matter of policy whether it is better, during the *individual* learning situation (as in a "consultation" or "control hour") for the teacher to sidestep the conflictual area in the student when it becomes apparent, or to try and deal with it somewhat from the student's personal point of view, with the hope of diminishing the intensity of the emotional block to learning.

There is some basis for proceeding cautiously with the latter approach as it may set in motion various complicating emotional currents in the student toward his teacher, so that the result may be a loss rather than a gain in learning capacity.

Workers in psychoanalytic group therapy have been frequently impressed with the relative freedom with which patients are able to talk about intimate and painful matters and with the degree of helpful discussion that takes place within the group.

It became apparent that in the *group* learning situation there were forces in play which facilitated such processes. . . . It seems that probing questions and painful interpretations coming from a sibling—or peer —figure have a different quality and invoke less anxiety than when they come from the group leader, who, most typically but not exclusively, represents a parental figure. There is no doubt that a given, more inhibited patient has occasion to learn from a freer patient in the group, that it is possible to bring up intimate material which, through discussion, can lead to new, useful insights. . . .

The question had to be faced whether a group of "normals" would tolerate a procedure similar in some respects to that used with psychiatric patients and. if so. would it be helpful.

## Basic Assumptions

Certain assumptions are made implicitly throughout. The group approach is founded on the belief that insight is good. Another way of saying this is that the more we know about ourselves and other people, individually and in groups, the more likely we are to be able to establish and maintain an atmosphere that will facilitate our professional goals. We are aware that this idea, while often commended, has never been acceptably validated.

Another assumption is that the groups are for the purpose of helping members achieve a measure of objective clarity about themselves and others so that they in turn may be more professionally useful. This almost "pollyannish" claim implies good will on the part of group leaders and group members. We are not so unsophisticated as to believe that such good will is unfaltering. However, it is our conviction that whatever unconscious conflicts may exist, the people who attend the groups prefer, when possible, to help rather than hurt the people for whom they have a responsibility.

We also assume that while it may be helpful to be tuned in on various emotional wave lengths, it is no substitute for knowledge. To be a good teacher or a good nurse or a good doctor requires a great deal more than good will or dedication. The knowledge and understanding gained in these groups may broaden and deepen the effective use of one's capacities to work productively.

It is here especially that we do not wish to be misunderstood. An unfortunate experience that occasionally befalls the presentation of this material at meetings or staff conferences is for the listener to misinterpret our assumptions. Listeners hear us saying that the educator's responsibility may in many situations be broader than, say, to improve the student's knowledge of history, and they interpret this to mean that we feel that the educator's chief function is what may be described as a therapeutic one. Our wish is to broaden the stereotyped definition of teaching or patient care, not to replace it.

Some educators and school administrators who are prone to be critical or even rejecting of group approaches like these cite the "therapeutic" elements as a negative characteristic. They state that individuals who participate in such groups are obliged to expose themselves unduly by talking about their personal background, experience, or personality. They feel that groups like these are aimed toward greater self-exploration and understanding than would be appropriate in a school or other educational institution.

It is true that discussions get into typical modes individuals have of responding to others, as well as into their emotional reactions. Many educators are inclined to see this kind of material as appropriate only to the home environment of the student or, in certain instances, to such special adjunctive services of the school as a counseling service or mental hygiene clinic.

In the same way, educators often criticize psychiatric methods for not teaching skills and information rather than for emphasizing feelings and human relationships. Some of the current writing on science and teaching and on educational methods in general derogates the importance of human relationships in education.

Psychotherapists, in contrast, may tend to view group approaches like these in terms of their educational content and significance as well as their therapeutic implications. This point of view goes back to the origins of the group approach in medicine in its attempts to use group discussion for teaching medical psychology, as well as in attempts by psychiatrists and psychoanalysts to apply their theories and techniques to problems of education, adaptation, and work.

Recent developments in psychoanalysis and psychiatry place a greater emphasis upon the functioning of the normal personality, and it is for this reason that applied group approaches have generated a great deal of interest. On the other hand, some practitioners have tended to be critical of group approaches because of a suspiciousness of the "educational" elements and emphasis. Their attitude is expressed in the words of one: "No matter what you call it, it is only therapy that counts or that would bring about any important change."

### Therapy versus Education

It would seem, then, depending upon one's own frame of reference, that the group approach may be placed in the category of education or in the category of therapy. We place it in the middle of such a continuum.

Therapy at its best is not necessarily different from education at its best, especially where we take the latter to mean the bringing forth or the maturing of capacities in individuals. Education stresses the learning of new information and new material, while therapy accents the understanding of personal and social modes of adaptation which have been interfered with or blocked; yet this distinction is not a sharp one since no individual comes to any situation without a background of previous experience and development.

There may be a point where it is difficult to distinguish formation from re-formation in education. In other words, any educational method must consider the individual and his capacities to learn.

The learning process, whether it takes place in an educational context or in psychotherapy, requires, among other things, that the person allow himself to open up to a new situation and to a new set of problems. Foremost is the ability to form a relationship with the person having the defined role of therapist or teacher.

The student or the patient has the goal of augmenting his own knowledge, not only of the outside world, but also of his internal response to the environment, to social situations, and to people in general.

The knowledge acquired in education may or may not be functional; it may serve directly in the initiation of new kinds of activities, new ways of perceiving things or people, new ways of finding gratification. Effective teaching or effective therapy allows one to do, feel, or perceive what he could not do before.

The importance of the relationship established between teacher and student is not always acknowledged by educators who stress the specific content and mechanics of learning, often without regard for its motivational underpinnings.

In therapy, it is through the analysis of the relationship established between therapist and patient, and especially the resistances of the patient to treatment, that psychotherapy is effective. Such analysis on a personal level does not occur in most educational settings; but whether the context be therapeutic or educational, with a *group* of students or patients the situation is made more complex. Can each person in a group have the desired relationship with teacher or therapist, a relationship uniquely catered to his needs and personality?

A teacher has to make the same kind of decision, whether explicit or implicit, as to how far he or she will go in dealing with individual needs and motivations. Some teachers can only teach certain kinds of students and are not equipped to deal with special problems. Others refuse to modify their procedures and rather feel they can reach *only so many* students effectively. These questions touch on the values of the teacher and, indirectly, on his or her personality. One of the purposes of discussion groups for educators is to provide the possibility for examining the teacher's motivations, interests, and perceptions so as to help extend his operations and negotiations with students: for example, to reach students with whom he is not usually capable of dealing.

As to the leader in the group approach discussed here, he uses a very special technique throughout the course of his seminar. Despite the resistances of a group as a whole or the resistances of individuals, he persists in maintaining the basic orientation.

There is little modification of this structure. That is, the group meeting is a place to take up a person's interpersonal feelings and reactions, whether prompted by events in the work situation or in the group situation itself, by personal experiences or by professional encounters, by individual feelings or by group relationships.

Perhaps a major virtue of the orientation is its attempt to relate group content and process to important individual and external content and process, so that problems on the job do not have to be seen as being distinct from personal problems, individual experiences not distinct from group experiences, and, to some extent, therapy not completely distinct from education.

In some discussions, the group leader may point out, where appropriate, that hostility between members of a professional organization has its impact on the quality and quantity of teaching care given. Hostilities between teachers or between teachers and principals or supervisors may have their direct effects on pupils, for if the pupil realizes there are ill feelings among the staff members, he may find himself in the position of playing one against the other, or of suffering the possible consequences by being the butt of staff hostility.

In the actual group work, it may be possible for the group leader to point out that it is very common for groups to direct hostility onto a specific target, either internally or externally, instead of tolerating the hostility directly. Groups often seek an external target for their hostility, a scapegoat, the out-group, an external enemy, and it is possible for a group leader under certain conditions to clarify this group process for the participants.

It is likely that the unique quality of the groups has a lot to do with their involving character. Novelty and surprise seem to be important dimensions in any kind of learning situation, and the groups provide these to a great extent. They challenge one's conventional ways of approaching things and of seeing things. At the same time, they provide support so that it is possible to explore not only realistic points of view but also fantasies, fears, and anxieties.

One may regress constructively to an earlier mode of adaptation or perception and in so turning back to earlier modes of reaction he may learn more about one's reactions to present situations, and perhaps learn how to achieve personal and professional goals more effectively.

### Group Case Study

At this point, an example from a group might be of help to clarify how the connections are established for the group participants between personality traits, individual personal experience, and increased professional sensitivity and competence. The example is taken from an educators' group of twelve members, meeting for the eighth of fifteen sessions.

The group members were from city-wide public schools, and none had known each other before. Typically in such a situation, it takes a few sessions for the members to get to know each other, and half-way through, if all has gone well, is the time of the most intense work.

One member of the group, Mr. A., was principal of a school in a rather wealthy outlying section of the city. By this time he had established himself in the group as a thoughtful, intelligent person respected by other members. He was just a trifle distant in commenting on the contributions of others. In this session the conversation turned to the issue of public vs. private school as educational instruments.

This was a valid continuation of discussion from a previous session concerning the problem of Miss R., whose school had begun to draw a socially lower-class group of students than previously and who felt that she was becoming less useful as a teacher to this group of students.

From one or two of his comments, the group leader was sure that Mr. A. believed that Miss R. suffered partially because she felt lower-class children lowered her status. Other group members had also questioned Miss R.'s personal feelings about this shift in the school, but she had steadfastly maintained that she loved these new, more waif-like children, but because of her own lack was unable to teach them. Various others in the group supported Miss R. in what the group leader felt to be a denial by her of a hurt feeling at not having as well-prepared children.

This narcissistic injury led to a rigid continuance of her old way of teaching despite her undeniable knowledge as an educator that a change both in content and method was in order. The group was split but no one stated this explicitly.

It was with some surprise that the group leader heard Mr. A. vehemently decry private schools as undemocratic and as a source of trouble to public schools. In answer to a direct question from another group member, he admitted that after the sixth grade he had lost many of his better pupils to private schools, although his school ran through the eighth grade. He was aware of his resentment but insisted that this was not the reason that he disliked private schooling. He said that in some ways the transfers eased the burdens on the seventh and eighth grades and enabled him to have smaller classes and to try out educational techniques that could not be done otherwise.

Mr. A. stated he had made his position known in his community when the annual town meeting struggle about the school budget occurred. He had reason to fight because some of the town members who sent their children to private schools were reluctant to grant more funds, for which they would pay increased taxes.

The group leader understood quite well and sympathized with the difficulties of a man in Mr. A.'s position in his fight to get the best for his school. However, the group leader was impressed by the extent of Mr. A.'s annoyance with private schools and also noticed that Mr. A. put the chief weight of his arguments on the concepts of democracy rather than on the good that might come out of educational experiments. It seemed that Mr. A. fought a just fight on dubious moral principles rather than on the facts, and this led the group leader to wonder about an irrational personal involvement on the part of Mr. A.

A curious split now developed in the group. One subgroup, who had tried to get Miss R. to see that her position was not the best one for a teacher, and who had more or less seen Mr. A. as their leader, were now slightly bewildered and quiet. Another subgroup who had felt that Miss R. should, to quote one, "teach as best she could and if they [the pupils] didn't get it, that was their problem" now supported Mr. A. in his idea that democracy was at issue.

The group leader felt it necessary to intervene. First, for the sake of the group as a whole it was necessary to help those members who were temporarily out of it. Second, he recognized that the group was espousing an irrational idea, i.e., that "democracy" was the point at issue. The group leader felt that what was going on in the group was based on emotional conflict and not on an intellectual difference about abstract political philosophy or even the concrete concern about where private schools fit into our society.

He felt that the question of where principles such as democracy fitted into their classroom work and presentations was a source of anxiety for teachers. This concern, so much greater in recent years, made it especially important that the group leader clarify the possibility that this use of an emotionally laden catchword was a defense against facing some painful personal feelings. An acceptance of this distortion of an educational concept in the group would be seen as unfortunate. Third, Dr. N. felt that if Mr. A. could understand something more of his involvement in this question of private vs. public schools, he would be a more effective administrator.

Dr. N. entered the discussion for the first time by asking Mr. A. if he had gone to private school. When Mr. A. said no, Dr. N. persisted by asking if any of his friends had. Mr. A. smiled and said yes, and said he

came from a small town fifty miles from Boston and that his gang had
been split up when two of his closest friends had gone off to boarding
school. He continued by saying that he knew what Dr. N. had in mind but
he doubted if it affected his attitude toward private schools.

Dr. N. was then silent, and so was the group, for thirty to forty seconds.
Finally one of the members, who had been quiet as a result of the group
split, asked if Mr. A. ever saw his old friends. Mr. A. now began to look
a trifle more annoyed and said no. Several of the people who had supported
Miss R. and Mr. A. then talked slightly anxiously in general terms until
the end of the session.

The next meeting began rather desultorily with pauses and silences.
Finally Mr. A., who had been silent, said that he had given last week's
discussion a lot of thought. To his surprise he said he had been so angry
when he left that his wife had noticed it when he got home, but he couldn't
remember exactly what had set it off. The group leader said that he thought
it had been the question of whether he ever again saw the old friends who
had gone to private schools. Mr. A. said he guessed that was it, because he
really had been mad about it for years.

He then elaborated at some length on how the separation came about
in his youth. He had never connected that incident with his present attitude toward private schools, but he felt it might have some relevance. Two
other group members talked of experiencing the difficulties of the break-
up of youthful groups and sympathized with Mr. A.

The group leader then asked the group as a whole how they had felt
earlier after the difference of opinion about Miss R.'s position. Several
people chimed in together that it had made them very uncomfortable,
and they had even thought about not coming back the following week.
Miss R. then said that she had not known there was such a difference of
opinion. It seemed that the idea that she was a subject of controversy was
enough to hurt her feelings.

With Mr. A., the group leader had felt that he was dealing with a man
whose defenses were good and that had made it easy to be direct and personal. Miss R. seemed more fragile and easily upset so he merely stated
that in Mr. A.'s case it had seemed that the things that had happened to
him as a pupil might still be affecting how he behaved as a teacher and
a principal, and that some members of the group had questioned the same
sort of thing in Miss R.'s case but that others had felt that her situation
was a very difficult one in which to teach. Dr. N. purposely did not ask
her about any of her past experiences or feelings, as he might have in
group or individual therapy.

Miss R. was mollified by the group leader's answer and was quiet for a time. Several members who had previously been so interested in democracy did show that the point had been made by suggesting different teaching techniques that might be helpful to Miss R. if she wished to make changes in her teaching. The group leader felt that this intellectual interchange was very helpful as a lull because each group member had been deeply emotionally involved in the previous, more intense, personal revelations in the group.

Several sessions later Miss R. commented gratuitously that one of the technical suggestions had been very helpful and that she had used it with much success. The group leader refrained from commenting that this suggestion was one that she had undoubtedly come across previously.

We hope that this example illustrates a number of points. It shows the extent of the responsibility that the group approach puts on the group leader and how he operates differently in a "normal" group that comes as educators rather than as patients, than he would in a therapy group.

The intention is also to convey how deeply emotionally involved a group can get, if led with care, about subjects that psychodynamically speaking are relatively superficial and in another setting would lead to a casual discussion. The limited nature of the approach is such that no effort was made to go into the possibility of Mr. A. being envious or Miss R. being angry. Such feelings can be touched on in these groups when appropriate, but the direct expression of strong "basic" feelings is not the only group work.

The shift between interest in the individual and interest in the group is illustrated by how Mr. A.'s individual awareness of his preconscious feelings about his friends going off to private schools made it possible for the group to become aware of subgroup formations, the hostility between factions, and the discomfort that may accompany such a split in the group.

Finally, without in any sense making any outrageous claims of character change in individuals or that group leaders can be trained by this group approach, we hope that the example portrayed indicates not inconsiderable achievements.

It has since been reported by Mr. A. that he is more at ease with his school committee, and even before the group was over, it was clear that Miss R. had made an effort to be more flexible in her teaching methods, even though she was not aware of any new insight into her previous rigidity. Several other members of that group also reported advances of similar order, but it is unnecessary for this purpose to portray the entire group.

**Summary**

A group approach which attempts to help professional people who work with others to be more aware of how their emotional reactions influence their professional function is placed in a continuum between therapy and education. The capacity and training of the educator, or nurse, etc., is assumed to be enhanced but not replaced by this increased understanding. Therapy and education have in common the relationship with a central figure and the attempt to enlarge a horizon.

A clinical illustration attempts to emphasize the difference between this group approach and group or individual therapy and, within this limited framework, to show the potential usefulness of increased understanding.

# A Group Approach to Nursing Education

NORMAN E. ZINBERG, M.D.

DAVID SHAPIRO, PH.D.

WALTER GRUEN, M.D.

FOR A LONG TIME, it has been recognized that many professional persons, whose work brings them face to face with the emotional reactions in others —and in themselves—can be helped by a deeper understanding of the nature of these reactions. In an effort to bring such understanding to nursing students at Beth Israel Hospital, in Boston, a research project was begun with the students and faculty, using a group approach based on psychiatric concepts but remaining within an educational framework. . . .

The chief medical resident and the dietetic supervisor at Beth Israel asked the psychiatric service for advice about several nursing students who had become grossly overweight since entering the school, and suggested that Berman's group approach (Berman, 1953a, 1954), which they had heard about, might be helpful to these students. . . . A project was planned.

An announcement was posted in the nursing school indicating that personality conflicts might be a factor in weight control. It further suggested that a group approach might help the girls understand such conflicts and that weight control might be easier and more successful if they knew more about what made it necessary for them to overeat. The medical resident brought this notice to the attention of eight obese students, four of whom joined the group. Nine other nurses of average weight also joined and attended regularly, because they had trouble with weight control— tending to be either overweight or underweight.

The group continued for eighteen sessions, but complications arose about attendance because of the students' tight schedules and their fre-

Reprinted, in abridged form, from *Nursing Outlook*, 10: 744-746, 1962.

quent absence from the hospital while on affiliations. The nursing school did not officially sponsor the group project, so the students came on their own time.

From this group of students, the project staff first learned about the unusual tension in nursing schools and gave much thought to the further application of the group method within the nursing profession. There had been much subjective evidence of the success of this group approach and some minor efforts at validation had been attempted (Buckley, 1954; R. J. Margolin, 1953). It was felt from the beginning that the special atmosphere of nursing might provide an excellent setting for further research on this group method.

The difficulties the girls in the obesity group had in getting time to attend, pointed up something learned earlier from educator groups: Tension being discharged at a lower echelon of the hierarchy can be alleviated if some understanding is achieved by higher authorities. If the teachers in one phase of a group began to discharge aggression at a principal or his assistant, who was not a group member, unless that authority was aware of it as a phase with constructive features, and unless he had support in tolerating this affront to his dignity, he might clamp down authoritatively and ruin the group sessions. Therefore, the official support of the nursing faculty was vital to the successful continuation of group sessions with nursing students.

### The Nursing School Faculty

The participants in the first group reacted favorably to the sessions, and this led to a request from the junior nursing faculty to have psychiatrists meet with them to help them understand more about their problems with students and the nursing education program in general. This faculty group consists entirely of head nurses, all of whom teach the students at one time or another. At their invitation, the psychiatrist who had led the obesity group met with them during one of their regular weekly meetings.

Many of these head nurses felt that times have changed, that student nurses have become more restive, have a greater tendency to be snippy, and are harder to handle than the students of their day. They also felt that they, themselves, became excessively upset by student behavior and wondered how they could better cope with difficult students and their own reactions. In reply and partial explanation, the psychiatrist discussed how educators in other disciplines had brought up similar problems regarding relationships with their students.

Two weeks later, the psychiatric service received an official request from the nursing school to conduct a "seminar" for head nurses. This led to regular group sessions for a year, followed by formation of more groups in two successive years. The junior faculty was most enthusiastic and pressed for still further sessions. Their leading satisfaction was in the improvement of communication throughout the hospital.

This interest encouraged Berman and his associates to apply to the National Institute of Mental Health for a grant to study the effect of this group approach on the formation of a professional identity in student nurses. An earlier project in which group sessions were held for regular or senior nursing faculty had received NIMH approval. In that group, the faculty had shared experiences with each other and a psychiatrist in an attempt to arrive at a consensus of what they could expect realistically from the students, and what the students could expect from them. The more consistent attitude evolving from this group helped faculty members feel more at ease with their roles as models for nursing students. The directors of nursing and of nursing education met with the director of the research project every other week to keep informed about the progress of the group without in any way violating the confidentiality of the meetings. Their sympathy and co-operation were necessary from an administrative point of view, as well as to enable them to be ready for any shifts in emphasis in the curriculum that might evolve from this new approach to nursing education.

As we on the project staff learned more about nurses and nursing, we became more concerned about the effects of the group approach on the entire social system in the nursing school. Because we knew that improper handling could make such meetings more of a hindrance than a help to the students and to the school, we stressed that the sessions were for educational and not for therapeutic purposes.

Material gathered from the weight control group and the first nursing faculty group helped us develop a clear appraisal of the role of the nurse and the possible usefulness of a group approach in nursing education. At this time, however, we had insufficient understanding of the special pressures on a young girl in nursing as compared, for instance, to the pressures on a girl in college.

### Special Pressures in Nursing

We began our project with the cooperation of the school of nursing staff. Experience having shown that groups up to fifteen can work effectively, we divided the freshman class into three sections of twelve to fifteen members each. Two sections were to be experimental groups led by a psychiatrist, the other, a control group taking a lecture course in psychology.

Only volunteers were accepted in the groups and, when we made this known, the entire class volunteered, which indicated to us the students' fear that the authorities expected them to participate. When the voluntary nature of their attendance was emphasized as the groups got under way, many girls absented themselves from time to time, obviously to see if the group leaders were telling the truth. When no reprisals occurred, almost all of the students chose to remain. It was necessary to stress repeatedly that these were not therapy sessions. They had a limited goal: to help the students understand something about themselves as people in a professional role and how they function in a nursing situation with peers, patients, and superiors.

The leader met with each of the experimental groups for fifteen weekly sessions of one-and-half hours each. Group members were asked to describe situations and incidents from their daily work in which undue or untoward reactions arose. These were then discussed, with the goal of clarifying some of the subjective and objective components which helped bring about these reactions. Sometimes the discussions led to a limited and selected exploration of pertinent adolescent or childhood situations but, as the group's development proceeded, increasing attention was paid to the emotional reactions of group members to one another and to the group leader. An effort was made to relate these reactions to the psychological factors which interfered with the professional growth and development of the persons involved. At selected points in the discussion, the group leader used some of the interactions which occurred during the group sessions as illustrations of various psychological phenomena. These often are difficult to grasp in a meaningful way if they are abstractly presented.

### Nursing Students' Anxiety

The most striking finding of the work with freshmen students was the low anxiety threshold manifested in the experimental groups. Their necessity to discharge tension by giggling, generally acting up, and showing poor control over their reactions was understood on two bases: the accumulation of tension brought about by the difficult situation of being a nursing student, and the relatively permissive leadership of the groups in marked contrast to the discipline of the classrooms, wards, and living situations of the students. While this kind of group behavior had its difficult aspects, its nature permitted the group leader to make certain comments about the little girl still present in each nurse. Recognition of the childish nature of their behavior was inescapable, and many of the girls saw as the most important aspect of the entire group their further understanding of the pull in them away from maturity and responsibility.

The groups continued for two years at Beth Israel Hospital School of Nursing. The data collected is being further studied; the results will be presented as an experiment in education.

### Some Generalizations

At this point, we believe we can make certain tentative generalizations about the usefulness of the group approach in nursing education. It is necessary to keep in mind the complexity of the group approach: the attempt to use modified therapeutic techniques for educational purposes; the fine balance of attention to the group as a whole, and at the same time to each individual in the group; and the use of some personal material in a professional setting with emphasis on professional goals. All these aspects require of the group leader enormous skill and rigorous training.

Other group approaches that have been attempted, while professing slightly different goals, seem to be designed to permit the leader to fit more directly into a concept of a faculty member. For instance, Rosenberg, while specifically differentiating herself from the faculty, used techniques that permitted the student to see her as a more recognizable figure than the psychiatrist in the "seminar" we are describing (Rosenberg & Fuller, 1955, 1957). This distance of the psychiatrist is shown by our study to be both a strength and a weakness. It should be restated that, while in this group technique the group leader is somewhat distant, in no case does he behave like the old-fashioned, stereotype of the silent, "reflecting mirror" of the psychoanalytic cartoons (Berman, 1950, 1953a, 1956).

The control group subjects appeared to change in the direction of becoming relatively more formal and distant in interpersonal relationships, less active in social groups, and relatively more authoritarian when compared with the members of the experimental groups. It seemed, also, that the group approach in the experimental groups served to soften the tendency of the nursing student to become "cynical" or overly professional. The research interviews conducted with students showed a higher level of personal involvement in the group experience on the part of the experimental group members. No shift in the percentage of girls leaving school for scholastic or other reasons could be demonstrated as being associated with the groups, and no significant differences in academic standing could be demonstrated between experimental and control groups.

While impressed with many of the results of the group approach in work with freshmen nursing students, the research team was anxious to experiment further with the technique with groups running for thirty or even more sessions; with important modifications in the approach; and with women rather than men, as group leaders. Unquestionably, nursing students seem to need something in the direction of an opportunity to understand further the nature of the reactions stirred up in them by their education.

While there is some uncertainty about the use of the group approach in nursing education, few of the same doubts seem justified in the work with nursing faculty as educators. In the twelve groups of faculty members, no rigorous research design was used to study the impact of the sessions on participants. Members of four of the groups were interviewed before their sessions began, however, as well as immediately after, and one year later. The responses were uniform, and confirm our subjective impressions, gained by informal discussion with the participants in those sessions in which no formal interviews were held. In none of the groups did all the participants feel favorably disposed toward the approach or that they had gained significantly from it, but in no group did more than two feel that the experience had been unrewarding.

The faculty members reported increased understanding of their students and of their own reactions in relation to the students. One comment repeated by most was about their newly acquired awareness of the extent to which their behavior toward students was dictated in some way by "the student" in each of them. They consistently reported enlightenment about group behavior which helped them in other meetings outside their faculty work.

Each group complained at times of not really finding an answer to a problem, were fearful of hurting feelings, and wanted more from the psychiatrist, but most of these difficulties had been more or less resolved by the end of the series for faculty.

It would seem to us that nursing faculty, as educators, have an unusually difficult task because of the emotionally charged nature of the problems with which they deal. Their field of work includes patients in whom illness creates an anxiety provoking situation, and students, who—having to deal with frightened patients—are themselves inevitably stirred up. This teaching milieu demands the utmost tact and understanding from faculty, and a group approach such as we have used seems effective—in the right hands—for helping teachers resolve a conflict without depending solely on regulations.

## Summary

The Berman Group Approach, after having been developed for use with educators generally, was tried with nursing students and faculty as an educational tool for helping the participants understand something about themselves as people in a professional role and how they function in a nursing situation with peers, patients, students, and superiors. The anxiety of the nursing student early in her educational program proved greater than anticipated and led to an understanding of the unusual stress such education represents to a late adolescent girl. The groups, uniformly effective with nursing faculty, highlighted the difficulty of their functions as educators.

# Some Vicissitudes of Nursing Education

NORMAN E. ZINBERG, M.D.

DAVID SHAPIRO, PH.D.

WALTER GRUEN, M.D.

NURSING STUDENTS USUALLY are girls in their late adolescence, a period of tremendous psychological and physiological turmoil in any case. Their mastery of essential primitive and childlike needs is still not complete, and dependency on the family is still very great. To them, the good will of family or surrogates is essential for the very continuance of life itself, as in earlier years, and certainly for any feeling of well-being. At the same time, there is a thrust for independence, a wish to prove that one can stand alone, and that one has the capacity to be viewed as an adult and to live up to the growing external evidence of maturity—that is, an increasing capacity to deal with childlike wishes and fears, an increasing ability to adapt to the outer world, and a growth of inner comfort and freedom.

Before discussing the pressures on these students, some mention should be made about the kinds of girls who seek nursing education. What influences a graduating high school senior to choose nursing school over secretarial school, college, or work?

Girls who choose nursing are oriented to the activity and diversity of life, as in a hospital, rather than to the more contemplative or more passive occupations. This is not to say that they are not bright; their high school grades usually have to be above average for acceptance to nursing school. The majority of them come from a lower-middle and upper-lower class socioeconomic background and have little sophistication or intellectual aspirations. In most instances, they have wanted to be nurses since childhood.

---

Reprinted, in abridged form, from *Nursing Outlook*, 10:795-799, 1962.

290

These girls usually have not been away from home for any significant period in their lives prior to entering the nursing school. In the group studied, several had been to camp for a summer, but we regard this as a special environment, not a true separation from home.

We found some evidence that there had been a serious illness in the family of many of these girls. This had a direct and powerful influence on their choice of nursing as a career, but it is impossible to determine statistically, at this point, how much more frequently they were exposed to such an episode than a similar group of college students. However, from our survey of various groups other than nurses, our strong clinical impression is that exposure to such an episode had a profound influence on their decision to enter a nursing school.

### Special Demands and Requirements

From the day they entered nursing school, these students lived more closely together, and were thrown into more intimate persistent contact with each other than is true in a college dormitory. Although rules in the nursing school have been eased considerably in the last ten years, they are still more strict than in a college atmosphere. The academic demands on these students—who are not primarily interested in such work—are impressive, and greater in many ways than the demands on college freshmen. In fact, to several of the members of the project staff, who worked closely with nurses in hospitals, it was of great interest to find that the early academic aspect of the nursing curriculum was considerably more rigorous than had been their previous impression. The requirements are almost completely inflexible—if a girl does not get the exact passing grade, she fails; there is little room for deviation. This is not a criticism of the meticulousness of the nursing faculty; they try to help the students, and they encourage them to do well on the quizzes—but failure is failure. The stiff requirements are unusual in the extent of their rigidity.

In comparison, the college student faces many of the same difficulties and fears in some respects. In the following instances, however, the distinctions between the nursing student in the hospital program we studied, and other girls who leave high school to seek a career are not seen as analogous:

Within the first six months of their education, neophyte nurses are asked to handle bedpans, to bathe men and women of all ages, and in the case of the elderly and the handicapped, frequently to see and touch their genitalia.

Death is experienced at very close hand. The nurse has to prepare dead bodies for the morgue; attendance at autopsies is required.

The students are trained to give injections: at first they stick needles into each other, in order to learn correct technique; then, during these first six months, under careful supervision, they give injections to patients.

Student nurses are closely supervised by older women, both on the wards and in the classroom. in a way that is more intensive than the supervision encountered in the college or in the office situation where, moreover, men are usually in charge. Submission to older women has important implications for an adolescent girl, especially in view of her attempt to free herself from the domination of mother and to establish herself as an independent person.

At the same time that the essential authority over the student lies with the nursing instructor, from the moment she goes into a clinical situation, the student is aware that the doctor is in charge of the patient. This, then, is a complex authority situation which permits any previous family conflict between mother and father to reassert itself in the work situation, and is emphasized by the frequent initial idealization of the doctor. The intimacy of the working arrangements in many hospitals prevents the avoidance of some aspects of this triangular situation.

### Problems of Mastery of Impulses and Dependence on External Structure

In consideration of these daily rigors, one can more readily comprehend the significance of a nursing school's inflexibility. The requirements of the staff for the educational aspects of nursing in the hospital contribute an external structure which may facilitate for some students the mastery of basic impulses stirred up by the training experiences.

Now, we must carefully consider what happens to a girl in this period of her development, when she is faced by the tensions and pressures just described. Her sexual and aggressive impulses, and all her defenses against them are activated. To indicate more clearly what makes the nursing student's situation so difficult, we shall contrast it with a college situation, treating the college as an ideal, to add emphasis to this comparison. We know that, in fact, such an ideal does not exist.

The college atmosphere is predicated on the proposition that in the course of living through their studies and associating with peers and teachers, the student will experience a gradual and careful awareness of the mixture of child and adult relationships and feelings. Efforts are made so that impulses will not be stirred up too quickly either by excessive stimulation or excessive restrictions, the latter often having the same effect as the former. Dating practices are, to a certain extent, regulated by one means or another so that sexuality, if possible, is held at least to a pace that accentuates social growth and minimizes unusual stimulation. Too much bitter argumentation, too much overwhelming competition, too much vicious provoking of the kind of aggression that has to be strongly defended against, is avoided.

In this ideal college setup, the authorities try to help students identify with them as adults rather than dictatorial figures. Their aim is to permit students to feel that they are in control of their own relationship with the world and with their own impulses, that they have the strengths to deal with their aroused impulses in a manner that can both help them and be acceptable to those around them.

Beginning with the freshman year—when more emphasis is put on required courses, to the senior year when many more electives are possible—the accent is on a particular student's relationship with himself as a maturing person who can deal with most things. This ideal school tries not to serve as an auxiliary conscience, and the student who leans too heavily upon rules and regulations, who shows no capacity for individual development and attainment, is not considered the best.

In the nursing school where we conducted our study, the opposite is true. The students' basic impulses are stimulated excessively by their ward and classroom experience. The pressure of their academic curriculum and the restrictions placed on their private lives are far greater than they are for college students, even in view of recent changes. Rigid defenses become necessary in this situation, especially the defense of leaning upon the outside world and of not trusting one's self to master the kind of impulses aroused and present in an adult body and in adult situations. This leaning takes the form of accepting a rule as a rule, following the letter of the law. No choice is possible. No individual feelings are allowed in the frightening experience of caring for sick people.

This extensive inhibition of individual judgment and feelings results from the student's fear of her inability to master her instincts, and her exaggerated fears are reinforced by the reality of the hospital atmosphere. If a nurse gives an injection to a patient in the hospital and it turns out to be the wrong medicine, real harm can be done. This kind of responsibility is great, and hard for anyone to accept without recourse to unusual means of neutralizing the natural and extensive anxiety.

As we understand it, what happens to the nursing student is complicated by special factors. She finds it hard to guard against error by the simple learning of useful precautions that can become automatic. These situations stimulate her own feared impulse to hurt rather than to help, so that the fantasy of making a slip in giving an injection might make her a murderer. The towel has to be placed exactly when a patient is bathing because making a slip and uncovering a part of the patient that "should not be seen," arouses the nursing student to accuse herself of voyeuristic impulses.

These examples are given in an attempt to illustrate how the reality of such things as the handling of potentially destructive drugs and exposure of genitalia lend themselves to exaggerated fantasies of being bad that are present in nursing students. They use a very natural and available defense—they turn to the school authorities for a rule to follow in order to avoid being harshly judged by their consciences. If one follows rules, one is acquitted; if one breaks rules, one can be guilty of all manners of evil.

### Disillusionment and Cynicism

To understand the nursing students' adherence to the school's rules and regulations, and why they lean on the outside world for structure in order to deal with their inner lives, one has to consider the inevitable concomitant of such dependence—disillusionment.

No instructor or doctor could live up to the expectations of the beginning nursing student. We have a wealth of material to indicate that the girls enter nursing school with an overvalued concept of doctors and nurses as people who help, rescue, succor, or mother. We are aware, also, that because they are adolescents, they are caught up in the struggle to establish themselves as independent persons, and that their feelings about it all are highly mixed. They yearn for early dependency relationships, while they have, also, a great fear of dependency—a fear of a loss of identity if one gives in, even for a moment, to such yearnings. This is projected onto the outside world, so that the girls see the nursing school and its faculty as making demands on them, either for dependency or for independence. It is a reflection of their relationship with parents; it is often the case that adolescents repeat a very early struggle with trust versus mistrust of adults (Erikson, 1950).

The material from the groups and from the individual interviews gives us the conviction that earlier more primitive relationships with parents, especially with the mother, are reactivated in nursing, and that the students become preoccupied with whether or not they are good or bad persons as totalities. The infantile dichotomy of the good and bad mother is revived by using certain faculty members to represent each side of the dichotomy. It is striking to see the extent to which the students achieve one-hundred per cent idealization of a nurse or teacher, of how totally they might "destroy" a faculty member because of a mistake. We know that this process is characteristic of adolescents, but it seems to differ here in the extent to which it is operative.

Members of the faculty who adhere to and embody the rules and regulations are most often idealized. This idealization often lasts throughout a nursing career. In fact, one of the head nurses groups took up almost the entire seminar with it (Zinberg, Shapiro, & Gruen, 1962).

Miss S., a member of this group, was in charge of the female medical ward which was universally accepted as the most difficult nursing job in the hospital. She was an unusually efficient, capable person whose ward ran like a clock. A stickler for detail, she brooked no excuses for lapses and was never caught without necessary supplies. On the other hand, the house officers felt that she was rigid and unyielding in clinical situations, and even mildly sadistic in her dealings with the patients. At the beginning of the sessions, several of Miss S.'s colleagues were deferential toward her, and when she was absent from the third session, they agreed that she was their ideal.

As the group progressed, Miss S. expressed a strongly authoritarian, and even punishing, point of view toward the student nurses, which the other group members were clearly unable to challenge. When the group leader realized that no one else in the group could oppose her, he took up the question of whether her expressed attitude was not unnecessarily harsh. Miss S. was at first furious, and later hurt and insulted; the rest of the group was paralyzed. Basically, they disagreed with Miss S.'s position, but were so much in awe of her that they couldn't express it. They were prevented from supporting her as a person apart from her attitudes, partially, as stated later, because recognition of her own need for support was to see her as imperfect, which the group could not bear.

When Miss S.'s attendance in the group became irregular, several of the members expressed annoyance with the leader for driving her away. When he pointed out their impotence in the situation, they were loath to accept it. They expressed fear of seeing Miss S. as a real human being rather than as perfect, a person without doubts, who would save them from their own uncertainties, anxieties, and frightening daily decisions—especially if they had some of her abilities. They saw themselves as very small children and Miss S. as the ultimate omnipotent mother.

The converse of this example was revealed in another situation discussed by the students.

One of their most admired instructors came to a student party just a little "tight"; she was a trifle raucous, a little crude, her voice just a shade too loud. The following week the girls in the group "destroyed" her, and even her former most ardent admirers raised barely a voice in her defense. They were willing enough to admit that they and others might, and often did, behave far worse, but they could not accept it from one so revered. They even expressed openly that feet of clay made a worthless statue.

This material is suggestive of the very early concrete relationship with parents or parental surrogates in which the child attempts to take over completely what the parents represent in order to be themselves whole, perfect, or good. Failure in this attempt means to be defective, bad, and even dangerous, and there are no middle grounds. The students seem to be dimly aware of their difficulty in utilizing the relationship to the faculty as a source of growth and synthesis, and to rationalize and justify this introjection in terms of what is expected of them by the school and hospital. They want so much to avoid any derivatives of their now rampant instinctual strivings. The inevitable end result of the projection of adolescent conflicts, and the corollary elevation of nursing faculty members into positions of idealized parental surrogates, is disillusionment when the idols do not and cannot live up to such expectations.

It seemed to us that the faculty had tended to miss the importance of this conflict and to accept the girls' responses to faculty as factual. This led to confusion in the faculty's minds as they became more aware that they were somehow misunderstanding the students (Zinberg, 1959). These authority figures wished to avoid co-operating in setting up the cynicism and disillusionment which is inevitable in the reality situation. That is, they strive to be the ideal figures the students envision them.

This incorporative mode of relationship is inevitable in these students, who have chosen nursing for a variety of reasons—some conscious, some unconscious. Among the less conscious wishes of this unsophisticated, nonintellectual—but bright adolescent—group, are the wish to mother, the wish to rescue, the wish to be close to other people of one's own sex, as well as the wish for heterosexual contacts. These girls come with high hopes that their deep-seated fantasies will be gratified—but in a way that is completely acceptable to their system of values and unknown to themselves and to the world. In their previous existence at home and at high school, they probably shared with other adolescents the alternate deprecia-tion and exaltation of the same adults (usually teachers and parents). On coming to the hospital world, they seem uniformly to overvalue some of the older nurses or doctors to almost Olympian status.

This overvaluation is of special importance inasmuch as the hospital world is different from the college world, where other adolescents work out similar problems of becoming adults. The very code which doctors and nurses use, and the fact that so often the members of these profes-sions are concerned or preoccupied with life and death, makes them seem like gods or devils. In contrast, the college professor deals with books, materials, and ideas. Thinking is terribly important; the girls in nursing school, as well as those in college, do not necessarily minimize or denigrate those who are learned. But it is not accidental that the surgeon is often "king" in a general hospital setting. The more dra-matic, the more direct, the more Olympian the relationship with Eros and Thanatos, the more overwhelming the impact. Actually, the outer world contributes in a massive way to the fantasies these girls have on entering nursing—as the current popularity of certain television pro-grams indicates. When the students accept as law hospital rules and regulations or what the doctor or nurse have said, when this is some-thing to be followed to the letter, it serves to avoid inner preoccupa-tions in accord with the dictates of the hospital world. If one violates sterile procedures, germs will creep in; the patient may die because hands are washed or forceps picked up incorrectly. This cannot be underesti-mated or taken lightly.

Many readers who have been patients will remember, no matter how they tried to deal with it or deny it, that there is potential terror in walking into a hospital and, in essence, turning over your life and well-being to the people there. As the students become acquainted with hos-pital settings, however, and turn—out of necessity and fear—to the rules and regulations, and to the things that nurses stand for, do they find that the rules and regulations are obeyed? Are the commandments that come down from above observed meticulously enough so that the lives and well-being of the patients are safeguarded to a point which is suf-ficiently pure for the worshiping student? No. Far from it. Laws are often observed in the breach, and the necessity for the use of something like sterile procedures on the wards is occasionally clouded.

Their need for strict rules helps explain why many student nurses find the operating room a favorable place to work; it is one area where the rules are closely adhered to and where great care is exercised. On the wards, where the students' initial experiences are in supplying dressings and giving injections, sterile procedure may not be followed precisely, because it is of much less importance. In things that are more essential, exactness in procedure is followed and accepted, such as the quantity of medicine in the injection. In these matters, nurses and doctors are, in fact, very meticulous, even though they may use their hands rather than sterile forceps to pull out the piece of cotton with which one dabs the patient's arm. The young nurse coming on the wards for the first time cannot discriminate readily between the essentials and the incidentals. All she knows is that the Olympians are not living up to their godhead.

What emotional recourse has the girl in such a situation where her idols have crumbled, have shown themselves to have feet of clay? Remember, she has, in our opinion, used these Olympians to fortify and even replace her own inner structure. She cannot trust herself to a contemplative assessment of the situation because to reflect would be to throw herself back on her inner resources which will threaten her with stirring up frightening impulses. The outside world, therefore, has proved itself unreliable to a certain extent and not to be trusted, contrary to what the student has longed for. But, she has no other place to go, so that the result is the cynical attitude which we see so often in senior nursing students and in some graduates—the attitude which gives rise to the saying, "It would melt the heart of a trained nurse."

At the same instant that the neophyte nurse surrenders to this dependence on the concrete, she also gives up her belief that rules can be helpful to her in any way. We say this because her capitulation to the rules represents the feeling that her independent judgment and emotional resources have failed her, that she has no recourse except to this intellectual straightjacket. She therefore mistrusts, fears, and even hates, the very thing to which she feels forced to cling. It is this unresolved ambivalence, the need to abide by the rule to the letter, and the cynical mistrust of the very law to which they subscribe, that seemed to us to be a most pernicious attitude in nursing, and one to which the groups could be properly addressed.

### Student Nurse and Demands of Hospitalized Patients

Another very important factor which cannot be overestimated in the nursing students is their perception of the patients' feelings and their own reactions to coming into contact with a sick person. A sick person entering a hospital is usually frightened and angry because he does not know what is wrong with him; he is putting himself into others' hands, and he wonders how well he can trust them. These feelings go back to childhood where the individual is truly dependent on his parents' devotion for the maintenance of life itself. By adulthood, these feelings have been pushed aside as one becomes independent to a degree and capable of handling his own life, but illness destroys the individual's capability, and the sick must once more depend on others—usually, doctors and nurses.

Patients, themselves, do not really know what goes into every injection, no matter how often it is told them; they must trust the person who is giving it, and this frightens them. They are frustrated and often angry because of the extent of their dependency in this situation. To badly need another human being with good intentions is very difficult for most of us, and patients are apt to express their anger overtly or covertly. Roughly, we might say, if, in the face of unresolvable conflict, a person usually regresses by being dependent, he will be ten times more dependent as a hospital patient. If he tends to be angry, he will be ten times more angry. If he tends to be cautious, he will be ten times more cautious.

When the student first begins to work with hospitalized patients, she has no awareness of the extent of this necessary regression (Kris, 1952). She has been unaware, also, of the extent to which the hospitalized patient has depended upon the outside world for certain responses in order to maintain his personality in its usual state of well-being; the hospital patient is deprived of every aspect of this "stimulus nutriment" (Rapaport, 1951). His clothes, his outside role, his dignity, in a sense, are taken away from him. His usual capacity to be competent in his habituated roles is impaired. The usual give and take of his interpersonal relationships is disrupted and almost destroyed. Even his family and friends, who care about him and love him, treat him as a patient differently from the way they treat him when he is well and functioning unscathed. The brunt of his reaction to this unusual situation often is dumped onto the nurse. It is her job, also, to spend time with him for the innumerable details that are easily negotiated by people not ill but which become crises for the hospitalized (Zinberg, 1959). The patient feels his loss of social identity very keenly, in part as a result of this deprivation of incoming stimuli. He turns to the person who is closest to him, who has the most personal contact with him, and who is most immediately available—the nurse. He also expresses his resentment in terms of his relationship to the nurse and the constant demands he makes upon her.

The nursing student, therefore, recognizes early in her education that she is called upon to take part in an intense human relationship, more intense again because of the special black and white character of the patient's fears, angers, and preoccupations. It may even be more intense than other intimate human relationships one may be called upon to endure in a professional capacity. It is a hard concept for an adolescent to accept.

## Summary

We know that nursing educators have puzzled for some time about the difficulties faced by adolescent girls entering the world of the hospital, as exemplified by the dropout rate and the high ratio of psychiatric referrals when such facilities are available. It is our contention that some of this is explained by the recognition of how much unconscious conflict is stirred up by the realities faced in nursing education. These are far different from those of the college student, and the extent of the anxiety generated in nursing schools calls forth in many girls unusual rigidity and dependence on rules. This dependence, plus excessive expectations from the story-book "men and women in white" leads to disillusionment. Too, the patients, by virtue of being ill, are permitted emotional reactions of unusual intensity. The neophyte nurse is faced with the reality of a professional lifetime requiring an appropriate emotional response to a remarkably demanding relationship. It is our hope that the reports of our research project will help nursing educators as they plan not only the curriculum in nursing schools, but the atmosphere in which the education is offered.

# A Group Approach to Predelinquent Boys, Their Teachers and Parents, in a Junior High School

EDWARD M. DANIELS, M.D.

BENSON R. SNYDER, M.D.

MAX L. WOOL, M.D.

LEO BERMAN, M.D.

AGREEMENT EXISTS AMONG those working with problems of delinquency that much study and experimentation is necessary to improve our effectiveness in working with delinquents. It is well known how difficult it is to treat such young people. Evaluation of our previous psychotherapeutic experiences and of reports in the literature led the authors to consider the use of a psychoanalytic group approach with boys in a junior high school who were regarded as predelinquent. As a second phase of the experiment a similar group approach was introduced for use with the faculty at the same school in order to increase psychological understanding among the teachers of the boys. The third and most recent phase of the work has involved group sessions with parents of students in the school. All three areas are now under concurrent investigation.

The project began in 1955 when work with two groups of boys in a junior high school of a Boston suburb was undertaken. Adolescent boys with delinquent or predelinquent problems do not take kindly to suggestions that they go to a clinic or guidance center. It was, therefore, decided to explore the possibilities of carrying out our group-psychotherapeutic approach in a more familiar locus from the boys' point of view, namely in a classroom-like setting within the school, during regular school hours. It was hoped thus to minimize some of the objectionable aspects of being treated in a clinic setting. Further, we thought that the psychiatrist in the school would be in a position to make direct observations on the school's structure and function and, conceivably, such knowl-

Reprinted from *The International Journal of Group Psychotherapy*, 10:346-352, 1960.

edge might be useful in his work as group leader. His presence might also make it possible to exert some favorable influence on the school environment as a whole.

The project was carried out as one of the current group projects undertaken by the Unit on Psychoanalytic Group Psychology of the Psychiatry Service at the Beth Israel Hospital in Boston. The community selected was a Boston suburb in which one of the authors (L.B.) had worked with groups of educators in the Public School system over a period of years. Throughout the work the school administrators and the school guidance department have been actively co-operative. Without their assistance the project could not have been carried out.

### Early Resistance to the Project

The earliest approach to the school community made by the group leader of the boys (E.M.D.) was met with unmistakable signs of resentment from both students and teachers. This occurred prior to any suggestions from psychiatrist or teachers that there be a group of teachers for discussion purposes. The 27 seventh- and eighth-grade boys with whom the project was discussed in a large group session, and who were invited to participate as members of the group, were openly hostile that they should have been selected for any such project. Their hostility was reflected in boisterous defiance of the group leader and the school authorities in the early months of the group work. This behavior led to antisocial manifestations during the group sessions which tended to carry over into the classroom after the sessions. This evoked strong resentment on the part of the teachers who felt that the group sessions being conducted with the boys were unstructured and disorderly and could not possibly yield beneficial results. Their resistance took the form of protests, both official and unofficial, to the guidance counselor and to the school principal.

From the beginning of the work with the boys, the teachers resented being excluded from the groups. A number of the teachers expressed concern that their methods were being undermined, that the very core of school discipline was being uprooted by the invading psychiatrist. They apparently felt accused of failure because a person who did not belong was brought in to cope with school problems. They seemed suspicious of any methods which were in any way a deviation from what they, as teachers, were familiar with. They resented mostly the secrecy surrounding the actual sessions with the boys.

Because of the tentativeness with which the boys received the group leader, it had been felt that the leader could not risk being identified with teachers and administration. Therefore, contact on the part of the boys' group leader with teachers and principal was reduced to a minimum, and was always discussed with the boys. Seeing the boys in the groups in what they felt was a favored position increased the feeling of hostility on the part of some of the teachers. Need for the establishment of a teachers' group, quite apart from our original theoretical considerations which led us to plan to offer separate discussion groups for faculty and for parents, became evident. It will be recalled that the value of the group approach with teachers was already known to us in view of the earlier work of two of the authors (L.B. and B.S.) with educators in the same community.

When the teachers met for the first time with the group leader of the boys, their hostility was obvious. The boys' groups had been in progress for over a year and the initial appearance of the psychiatrist at a regular weekly meeting of the teachers was the first response they had seen to their requests for a discussion of the work with the boys. In this initial meeting the boys' problems were discussed with them in general terms. Later in the meeting, their participation in a group seminar of their own was invited with another psychiatrist (B.R.S.) as their group leader. The psychiatrist expressed his conviction that such group sessions would prove helpful to them personally and also in their work at school as it involved their students, their colleagues, and their supervisors. The general response of the group was favorable. The group came to consist of 15 of the 28 faculty members, who met weekly for seventy minutes on a voluntary basis on their own time at 7:30 in the morning. This group has met for 30 sessions over two academic years with definite favorable changes in the climate of the school, as the teachers have become more constructively involved with the boys.

A rather extreme example of a teacher who objected to the boys' groups was Mrs. Smith, an older teacher of some thirty years' experience, who often had been the object of the boys' resentment. She, too, had felt the psychiatrist was unable to maintain discipline and that everything that the school stood for was in danger of being undermined by the antisocial activity of the group. Mrs. Smith, who was a stern disciplinarian, was resented by the students who went out of their way to poke fun at her, to perform poorly in her class and, when possible, to be transferred from her division to another. On several occasions during the first two years of the group work with the boys, Mrs. Smith left her class to complain to the principal or directly to the group leader about the noise and the unruly behavior of the groups. She treated the group leader much as she was reported to treat the students, with scornful resentment, as if he, too, were a wayward young boy.

The favorable change in Mrs. Smith is well borne out in two specific areas by the different remarks which the students made about her and by her changed manner toward the boys' group leader. Whereas formerly this teacher had been openly disliked and criticized in the boys' group sessions, there has been no hostile mention of her whatsoever in over a year of group meetings. She is now more favorably regarded as "strict but fair." In her last meeting with the boys' group leader she was cheerful and friendly and carried on a rather lengthy conversation with him in contrast to her earlier gruff, critical manner. She volunteered the information that there was a marked change in the behavior of the current groups as contrasted with the first several months of group meetings, stating that the present groups were "no trouble to anybody." She added later in the conversation that "we don't even know when they meet any more."

### Changes in Reaction to Authority

Our findings suggest that certain changes have apparently resulted from the influence of the group sessions on the teachers and on the boys. The principal and guidance counselor of the school have reported that certain boys in the groups are "easier to live with." No longer do the boys find it impossible to sit through class and they do not come as often to the guidance counselor for excuses from class as they did previously. Acts of vandalism by group members have also been unknown for the past year. Previous to this year there had been a number of destructive acts such as flooding the boys' room and tipping of the fire extinguisher in the science laboratory. Infractions of school rules resulting in banishment from class to the principal's office have also been quite rare. In addition, the teachers have felt generally that the group members are more relaxed in class and are not disruptive to the classroom activity.

Stanley, a group member for two and a half years, reported to the group that he thought he became a winning pitcher for the school baseball team through his participation in group meetings. He also said he no longer became tense and frightened in a baseball game. Another boy, Jimmy, who joined one of the groups six months after it began, had come to the attention of the guidance counselor shortly after his arrival at the school because he daydreamed in class and was taunted by the other boys. His early attendance in the group was stormy; the already functioning group continued to exclude him and to take advantage of his passivity and slowness. Gradually, he was accepted into the group, through the efforts of the most aggressive of the group members, Bob, who defended him and became his constant companion outside the school. Grateful for a new friend, Jimmy allowed himself to be exploited through inclusion in acts of an antisocial nature. He took the blame more often than did Bob, as the latter gradually urged him to be more aggressive and to look after himself better. Bob's strength helped Jimmy, but a major effort of the group work this year has been to help the group become more aware of the true relationship between Bob and Jimmy, so that they could better help Jimmy to see his masochistic tendencies.

Jimmy, who has very strict parents whom he fears, and who had run away from home and other schools on previous occasions, changed his report card because he was afraid to take it home with two low grades. He then returned it to the school, after signing it himself, instead of showing it to his parents. The boys' group, informed of this by Bob, bluntly showed Jimmy how he was exposing himself to the wrath not only of his parents but also of the school. Detection was certain. They urged him to talk to his favorite teacher about it and get help in working it out. The group took Jimmy to the guidance counselor, a key person on both faculty and administration and a bulwark in the entire project thus far. The counselor and Jimmy visited the division and home-room teachers after the counselor had obtained Jimmy's permission to acquaint them with details. Each teacher approached Jimmy sympathetically but realistically supported the position taken by the group and showed willingness to help him. He was given another report card to take home; the guidance counselor prepared his mother for poor grades, and helped her to react realistically but supportively.

This experience proved to be very helpful to Jimmy. He expressed amazement and gratitude at the help he obtained. His general patterns have certainly not changed remarkably but he is able to recognize the friendliness of some aspects of his school life. The guidance counselor, in discussing the elements of the incident, stated quite simply that the faculty attitude toward such students and events is changing, that he now finds that teachers with increasing frequency look for and discuss the significance of antisocial acts and a constructive approach to them. This contrasts with the resentment which was expressed when the psychiatrist first came to the school, when the group was labelled "no good" when difficulties arose with any of its members.

## Parents' Groups

Attempts to initiate group discussions with parents of the boys met with strong resistance from both parents and boys. The boys stated quite openly that their success as culprits depended upon preventing communication among teachers, parents, and leader. As the boys became more concerned about and better able to focus on their difficulties, they agreed that their lives at home might be more pleasant if their parents talked things over as they did.

The response from the parents was discouraging. They resented being contacted and most families did not respond to the invitation to meet for discussion with a psychiatrist. Finally, representatives of 5 out of 23 families appeared at a meeting. They were angry, blamed the school for the difficulty of their children, and disclaimed any responsibility for their sons' problems. They reacted defensively as if they were accused of being "bad parents," exactly as the boys had responded when they felt singled out as "bad boys."

These parents were unable to arrange for group meetings. It was decided to explore the possibility of a group comprised of parents of children who were not group members. The response to a Parent-Teacher Association talk by the group leader of the parents (M.L.W.) was enthusiastic and 18 parents responded. This group continues to function and indications are that it will develop into an effective discussion group.

Resistances are active in this group, too. Denial was obvious in the earliest meetings as these parents said that their children presented no difficulties, that all was well. They were chatty, sociable and polite. Gradually, however, they have begun to discuss discipline, shyness, and social problems among their children and have begun to help each other by giving advice. In the more recent meetings they have also pointed out to each other certain violations of the law, such as speeding, and one parent has asked another directly how he expects his children to obey when the parents do not. An opportunity for further exploration of this basic point developed when two parents began to smoke immediately after the custodian of the school building in which meetings are held had asked another parent to douse her cigarette. It is our feeling at the present time that this group is on the verge of recognizing the influence that parents have in the school problems of their children through the recognition of their difficulties as demonstrated and reported in the group.

### Concluding Remarks

Selected areas of a pilot project have been described in which a psychoanalytic group approach was utilized in treating groups of junior high school boys with delinquent tendencies and in meeting with a group of their teachers and a group of parents. Slowly, favorable changes are occurring in the boys, the teachers, and the school as a whole, and it seems that these changes can be, in part, attributed to the group sessions.

Further plans are being formulated for an expanded long-term project with additional personnel in order to study the backgrounds of the individuals in our groups, to evaluate more carefully the changes in the individual group members, and to formulate the influence of these changes on the school as a whole.

# The Use of a Psychoanalytic Group Approach With Teachers at a Junior High School

BENSON R. SNYDER, M.D.

LEO BERMAN, M.D.

A GENERAL CONCERN of those working in mental health fields is to develop methods of communicating certain basic psychological knowledge to parents and teachers. Means must be found so that such knowledge can be both understood and integrated into the individual's attitudes and behavior. To phrase this as a specific question: Can we find a method short of personal psychoanalysis which will help teachers gain further insight into their work with students and into their relationships with their colleagues? Such methods should lead to an appreciation of preconscious, and to a lesser extent, of unconscious forces which are at work both in their students and in themselves.

The goal of increasing psychological and, specifically, psychoanalytic understanding for mental health purposes has been a part of the history of psychoanalysis since the turn of the century. Only in more recent years have experiments with specific and carefully planned group approaches of various types for use in schools been receiving more attention in psychoanalytic literature. For example, a report of 1951 of the Group for the Advancement of Psychiatry (1951) summarized and evaluated four such approaches: the Bullis, the Force, the Ojemann, and the Forest Hill Village projects. This paper will be limited to a description and preliminary discussion of a type of psychoanalytic group approach which we have been using with educators and others since 1949.

This paper describes a junior high school faculty discussion group which met for its first introductory year of work during the school year

Reprinted from *The American Journal of Orthopsychiatry*, 30:767-779, 1960.

1956-1957. Most of the members of this group participated in a second year's seminar. This group was part of a research and service project in a junior high school of a suburban public school system. The project, reported on in 1957 by Edward M. Daniels and Leo Berman at the Annual Meeting of the American Orthopsychiatric Association, is concerned with the application of a psychoanalytically oriented group approach with groups of predelinquent boys, their parents, and their teachers. This project was one of the group projects undertaken by the Unit on Psychoanalytic Group Psychology of the Psychiatry Service of the Beth Israel Hospital.

The faculty in the same school where Dr. Daniels had been meeting with two student groups since the Spring of 1955 was offered the opportunity to become members of the discussion group, with a psychiatrist (B.R.S.) as group leader. It was explained to the faculty at a regular faculty meeting that the discussion in the group would provide an opportunity for them to deal with their classroom problems. The group leader specified that their problems with students, students' parents, colleagues, and superiors might be of primary interest to them. Fifteen out of 30 teachers on the faculty eventually joined the group, 8 men and 7 women. They were representative of the faculty in terms of age, tenure, grades taught, and academic fields.

There were 18 weekly meetings lasting approximately 70 minutes each. The meetings will be briefly summarized. The special complexity of the resistance in such a group will be discussed and reference will be made to the ways in which these resistances, in part, were resolved. The following themes came up for discussion: "hard" versus "soft" attitudes regarding discipline in classroom; liberal versus conservative educational philosophy; economic, social and racial prejudices; reactions to Dr. Daniels' groups; reactions to the principal, to authority in general, and to the group leader. The psychosexual problems of masculinity and femininity, as well as sadomasochism, came up in a somewhat less direct manner.

### Selective Summary of the Group Sessions

This section is intended to give a broad view of the sessions and of the group as a whole and to describe the ebb and flow of various key themes which concerned the group. In addition, some concept of the group leader's function will be presented.

The relatively long introductory period consisting of the first three sessions was, in part, a reflection of the complex resistances inherent in the situation. The group met in a classroom in the school where they all taught. The members were on the same faculty, teaching together under the same principal. Further, Dr. Daniels had for the past two years been working with two groups of predelinquent boys in this school. It developed that many teachers had strong reactions to these groups.

The leader, during this phase, offered much support to the group. No pressure was put on them to enter into charged personal material. There was some clarification, by means of restatement, of faculty misgivings concerning the seminar and the psychiatrist leader.

The first meeting, scheduled for 7:30 on a Monday morning, attended by 25 of the school's 30 teachers, began with a teacher's defensive suggestion that they discuss hypothetical cases. This comment received almost no support. The time and place for the seminars were then considered briefly. A teacher asked if they could receive credit from the State Education Department for attendance.

An older teacher requested a list of the students' grievances against the faculty that might have come up in Dr. Daniels' "therapy group." A young woman doubted their need to get to school more than an hour earlier than usual "to gripe about students," and suggested instead that they explore their own feelings about teachers and students. Supported by a general nodding of heads, the same teacher spoke of a recent episode in her classroom. The school administration had not taken her position into account sufficiently; "they" (the administration) were more preoccupied with public relations than with the faculty's opinions.

It was in this context that the group first turned to the leader and asked him what was he "doing here." When the question was turned back to them, they discussed Dr. Daniels. Initial confusion and dismay had been a common reaction among the faculty to the students' behavior during and immediately following their group "session" with Dr. Daniels.

One of the teachers remarked, "We can understand the students, but this does not gives them permission to clonk one another over the head just because they had an unhappy childhood." Several teachers, in a defensive mood, wondered if they might be doing the "wrong thing" with their students. It was evident that many of the teachers had initially thought of Dr. Daniels' group as unstructured, without limits, and had reacted with annoyance and some apprehension.

The leader, using the group's phrase, "blowing their tops," asked them whether their reaction to the students' groups did not also indicate some concern about the possible consequences of the current group discussion. Following the general laughter, he went on to point out this was not therapy, but that they could still profitably explore their own feelings in relation to their problems in school.

In the second meeting, the leader suggested that they bring in problems from daily work in relation to students, colleagues and administration, and parents. In discussion, the group could consider the variety of subjective and objective factors that went into these problems. The leader also commented that they would probably learn various things about themselves from their reactions to each other's behavior in the group. He suggested that there was a middle way open to the group, a way which lay between the emotional detachment often apparent during an academic discussion, and the more personal type of discussion which occurs in group psychotherapy. There followed a brief discussion of confidentiality and an extended discussion of the time for meetings.

The third meeting began with a request by one of the men for the leader to "take over." A younger woman said this was purposely "unstructured" and wondered where it could lead. In this context the group was asked to consider their expectations for the seminar. There followed, from a teacher with twenty years' experience in the school, a request for specific assignments for the group. She also referred to the students' group as an experiment. When the leader noted this mention of "experiment" the group politely denied any uneasiness on this point but proceeded to discuss whether the content of the meetings should be confidential. They were almost equally divided on this issue. The younger members felt that complete confidentiality within the group was essential, while the majority of the older teachers, together with two of the younger men, took the position that anything said in the group could be said to the principal. A suggestion was made that the principal be invited to join the group "so that we won't get our hands dirty." A heated interchange developed between the factions. The leader attempted to clarify the group concern that the meetings "might get out of hand" and wondered if the principal would not act as a limiting factor in helping the group to keep its "hands clean." The group was asked if this was what they wished. It was pointed out that there appeared to be some uneasiness in the absence of clearly defined limits.

There was much excitement and general talking as the group left the room with this issue still unresolved. It was apparent that they were not simply seeking an external limit on the expression of affect in the group in their suggestion to include the principal. The anger of some group members, directed at the administration, appeared to be related primarily to feelings of not "being backed up" or "supported."

The material of the fourth hour illustrated this annoyance with administration, particularly in the comments of the teacher who felt
"dragged" because he was "not backed by upstairs" (meaning the principal. As he said: "They don't want to take the responsibility for discipline. The teacher is marked down if he sends a student to the office."

Another recurring series of comments first appeared in the fourth
meeting. "The good old days" referred to a time when teachers taught
without problem students, and were themselves free of tension. The
group in the classroom was homogeneous then, where it is now heterogeneous. Homogeneous was defined as meaning that all students were
on the same intellectual level. The administration now strongly supported heterogeneous grouping in the classroom. These terms, homogeneous and heterogeneous, used by the group to describe an educational
point of view, could also be applied directly to the "good old days" controversy. The social structure of the city had changed considerably since
World War II. Now there were fewer Yankees, more Irish, Italian, and
Jewish. The group was wary of the direct discussion of this theme, but
it recurred frequently in indirect ways during the meetings.

Four of the older teachers spent the major portion of the fifth hour
describing the changes in the school and in the community, with particular emphasis on the "lack of culture in the new elements." One of
the teachers observed that the present group was equally divided between teachers who had been in the school system more than ten years
and those who had been in the school less than ten years. He observed
that the "new teachers" were sitting on one side of the room and the
"old teachers" on the other side. Laughter and the comment that parents expected too much to be done for their children these days brought
the "new" and "old" teachers together. An older teacher, who had expressed herself strongly in favor of a firm, hard approach with the students, told of her feelings of depression and discouragement with teaching approximately four years ago. She felt lost when the former principal
had retired and saw all of her teaching techniques as outmoded and no
longer acceptable, but added that perhaps there was some hope now. She
was willing to learn "the new ways." The former principal had, she went
on, taught her "all" she knew about "holding" a class.

In the seventh and eighth sessions pressure on the leader mounted for
specific answers to the group's questions. They wanted to know the
"right thing to do." They explored the merits of a firm versus a soft
approach toward a boy who was caught stealing. They wanted to know
what should be expected from teachers; should they be therapists? All

of the group felt under pressure from the administration and from the parents to function somewhat like psychiatrists or, stated more generally, to be something they were not.

Discussion in the eighth meeting began with curiosity and concern at how to deal with disturbed students. Dr. Daniels' student group, in the beginning, had led to minor upheavals. For example, one boy returned from his group meeting and proceeded to swing from a light fixture. Several of the teachers defended Dr. Daniels' group and pointed to the improvement in individual students and emphasized that "wildness" was no longer a problem. They were troubled because they knew no certain method of coping with the difficult student. Giving such a student a lower grade was patently ineffective. In a characteristic manner, the teachers moved from blaming themselves to a search for a "scapegoat." In this instance, the changes in the community were the first target, which led directly into the second, that certain delinquent girls were at the root of "the problem." These girls stirred up the boys and sat quietly back watching the trouble unfold.

From the more general discussion of the previous meeting, in the ninth session they considered in detail the problems of a student called John. This student refused to do any homework. A young teacher with three years' experience asked what he should do about this situation. The many suggestions can be divided into two categories, those representing a "hard" or "firm" approach and those representing a "soft, understanding" position. When it was learned that John had a severe cardiac disability, the discussion became even more lively. One of the older women said that we do a disservice to the handicapped by not demanding enough from them. As the session ended, she told the leader that when she was a child, she suffered from a physical impediment which was "incurable." By will power and hard work she overcame it.

The tenth session began with a follow-up on John, who received a D in the course which was taught by the teacher who presented his problem. The faculty wondered how the administration would react. The discussion moved from the school administration to parents who had put pressure on them. The "worst offender" turned out to be a parent who was high in the administration of the school system. For the second time, they turned from their feelings of being blamed to blaming the "bad girls" who, they felt, were responsible for the "bad" reputation of the school. In this meeting, the following sequence of events was clearly evident. The teachers felt guilty and depressed when the principal or parents disapproved. They then often reacted with anger and handled their own feelings of "having failed" by blaming students. It was impressive that they tended to blame a few girls from the "wrong side of the tracks." There was almost no mention, in this connection, of the boys in Dr. Daniels' group.

A concern which had been implicit in the previous three sessions came up directly in the eleventh meeting, namely, the pressures for a teacher to be a therapist in the classroom. This was felt most acutely by those who had some guidance responsibility, but all of the group described varying degrees of confusion about their role. This was again expressed in terms of hard versus the soft approach toward students. Should the teacher be hard, distant? Does he become soft if he makes an effort to understand the student?

In the twelfth session, one of the older men stated with emphasis and finality that what really concerned him was how to maintain order. "Are we doing too much for the students?" he asked. He then spoke of his own experiences when he had been a student in the same junior high school. There were no problems in the classroom in those days, but he had to "fight his way home every afternoon." The fighting began in the kindergarten or first grade. "I was almost a nervous wreck until I got my own organization. You either ran faster than the other gang, or stayed and fought it out." In direct association, two of the women who had been in the school for over twenty years spoke of the different problems in the first, second, and third generation foreign-born. They were not all bad, some of the "worst offenders" come from "up on the hill," the wealthy section of town.

The shift in the teacher's role in the past five years was further described by several teachers in the thirteenth session. So much more, they claimed, is expected of them now. Before, one only had to understand what one was teaching, and if a student misbehaved he was "isolated" by being sent to Latin class or to the principal's office, though the problem was shifted outdoors to fighting after class, or gang wars. The group was concerned that the disturbed child interfered with the learning of the other students. A young man told of his technique for "treating" such students. He attempts to win them over and then, when he has them on his string, keeps them guessing. He had more to say about this technique in a later hour. The leader made an effort to shift the discussion in the direction of personal and meaningful experiences which, it was suggested, would enable the group to understand more effectively their own attitudes toward the question of discipline.

The fourteenth session began with a suggestion for more "structure."

This met with general disapproval. Most thought they were getting somewhere though they found it difficult to be more precise. Two teachers wondered whether the leader was interested in how their "personalities" reacted on the problem boys. There was an implication in this that the psychiatrist possibly considered the teachers "responsible" for the boys' problems. The two guidance teachers stated that they did not see the purpose of these meetings as primarily designed to further group work with students but as helpful for the faculty. There were other comments about how they had gotten to know each other much better and talk more about things that they had never talked over together before. The several references to "experiment" and "experiment on teachers" were not pursued by the group even when called to their attention by the leader. They closed the hour in a statement of solidarity and indicated that they were really a cross section of the faculty representing all points of view as well as all levels of experience. They were pleased "to be in this together."

During this meeting the leader made several comments regarding their reaction to the group and the group leader. There were no direct negative statements, and they spoke of their positive feelings though the leader stressed the possibility of negative aspects. At the end of the meeting they took what amounted to a standing vote "to go further in the same direction."

There was greater spontaneity in the fifteenth meeting, with fewer pauses, and all members of the group appeared to be more at ease. One of the older members of the faculty remarked it was becoming easier to talk and "ventilate." He didn't expect any answers, and with a smile added that he didn't recall the leader's having offered answers. Another teacher asked the group why they hadn't talked more in detail about some of the problems that had been discussed. The leader picked this up and suggested that there might be a connection here with their attitudes toward the meetings or toward the leader. They denied this, saying there was just not enough time for details. With considerable heat one of the newest members of the faculty suddenly asked the group what they thought of "capital punishment" for students. It was almost a full minute before he realized his slip, and corrected himself to "corporal punishment." There was much laughter. Mrs. Smith, one of the most experienced on the faculty, told of her first years in teaching "a long time ago" when she had whipped a colored student with a rubber hose for writing dirty notes. Her principal had praised her for this and told her that he wished he could have been a fly on the wall to watch the episode.

She went on with increasing agitation to describe four girls who had cut their boy friends' initials in their arms. She was shocked with this behavior and had apparently been instrumental in having the girls suspended from school for a week. The severity of the punishment and the extent of her feelings troubled the group but presently led to a clarification of her attitude. She had reacted to this "self-mutilation" apparently, as a form of masturbation. "They did it to have the sensuous sensation, it's not nice." The majority of the younger teachers wondered if she might have misinterpreted the situation. It was simply not "that significant." There was a persistent doubt whether this behavior should have been dealt with so severely.

One of the men began to talk, raising his voice and becoming flushed. He prefaced his remarks by saying that digressions and infractions of rules should be stopped when they are minor. It developed that three years ago a boy in one of his classes had been "misbehaving." On several occasions he had asked the principal to speak firmly to the boy but reported that he had been told to handle it himself. One month after the teacher had discussed the situation with the principal this boy, in a tragic accident, shot and killed the student sitting in front of him. The teacher had difficulty in controlling his rage at the principal. The more he blamed the administration's attitude for this accident, the more uneasy the group became. They appeared to isolate themselves from him. No attempt was made to clarify the projection of the teachers' guilt onto the principal, but rather their defensiveness was pointed out to the group, and they were asked what their feelings were concerning these incidents. They ignored the shooting episode and returned to the girls who had cut themselves. Four of the younger teachers jokingly commented that as kids they had pricked themselves with pins to make tattoos.

In the sixteenth session it was reported that in the past week a boy who, like the girls, had cut himself, had not been expelled. There were many recriminations about the inconsistency of "the front office" though the teacher who had been instrumental in the girls' suspension maintained that the group was not aware of all the facts. Girls, she implied, were worse than boys. They discussed using the public address system of the school so that they could "know what was going on." The teacher who in the last meeting had described the shooting episode asked the group to help him with a problem girl in one of his classes. She teased him, for example, by provocative requests to be sent to the principal's office. The methods the other teachers used to cope with the same girl were discussed. A teacher who had remained almost silent during the meetings jumped to her feet and excitedly announced that this girl had finally begun to work in her class just a few days before. She contrasted this with the work which some teachers give their students to "keep their hands busy." The group was troubled. Many felt they did not have enough time to talk with their students to establish a relationship with them. Several then wondered whether more rules wouldn't "keep them in line" more effectively than cultivating a relationship with them. Toward the end of the meeting, the teacher who had complained of being teased launched a flank attack on the administration by referring to another student who, he felt, had been grossly mishandled. There was considerable excitement as the session closed. They all rushed in to take sides, a clear majority defending the administration.

The man who had been critical of the administration was absent the seventeenth meeting. Mrs. Smith, one of the older teachers, had felt personally criticized by his comments. The group supported her but were also unanimous in pointing out that she had misinterpreted the criticism of the week before as meant for her. This was the same woman who had throughout the meeting most staunchly maintained the need for rigid discipline and had also reported the girls who had cut themselves. She seemed to feel uncomfortable in accepting the group's assurance and "asked for more" by telling of a student that she was unable "to handle." Finally, one of the relatively young teachers pointed out that changes in the curriculum or school would not change students in a major way. She felt that they were all much too hard on themselves and that actually they did a rather good job. Referring back to the difficult problem students, one of the men suggested "the iron fist under the velvet glove. Be nice to him until he is confident of you and as soon as he steps out of line, whamoo." He added that it was fun to lead the students on to think you were a nice guy, "subtly direct them into misbehaving and then give them the business." He boasted about his own exploits as a boy and said that students today were "pikers" compared to him. The others smiled, but did not comment on this technique.

The next to the last meeting, the eighteenth, began with positive statements regarding the group experiences. The question of discipline was considered to be much more complicated than the group had realized before the meeting. The teacher who had been most critical of the administration, and who had been teased by the girl, complained of having been ostracized by the faculty five years ago because he had "continued to harp on discipline," when discipline was no longer fashionable. The rest of the group did not think that he had been ostracized. Several commented that it was valuable to talk things over to find out what others think. Most of the older teachers described the faculty as having been a "happy family" in the past, a situation which no longer obtained. They felt that the administration was too busy and did not have time for them. There were many expressions of feeling "left out on a limb," "not getting support," with "no one to turn to." It developed that four years ago an officer in the administration was quoted as having said that this particular school was a "country club" for teachers. Many of the older teachers were angry about this. It now looked to them more like a country club for students. This attitude was tempered by an account of the principal's insistence on silence in the library; they were pleased that he was taking a firm stand.

The nineteenth and final session began with an old New Englander's asking to what extent teachers should control their feelings. He had seen in the group that they all had strong feelings, but wondered if teachers were under more pressure than other groups to inhibit these feelings. He asked if emotional illness can result from holding back feelings over a long period. This had been his personal method of dealing with tension and disappointment. Resentment with externally imposed controls was expressed by several group members. In association to this, the change in school administration four years ago was brought up. Several teachers spoke of not knowing where they stood, though they were clear that their own attitude toward discipline, i.e., a soft or hard approach, had not necessarily shifted with the new administration. Several connected their current approach to discipline with their own experiences as children. There were many comments about continuing to work next year. At the end of the meeting the group applauded.

### Favorable Change in a Group Member

As one would expect, there was a wide range of responses to this group seminar among the individual members. We thought it might be helpful to describe some of the observable changes in Mrs. Smith, one of the group members who seemed to show some significant positive changes. Impressionistically, it can be said that most of the members showed some favorable responses, and that none of them were hurt by their group experience. A more careful follow-up study of the effects of such group experience is planned for the future.

Mrs. Smith, a married, childless woman in her mid-forties, has taught science in the same school system for 18 years. She was born and grew up in Maine. Her friendly manner carries with it some restraint. Her speech is simple, direct, occasionally harsh. She is proud of her responsible role as a teacher and is dedicated to the profession. She holds an important position in the state teachers' association and is active on various school committees.

In one of the early sessions Mrs. Smith brought in a magazine article on mental deficiency, suggesting that the group discuss this. On one level she was uncomfortable with the departure from organized and directed classroom discussion and was making a bid for a return to this more structured academic approach. The other group members gave her little support in this though they treated her with deference. In the next session she expressed irritation with the current trend that paid "too much attention to problem cases in the classroom. In the past, rules and firm principals took care of these problems." She was annoyed with the suggestion that teachers "understand" students. Two meetings later Mrs. Smith stated that "present-day parents are not as cultured as they used to be." In association to this she complained that the parents expected teachers to do too much for students. In the discussion which followed she described her feeling of being under pressure from parents and school administration to be something that she felt she was not. With much feeling and admiration she went on to describe how "rules and a wall of discipline" had carried a woman she knew through a very critical period of her life.

The fifteenth session, in which the group had not gone along with Mrs. Smith's "harsh" treatment of the girls with the tattoos, can be seen as one of the points at which she began to show some change. It appeared to be very meaningful to her that the group had not reacted to the girls as she had.

In the next meeting it was reported that some students were afraid of Mrs. Smith. She was hurt and troubled by the prospect that she was viewed as "a rigid disciplinarian." The discussion which followed centered on the theme of "soft" versus "hard" attitudes toward discipline. Mrs. Smith gave an example of a boy she had befriended. With the support and encouragement of the group she decided that it was necessary to know more about what makes for problems in the classroom. In her characteristic way, it became a responsibility for her to be an understanding teacher. In the next to the last meeting, Mrs. Smith made a point of sitting with the men, joking that they were all one group. Several group members said that they had found the meetings helpful. Mrs. Smith then pointed out that it was a new experience for her to have time to sit down and talk things over. She had not known what many of the other teachers felt before. "It's helpful to find out what others think." While these words had certain defensive implications, they were also combined in the last meeting with her feeling that "seeing new points of view is helpful." She thought she might see where she gets "stuck" in her dealings with a student by learning why other teachers can deal with the same student without difficulty. She added with a smile, "especially in a discussion where no holds are barred." Mrs. Smith wondered what would happen to her if she had to teach Latin. Perhaps, she added, she used her subject matter to help control the class. She saw this as her "homework."

A suggestive indication of change in the teachers appeared in the report of the concurrent student groups. The students no longer complained of "raw deals." They singled out Mrs. Smith for comment: "She's a new person." "She's easier."

### Discussion

The group described a shift in the educational policy which had occurred four years ago at the administrative level, a shift from the more conservative to a more "liberal" educational approach. The impact of this shift on the teachers in the group has been suggested. All members of the group initially expressed approval of this policy, but reacted in very different ways according to the individual backgrounds of the group members. For example, anxiety and depression, reactive hostility and passive compliance were some of the underlying reactions which became evident in the course of discussion. Some of the effects of the administration's attitude on the teachers' self-image have been described. This was most apparent in their feeling of being called upon to be something other than a teacher.

Our material suggests that such a group approach, as introduced by one of the authors (Berman, 1950, 1953), is well suited to explore and deal with highly charged preconscious conflicts pertaining to the educator's daily work. In addition, the educational value and some of the unsolved problems of this psychoanalytic group approach are indicated. This seminar was in many ways a new experience for the participants. They described feeling a greater involvement personally than they might have with an academic approach. As with Mrs. Smith, the seminar appears to have opened the way for a different and improved level of awareness and understanding of self and others. Two factors might be mentioned by way of explanation of what might be referred to as the relatively superficial level at which the group leader (B.R.S.) worked: first, his relative inexperience in working with groups; and second, the composition of the group. As previously noted, all members were from the same school and had to work with each other for the rest of the week. The pressure is considerable to avoid "too much" personal material in such circumstances. The meetings of the second year (not reported in this paper) presented something of the opposite difficulty—an almost too great willingness to move into personal and highly charged material.

The question which is raised at the beginning of the paper can now be related to the particular material. Essentially, we are concerned with the extent to which, by way of the work done in the group under a specific type of group leadership, the group members are able to acquire a more personally meaningful understanding of their relationship to their students, to their colleagues, to their principal and to themselves. The strong positive statements, the applause at the end of the sessions and the request to continue the group for another year are suggestive of the favorable effects of the seminar, but they may also indicate exaggerated positive reactions to the group leader. A major goal for the future is to carry out a systematic evaluative study of the effect of the group experience on the individual teachers.

# The Psychiatrist as Group Observer:
# Notes on Training Procedure in Individual
# and Group Psychotherapy

NORMAN E. ZINBERG, M.D.

MANY FIELDS OF MEDICINE allow the student, in his early stages of training, to observe what the trained physician does and what happens when he does it. In psychiatry, the student learns by taking part in staff conferences and supervisory sessions and by observing the patient being interviewed in the presence of an entire group. The group situations which are to be described in this paper gave the student an opportunity to observe directly what a more experienced therapist does and then discuss what has happened with him.

The group sessions to be described in this paper were offered as "seminars" under the joint auspices of the Massachusetts Association for Mental Health and the Psychiatric Service of Beth Israel Hospital. Eight of these groups consisted of people in the educational field who were brought together in order to investigate their own reactions and to learn how irrational emotions might affect their relationships with pupils and colleagues, and even adversely affect the full use of their capacities as educators (Berman, 1953). Before being accepted for the seminars, it was ascertained that the applicants were functioning adequately or better. None was suffering from any gross malfunctioning or decompensation, and, although the question whether anyone was concomitantly in some form of psychiatric treatment was not raised, it is unlikely that many of them had sought psychiatric treatment.

The eight groups varied somewhat in composition. One was made up entirely of faculty members of a large university. In the others, there was a heterogeneous mixture of teachers from kindergarten to college level, including some principals and supervisors, guidance counselors, nurses,

322

etc. Each group contained from nine to eleven members and met once a week for twelve two-hour sessions. All groups included both sexes.

The ninth group included in this study was composed of seven women selected at random from the waiting list of the Psychiatric Clinic of Beth Israel Hospital, with the condition that their difficulties were primarily of a psychoneurotic nature. These women were invited by mail to participate in the group. The letter stated that the people invited were especially selected and that in the experience of the Clinic such groups had been found helpful to patients. This group was part of the Clinic's extended program of group psychotherapy and served the training program described here as a control group in order to illustrate similarities and differences between group psychotherapy and group seminars.

The group leaders were Leo Berman and four of his associates. Although the leaders had had varying degrees of training, all had had extensive experience in individual psychotherapy. All were psychoanalysts except for one, who was in advanced psychoanalytic training. The leadership technique of the leaders of the eight educator groups may be regarded as a blend of what he had learned as a therapist in group psychotherapy and as an instructor in educational seminars on psychodynamics (Berman, 1950; Redl, 1942).

All of these groups were observed by trainees of the Beth Israel psychiatric training program. Two of the educator groups were observed by one trainee in the same room as the group leader. The other six educator groups and the psychoneurotic group were observed from behind a one-way screen by from four to ten people. The seminars were offered twice a year so that the eight seminars discussed in this paper were offered during a four-year period. The first two were the ones observed by a single trainee. The four groups which met during the next two years were observed by members of the Psychiatric Staff of Beth Israel Hospital and a group research team from the Harvard University Department of Social Relations. The psychoneurotic group which met throughout the middle two years of this project and the two educator groups which met during the last year were observed by members of the Psychiatric Staff only. The staff members participating were principally psychiatric residents with an occasional senior staff member interested in being trained as a group leader, a psychologist, and a social worker. All observers agreed to continue with the group for its entire duration.

After each session, the group leader and the observer met for about forty-five minutes to discuss what had happened. These after-group meetings had several purposes. Principally, the purpose was to use the group observation situation to train group leaders. Secondarily, while training the psychiatric residents as group leaders, the problems posed by the group aided their training as psychiatrists with all patients (Eddy, 1951). The method of training required the observer trainees to report what they had observed and what inferences they had drawn from these observations. This organization of material indicated the depth and consistency of their knowledge and gave the leader of the after-group session (if a less experienced leader led the group, a better trained leader would be behind the one-way screen and would preside at the after-group meeting) an understanding of what areas of training needed to be emphasized. This method of teaching provides the secondary gain of building into the role of the observer a function which is of great help to the group leader and consequently, to the group participants. When the Harvard research team participated in the after-group meetings, a research orientation was introduced also which led to a research project.

Permission for the sessions to be observed and recorded on tape was obtained from each group by the group leader. Reactions to the initial request differed, but, in general, permission was granted with relative freedom. Group members turned and peered either at the observer or at the one-way screen, and some made facetious comments. In two of the one-way-screen groups, reactions of suspicion and anxiety were pronounced. This sample is too small to draw any conclusions regarding the observers behind the one-way screen versus observers whom the group could see, but two directly hostile reactions to being observed from behind a one-way screen are worth noting, both for the implications about people's feelings about being observed, and for the implications about good group leadership technique. In one group the members discussed the function of the observer directly with the leader. They asked what he was "up to" and expressed quite plainly the negative portion of their feeling that it was an invasion of privacy. The group leader explained carefully that some of the objections were excessive, pointing out that the observers were all professional people interested only in research. After some discussion, the group was mollified and accepted the observers. Later, when the group members expressed their feelings that the observers were "judges," striving to find out their faults and defects, the group leader was able to discuss these reactions as transference manifestations toward him. The group members were reminded of their earlier rational agreement to be observed, and with this in mind they accepted the group leader's comments with little resistance.

In another group, however, when the question of observers was brought up originally, the relatively inexperienced group leader was unaware of the extent of the group's objections and was rather peremptory. Several sessions later, the matter returned with great force. The group felt strongly that the leader had been authoritarian and had used the group for his own ends. The idea of the observers representing destructive critics who viewed the group almost as experimental animals was stated again and again. This feeling was difficult for the leader to work through, and was, in fact, never satisfactorily resolved.

The functions of the observer as an aid to the group leader and as a trainee will be discussed and illustrated below, as well as the subjective reactions of the observer. The data for the latter were obtained from the author and five other observers with whom these ideas were discussed.

## The Observer as an Aid to the Group Leader

The most obvious and characteristic way in which an observer may function is as an auxiliary perceiver for the group leader. This function in no way implies criticism of the leader. No group leader can possibly take note of everything, e.g., facial expressions, hand gestures, and verbal asides. To illustrate how what the observer sees can help the group leader:

At the end of a lively group meeting, one of the members engaged the leader in conversation. As this member had been relatively silent during the meeting, the group leader wanted to speak to her in order to learn her reaction to the discussion. The observer noticed that two other members, Mrs. B. and Mrs. R., antagonists during the group sessions, had become very friendly and were making plans to go out together following the meeting. Mrs. B. had just described in the session how, as a child, she had been extremely hostile to her mother. She felt that now she had achieved a purely friendly relationship. However, during this meeting, she had reacted to Mrs. R., an older woman, with marked asperity. The group leader had commented that this might indicate that not all of her childhood feelings had been completely resolved. In the postsession discussion with the leader, the incident noticed by the observer helped clarify points about the personality of Mrs. B. in the operational structure of the subgroups, and helped the group leader to achieve a more accurate idea of the effectiveness of the clarification he had offered the group. It can be argued that such an occurrence would sooner or later become apparent in the group session, but known in advance, it facilitates a sounder and more realistic evaluation of the group situation by the group leader.

Another frequent, self-evident, but important function of the observer is to convey to the group leader his impressions, working hypotheses, and hunches about individuals, cliques, and reactions that occur within the groups. Here, too, the observer's actual and figurative distance from the group may permit him a wider or a different grasp of a particular situation. The most frequent instance of the observer's relative freedom to see more than the leader occurs because a prominent difficulty for therapists who have little experiences as group leaders, but extensive experience in individual psychotherapy, is their tendency to work almost as if they were dealing with individual patients in therapy. When individual therapy of this kind occurs within a group, the group leader has much greater difficulty noting what other group members are doing. In such cases, an observer is useful in relaying to the therapist his inferences about what has taken place as in the following instances.

In one of the educator groups observed through the one-way screen by several observers, a young male teacher, Mr. R., who had been psychoanalyzed, was regarded by the other group members as a substitute or assistant leader. One evening, when Mr. R. was absent, several of the women in the group began to comment on how ineffective he was, that he really meant well and was a nice person, but just made no significant impression. The group leader was silent through most of this discussion and when he did participate, took up the individual problem of one of the women's denial of anxiety in her school situation. In the postsession discussion, there was agreement among the observers that the talk in the group about the ineffectiveness of Mr. R. was an expression of feelings representing transferences to the group leader. This information enabled the group leader, in the next session, to discuss these transference comments more directly and resulted in what seemed to be a more lively and useful session.

In another educator group, an inexperienced leader also lost contact with his group by going in the direction opposite from doing individual therapy in a group. He became extremely interested in what he considered the "group process." He perceived certain feelings of the group members that he felt were related to the group process. For example, when one of the members dropped out of the group, in attempting to get the other members to express their feelings about this incident he used words such as "grief" and "guilt." In the postsession discussion the observer's impression that many of the members of the group could not understand such "strong words" was considered by the group leader. In the next session he modified his words to "sorry" and "missed," and there was a more active response and a more useful discussion.

## The Observer as Trainee in Group and Individual Psychotherapy

In the training of psychiatrists in individual psychotherapy, an important problem is the way in which case material should be presented. Too frequently, in a case presentation or in a seminar, because of the specificity of the material presented, the inexperienced therapist tends to formulate everything in terms of unconscious determinants, grouped in broad general categories (e.g., oral, anal, phallic, compulsive, hysterical). In the observed group situation, the leader and the observer trainee have both seen and experienced the same situation, and such simultaneous observation permits a wide range of discussion. Both trainer and trainee can see how group members behave characteristically in their daily relationships with other people, and the individuality of each member of a group becomes remarkably clear. When groups are observed, it is possible to describe and to understand how each person in the group perceives the reality of a situation somewhat differently, based on his own individual perceptual deviations or lags, anxieties, and characteristic reactions to the situation and to the other people present (Erikson, 1945).

Another way in which group observation can be an adjunct to a psychiatric residency training program is that the observer trainees are able to watch experienced group leaders, who were also experienced as individual psychotherapists, rapidly assess the defense structure of group members. In individual interviewing, whether directly psychotherapeutic or not, the interviewer or therapist has at least a whole interview before he has to commit himself by an intervention to one concept of how a particular patient or interviewee operates. No such luxury is allowed the group leader under the conditions that are being described. In these groups the participants were not interviewed by the group leader before the groups began. Occasionally, for the sake of an individual member or for the sake of the group as a whole, the group leader was forced to comment to one member after having heard that member speak only once or twice. It is true that the group leader had had a chance to watch this member's actions in the group and, if it was past the first session, the observer might have provided him with auxiliary data. But generally speaking, there was still considerably less direct material available than would be desirable. In the postgroup session, the group leader summarized the reasoning that led to an intervention and what had gone into the assessment of the individual's personality structure and defenses. By being able to see how correctly the group leader had judged the situation and by being able to follow his reasoning from the skimpy data, the trainee learned much that he could use in his nongroup activities. The group leader may have made use of simple technical maneuvers which were so automatic that it never occurred to him to present them in a usual supervisory session. The observer trainee observed these techniques directly and could raise questions about them in the discussions that followed.

In learning how to make the transition from individual therapy to working with many people at once, it is most important to learn how to use the group as a therapeutic agent. For example, the observer trainee learns early that a remark by a peer may result in a different reaction in a group member than a similar remark made by the group leader. In individual psychotherapy, the novice therapist soon discovers that many clarifications cannot be offered to the patient immediately. The relationship between patient and therapist is such that the therapist's remarks have an unpleasant impact on the patient unless the latter is prepared and ready. In a group, however, group members, not the therapist, often make interpretations to each other and discuss them with relative freedom. The group leader in his comments is only underscoring ideas already expressed out loud. By focusing these ideas more sharply, he may shape the discussion without arousing the powerful defensive needs which would arise in individual therapy. The following clinical material illustrates this point.

A member of one of the educator groups, Dr. A., a clinical psychologist, happened to be the advisor of another group member, Mr. B., who was working for his Ph.D. It soon became apparent in the group that there had been friction between the two men, which had begun, according to Dr. A., when Mr. B. consulted another professor without letting him know of it. In addition, Mr. B. had given Dr. A.'s name as a reference, again without consulting him. Dr. A. felt that these actions had not been strictly "honest." To complicate matters further, he had been unable to get in touch with Mr. B. in order to discuss the letter of recommendation with him. For these reasons, Dr. A. had not written a favorable letter. Mr. B. was quite upset at hearing about this and responded in a rather aggressive fashion. Dr. A. said he felt justified in giving a negative recommendation, and denied that his rivalry with and hostility to the other professor to whom Mr. B. had turned had influenced the decision. Dr. A. insisted that a moral principle was involved, that Mr. B.'s flouting of protocol was the source of the judgment, and that personal pique had not been decisive. The group leader's problem was to know how far he could carry this discussion of a real life situation which might have serious consequences for Mr. B. Earlier in the session, Dr. A. had described at length his relationship with his father, stressing that he maintained a good relationship, although he felt his father had treated him harshly when he was a young man. From this and other observations of Dr. A., the group leader inferred the presence of a powerful reaction formation in Dr. A. against his hostile feelings toward his father. It could be directly observed that the attitude of Dr. A. toward Mr. B. was disappointing to other members of the group. Until that time, Dr. A. had been highly regarded by the group because of his position and intelligence. The group leader felt that if he forced a discussion of this subject, Dr. A., faced with the disapproval of his peers, might reconsider his position. If this were to happen he would then feel it necessary to make peace with Mr. B. The group leader then indicated to the group that discussing difficulties between group members that affect their lives outside of the group was a difficult and tricky problem, but one with which the group could work if Dr. A. and Mr. B. concurred, and thereby achieve some resolution and understanding that would benefit all. It was agreed. The group members then expressed their feelings that Dr. A., as the instructor, had the greater responsibility. They suggested that behind his dislike of "dishonesty," he might be concealing his annoyance and hurt feelings at Mr. B. for going to another professor "over his head." When Dr. A. was faced with these feelings by his peers, he became more conciliatory. At this point the climate of the group made it possible for the group leader to intervene. He agreed with the group that Dr. A. might have been more influenced than he was aware of by old personal conflicts, and that knowing more of Dr. A.'s relationship to his father might be helpful in explaining why Mr. B.'s turning to another, older professor had aroused feelings that Dr. A. might not wish to face directly. Now Dr. A. could respond to Mr. B., who was enabled, with the support of the group, to feel less anxious and less attacking. The group benefited by the continuing more general discussion of the use of a "moral principle" to cloak hurt feelings.

In individual therapy, patients are often convinced that the therapist and other people think as they do, especially about emotionally charged issues. Sometimes it is difficult to convince them that this is not true. In groups, this fact can often be graphically illustrated, as when five members of one group of educators each outlined a different way of criticizing someone. Mr. T. could only criticize those whom he liked; Mr. M. could only criticize those whom he disliked; Miss G., only those who liked her; Mr. V., those who disliked him; and Miss A. only felt comfortable criticizing strangers. Such a situation cannot, of course, be observed in individual psychotherapy. What it might emphasize for the beginner who has the opportunity to be an observer is that, when a patient describes the reactions of another person, he may present them so plausibly and naturally as being the same as his own that the therapist may not question the fact. In this way a valuable opportunity to help the patient to see more of an underlying attitude which expresses a characterological trait causing undue anxiety may be delayed or missed.

In group work it is necessary to assess not only each individual but also "the group climate." In individual psychotherapy the therapist's task of following just one unconscious stream of thought is certainly sufficiently complicated. In groups the situation is further complicated by the task of following, if possible, the individual stream of thought of each member, the resulting group interaction and resolutions into a group climate, and the complications resulting from the highly individualized and seemingly nongroup-related reaction of any one member (Berman, 1950). There are analogous situations in individual psychotherapy, when a patient who has been going along in one direction suddenly "erupts" in the next interview, or even in the same interview, in an unexpected way. In the individual situation, the therapist can focus on the patient; in the group situation, the leader must consider the other members of the group and, in his handling of the eruption, consider the possibilities of both harm and benefit not only to each individual, but to the group as a whole. An example of this type of situation has been taken from one of the groups.

Miss S. began discussing at length her problem with a child in her classroom. Miss S. was outwardly an aggressive, competent person, but was actually sensitive and easily hurt. The group discussed the problem presented by her, trying to take into account Miss S.'s personality. The group leader observed a growing resentment on the part of the group toward Miss S. This response was a reaction to her aggressive manner and her attempts to dominate the group. He began to work in the direction of making this apparent to the group without concomitant injury to Miss S.

At this point, Mr. G., who had been sitting quietly, suddenly began to speak with marked emotion. He complained bitterly about situations in which people who had done important work were afforded no recognition. Mr. G. was an older man who had expressed himself earlier as being interested in the group only to help others. At the beginning of the sessions, his remarks had indicated intense unconscious hostility to principals, school supervisors, and other authority figures. However, up until this time in the sessions, Mr. G. had attempted to force a close, friendly relationship between himself and the group leader, and to this end had made every effort to please and support him. It seemed clear to the leader that this present outburst was a specific reaction of Mr. G.'s which reflected his ambivalence to authority figures in general and his feelings toward the group leader in particular. However, it was not relevant to the worthwhile direction in which the group seemed to be working. The group leader was now faced with a dual problem. On the one hand, he wanted to help Mr. G. with his individual problem which was causing him considerable discomfort, and on the other hand, this would have to be accomplished without interfering with the progress of the other group members and the group process. The leader attempted to relate Mr. G.'s feelings that increased recognition might help him to feel more at ease and stronger in the group with Miss S.'s presentation of a school problem of the moment. Mr. G. refused to accept this intervention, denied that the feeling to which he was alluding was a personal one, and continued to rant. The group leader felt it necessary, for the sake of the group, to insist gently that this much expressed feeling must indicate a personal involvement in Mr. G.'s remarks. The group joined in, too vociferously, finding it easier to be annoyed with Mr. G., who seemed so far off the track, than to deal with Miss S. Before the group leader could step in and protect Mr. G., the situation had become tense and Mr. G.'s feelings were hurt. Although he remained in the group, he was relatively silent during the rest of the sessions, in spite of the group leader's efforts to make it clear that the attack had not been entirely a personal one on Mr. G., but a result of a complicated interaction with Miss S.

Let us examine a similar situation which also differentiates group therapy from individual psychotherapy for the observer trainee. In this situation, a group member accepts the general clarification of a problem from the group leader and considers it silently while the group proceeds on a more superficial psychological level. Suddenly, this silent member may respond at a much deeper level than the group is prepared for. In individual therapy, the therapist has the associations of the patient to help him gauge the direction in which the patient is proceeding. In group therapy, it is possible for a patient to work along silently so that the group leader does not have the opportunity to anticipate what may be about to come forth.

In the psychoneurotic group, Mrs. R. and Mrs. B. were discussing frigidity in their relationships with their husbands. The group leader commented to the effect that perhaps the group could look to their childhoods and earlier experiences for an explanation of some of this difficulty. The group, with the exception of Mrs. D., began to explore this, gingerly bringing up relationships with their mothers, lack of sex education, etc. Suddenly Mrs. D. burst forth with a tale of her mother's being a prostitute and on many occasions having witnessed her mother having intercourse with men. Mrs. D. then discussed her own marriage at age seventeen to an older man who forced her to have intercourse with him seven times on their wedding night. The effect on the group was electric, and the group leader was presented with the problem of how to deal with this extremely disturbing material of Mrs. D.'s and still preserve some integration of the group. The leader feared that this kind of shock material might frighten the other members of the group so much that they would shy away from the topic of sex completely. Although the previous discussion had been superficial, it was more useful to most of the members at this time.

Mrs. D. was the oldest woman in the group and obviously had the most disturbed background. She had achieved a superficial calm and knowledgeability, maintained at great inner expense. The group leader suspected that merely to ignore her problem might hurt her deeply and increase her feeling that she was not an acceptable group member. He began by sympathizing with Mrs. D., expressing his understanding of how terribly difficult such early experiences must have been for her. In essence, he invited the group to join him in this expression of sympathy. However, Mrs. D. had earlier aroused much hostility in the group by her "pollyannaish" responses. The difference between her earlier attitude of pseudo innocence and her present disclosures, which indicated how embarrassed she was about her experiences, was not immediately apparent to the group members. They simply felt anxious and, instead of sympathizing with Mrs. D., criticized her. At this point the group leader spoke up and, using material that had been discussed earlier in the group, showed two or three members of the group that they were expressing feelings toward Mrs. D. that had been carried over from childhood conflicts with their own mothers. In this way, Mrs. D. was enabled to feel that the criticisms of her were not directed personally, but were a result of the other group members' using her to help them with their own conflicts, and her feelings were spared. The other group members learned how easy it was for them to use a real life situation for the purpose of expressing some of their old forbidden feelings.

## Subjective Experiences of the Observer and their Implications for Training

An observer within the room seems to experience a more intimate relationship with the feelings of the group than does an observer behind a one-way screen. On the one hand, there is, of course, the physical proximity: the observer is seen and interacts with the group, even if this interaction is limited to "hello" and "goodbye." However, an even stronger kinship is created than this much contact would suggest. If the discussion is heated, the observer may think of his own reactions to the material under discussion as if he were a participant. It is as if he were a group member who would have his say next.

The observer's identification with the group leader is also probably more intense. When he is in the same room as the group, the observer experiences more strongly the feeling of "why doesn't he say this?" or "can he have missed that?" This increased intensity makes it necessary for the observer to formulate what are the present exigencies of the group situation. The fact that the observer has direct contact with the group makes him more aware of the possible hostility directed toward him either as a surrogate group leader, or as a person who represents a participant but who does not pay his way by actively responding and contributing to the group situation. This may increase the observer's anxiety and result in discomfort and possible interference with his ability to evaluate the situation. The feelings the observer may have toward the group leader, whether of rivalry, fear, admiration, or identification, have a tendency to increase. Again, this situation differs from individual psychotherapy, in which the trainee's relationship with his supervisor is more clearly structured.

Occasionally, a situation occurs in a group that would not occur in individual psychotherapy, and it requires a shift in the "set" that the trainee has learned in becoming a competent individual psychotherapist. A group leader may find it necessary to take something up with a single group member which may not be directly helpful to that member, but which is necessary for the continuance and furtherance of the work of the group. A clinical illustration of this situation follows.

Dr. J. was the best educated member of his group, and insisted that education was the prime standard by which to judge other people. The rest of the group held Dr. J. in some awe, and the group leader thought it necessary to challenge him about his attitude. He saw that, even if the other group members recognized that Dr. J.'s expressed attitude about education was irrational, none of them felt ready to disagree with so redoubtable an antagonist. The group leader sensed, or hoped, that Dr. J.'s defenses were good enough to handle such differences of opinion. The group leader also believed that he should show that he was not afraid to disagree with Dr. J. and indicate another point of view that was more reasonable and would help the other group members feel more at ease. The leader was convinced that if he were not able to do this the group would fall apart and he would be viewed as weak and as having nothing to contribute. He asked the group at large if it really made sense to judge people using any single standard and, further, he wondered how anyone decided when he was in a position to do the judging. After the leader's comment, the group was relatively quiet: Dr. J. said little or nothing. In this situation, the observer became so concerned about the welfare of Dr. J. that, after the session, he took the leader somewhat to task. But in subsequent sessions it became clear that this was the turning point in the group. Later, the group members expressed their feeling that without this help from the group leader they would not have been free to talk about other intragroup annoyances or about various feelings of inadequacy or superiority.

The experience of the observer who is in a separate room behind a one-way screen differs markedly according to whether he is alone or whether there are several observers. If the observer is by himself, he feels isolated, owing to the physical barrier which separates him from the group. Surprisingly, none of the observers polled for this report stated that their principal reaction at the physical separation from the group was of feeling more "at ease" or "secure." When several observers are behind the screen, there is a marked interaction among them. They make remarks about what is happening in the group, chat in quiet tones, and occasionally even laugh. The tendency to discharge tension may reach such proportions that conscious restraint becomes necessary. More interactions seems to occur when there are several observers of the same discipline and of relatively the same experience. The more diverse the experience and the professional specialty or subspecialty, the less the interaction. The groups which were observed jointly by members of the psychiatric staff and the research team from Harvard were relatively quiet. Later, when the groups were observed exclusively by psychiatrists, it became apparent that the latter were showing less restraint as observers. When this was recognized, the excessive reactions ceased.

A striking and uncanny example of the problems implicit in the role of observer occurs when a group member gazes into the one-way screen and the observer has the illusion that the group member is looking him directly in the eye. When this happens, the observer momentarily has the illusion that there is no screen. He has a feeling of embarrassment which may be at least partly explained by a certain feeling of guilt involved in the role he fills. The observation of an intense human relationship without participation seems to provoke such a reaction in many people. A similar, but less striking, instance occurs when the observer meets a group member whom he has observed for some time, on the street or elsewhere. The observer then has a tendency to nod before he recalls the situation, and when the group member stares back blankly, the observer feels embarrassed and guilty.

How does this feeling of guilt affect the observer's training? Tension may make it difficult to learn and may result in untoward reactions to the group leader, expressed in excessive criticism of the leader, or in finding the experience of observing arduous or even boring. Even more frequent is a kind of excitement in observing the situation that makes the observer experience it as a kind of soap opera, with more interest in "what will happen next" than in a professional evaluation of the situation which would lead to increased psychiatric knowledge and experience. There is no question that the above-mentioned tension must occur to some extent, and has certain positive implications, in that it is a measure of the observer's interest. However, it seems that if this reaction becomes too strong and the observer begins to feel that he is making use of the group members for his own pleasure, he loses his capacity for therapeutic objectivity and, more important, loses some of his feeling of dedication. He sees himself as a spectator being gratified by the group rather than as a professional person learning from it. The resulting guilt can lead to a degree of disorganization or a loss of interest in observing.

### Summary

The groups discussed in this paper were primarily groups of educators or nurses who were gathered together in seminars with an analytically oriented psychiatrist as group leader to investigate how their reactions might be affecting their relationships with their pupils, colleagues, and superiors. The observer sat silently in the room or watched from behind a one-way screen.

The role of observer is discussed and illustrated clinically. He functions as an aide to the group leader in that he reports incidents he has observed that it was impossible for the group leader to see, and reports to him impressions that his relative objectivity permitted him to make. The observer, who is a trainee in individual and group psychotherapy, is in a position to see more experienced psychiatrists in action. Both trainee and supervisor have the same material available for discussion. In a more usual case presentation by an inexperienced therapist, his supervisor may be hampered by the generality of the material, and the opportunity to discuss the patient as a person different from other people may be lost.

The problem of observing a human transaction in which one participates minimally has many implications for all sorts of professional situations. It is one of the points of this paper that there is no professional situation in which one has less opportunity to respond to the human beings with whom one interacts than in the situation of an observer. Even the second-year medical student who feels, as a general rule, terribly anxious about having to do an unnecessary physical on a patient, is permitted by the nature of his function at least to say "thanks" to the patient. The observer has no such opportunity. This may result, in a mild way, in a form of sensory deprivation; the observer participates in a one-way transaction in which he, in a sense, is deprived of the usual give and take of human relationships. The resulting tension makes observing an arduous task. It is necessary for the observer to be aware of his reactions to this role in order for him to be able to fulfill his functions as a student, as a researcher, or as an aide to the group leader. This phenomenon is thought to have many implications for all forms of research in psychiatry that use observers.

# References

ABRAHAM, K. (1921), Contributions to the Theory of the Anal Character. In *Selected Papers on Psychoanalysis, 1*:370-392. New York: Basic Books, 1954.

—— (1924), The Influence of Oral Erotism on Character-Formation. In *Selected Papers on Psychoanalysis, 1*:393-406. New York: Basic Books, 1954.

—— (1925), Character-Formation on the Genital Level of Libido Development. In *Selected Papers on Psychoanalysis, 1*:407-417. New York: Basic Books, 1954.

—— (1925a), Die Geschichte eines Hochstaplers. *Imago, 11*:355-370.

—— (1949), The History of an Imposter in the Light of Psychoanalytic Knowledge. In *The Psychoanalytic Reader Vol. I,* ed. Robert Fliess. New York: International Universities Press.

ACKERMAN, N. W. (1945), Some Theoretical Aspects of Group Psychotherapy. In *Group Psychotherapy.* New York: Beacon House, pp. 123-124.

ADAMS, W. R. (1958), The Psychiatrist in an Ambulatory Clerkship for Comprehensive Medical Care in a New Curriculum. *J. Med. Educ., 33*:211-220.

ALDRICH, C. K. (1953), Psychiatric Teaching on Inpatient Medical Service. *J. Med. Educ., 28*:36-39.

ALEXANDER, F. (1939), Psychological Aspects of Medicine. *Psychosom. Med., 1*:7-18.

—— (1953), Current Views on Psychotherapy. *Psychiatry, 16*:113-123.

—— & FRENCH, T. M. (1946), *Psychoanalytic Therapy: Principles and Application.* New York: Ronald Press.

AMERICAN PSYCHIATRIC ASSOCIATION. Psychiatry and Medical Education. *Report of 1951 Conference on Psychiatric Education.* Washington, D.C.: American Psychiatric Association, 1952.

AMERICAN PSYCHOANALYTIC ASSOCIATION (1951), Group Psychotherapeutic Techniques with "Normal" Leaders. *Bull. Am. Psychoanal. Assn., 7*:339-344.

APPEL, K. E. (1953), Putting the Family Back in Medical Education. *New England J. Med., 249*:397-399.

BAERWOLF, H. (1961), One Year's Experience in Psychosomatic Group Training of General Practitioners. In *Advances in Psychosomatic Medicine*, eds. Arthur Jores and Hellmuth Freyburger. New York: Robert Brunner.

BALINT, M. (1954), Method and Techniques in Teaching of Medical Psychology. II. Training General Practitioners in Psychotherapy. *Brit. J. Med. Psychol., 27:37-41.*

—— (1957), *The Doctor, His Patient and the Illness.* New York: International Universities Press.

—— (1961), Training for Psychosomatic Medicine. In *Advances in Psychosomatic Medicine,* eds. Arthur Jores and Hellmuth Freyburger. New York: Robert Brunner.

BERLINER, B. (1941), Short Psychoanalytic Psychotherapy. *Bull. Menninger Clin., 5:204-213.*

BERMAN, L. (1948), Depersonalization and the Body Ego, with Special Reference to the Genital Representation. *Psychoanal. Quart., 17:* 433-452.

—— (1949), Countertransferences and Attitudes of the Analyst in the Therapeutic Process. *Psychiatry, 12:159-166.*

—— (1950), Psychoanalysis and Group Psychotherapy. *This Volume,* pp. 264-270.

—— (1950a), Personal Communication.

—— (1953), Group Psychotherapeutic Technique for Training in Clinical Psychology. *Am. J. Orthopsychiat., 23:322-327.*

—— (1953a), Mental Hygiene for Educators: Report on an Experiment Using a Combined Seminar and Group Psychotherapy Approach. *This Volume,* pp. 253-263.

—— (1954), Mental Health of the Educator. *Ment Hyg., 38:422-429.*

—— (1956), The Educator and Mental Health. *Am. J. Orthopsychiat., 26:204-207.*

BERRY, G. P. (1953), Medical Education in Transition. *J. Med. Educ., 28:17-42.*

BIBRING, E. (1953), Unpublished manuscript.

—— (1954), Psychoanalysis and the Dynamic Psychotherapies. *This Volume,* pp. 51-71.

BIBRING, G. L. (1947), Psychiatry and Social Work. *J. Soc. Casework, 28:* 203-211.

—— (1949), Psychiatric Principles in Casework. *J. Soc. Casework, 30:* 230-235.

—— (1951), Preventive Psychiatry in a General Hospital. *Bull. World Federation Ment. Health, 3:224-232.*

—— (1956), Psychiatry and Medical Practice in a General Hospital. *This Volume,* pp. 75-87.

—— (1959), Some Considerations of the Psychological Processes in Pregnancy. In *The Psychoanalytic Study of the Child, 14*:113-121. New York: International Universities Press.

—— (1960), Work with Physicians. In *Recent Developments in Psychoanalytic Child Therapy*, ed. J. Weinreb. New York: International Universities Press, pp. 39-52.

——, DWYER, T. F., HUNTINGTON, D. S. & VALENSTEIN, A. F. (1961), A Study of the Psychological Processes in Pregnancy and of the Earliest Mother-Child Relationship. In *The Psychoanalytic Study of the Child, 16*:9-45. New York: International Universities Press.

BINGER, C. (1954), Aspects of Psychotherapy in Everyday Life. *J. Med. Assn. Alabama, 23*:219-226.

BRACELAND, F. J. (1950), Symposium on Psychiatry and General Practitioner: Psychosomatic Medicine and General Practitioner. *Med. Clinics North America, 34*:939-955.

BRUCH, H. (1952), Psychiatric Aspects of Changes in Infant and Child Care. *Pediatrics, 10*:575-580.

BUCKLEY, F. M. (1954), An Investigation of Outcomes in the Use of an Analytic Group Discussion Method in Working with Teachers. Cambridge, Mass.: Harvard University (Ph.D. Dissertation).

BURCHARD, E. M. L. et al. (1948), Criteria for the Evaluation of Group Therapy. *Psychosom. Med., 10*:257-274.

CHASSEL, J. (1953), Report of Panel on Psychotherapy. *J. Am. Psychoanal. Assn., 1*:550-561.

COHEN, SIR H. (1953), The Balanced Curriculum. *New England J. Med., 249*:871-875.

COMBS, A. W. (1948), Some Dynamic Aspects of Non-Directive Therapy. *Annals N. Y. Acad. Sci., 49*:878-888.

DANIELS, G. E. (1940), Treatment of Ulcerative Colitis Associated with Hysterical Depression. *Psychosom. Med., 2*:276-285.

DEUTSCH, F. (1936), Euthanasia: A Clinical Study. *Psychoanal. Quart., 5*:347-368.

—— (1939), Associative Anamnesis. *Psychoanal. Quart., 8*:354-381.

—— (1940), Social Service and Psychosomatic Medicine. Mimeographed by the American Association of Medical Social Workers.

—— (1953), The Application of Psychoanalysis to Psychosomatic Aspects. In *Psychoanalysis and Social Work*, ed. Marcel Heiman. New York: International Universities Press.

—— (1955), Minutes of the Workshop on the Theory of the Conversion Process. Boston Psychoanalytic Society and Institute.

—— (1959), Symbolization as a Formative Stage of the Conversion Process. In *On the Mysterious Leap from the Mind to the Body*, ed. Felix Deutsch. New York: International Universities Press.

—— KAUFMAN, M. R. & BLUMGART, H. L. (1940), Present Methods of Teaching. *Psychosom, Med., 2*:213-222.

DWYER, T. F. & ZINBERG, N. E. (1957), Psychiatry for Medical School Instructors. *This Volume,* pp. 88-97.

EBAUGH, F. G. (1952), Applied Psychiatry in General Practice. *Canad. Med. Assn. J., 67*:613-619.

EISSLER, K. R. (1950), Ego-Psychological Implications of the Psychoanalytic Treatment of Delinquents. In *The Psychoanalytic Study of the Child, 5*:97-121. New York: International Universities Press.

—— (1955), *The Psychiatrist and the Dying Patient.* New York: International Universities Press.

ERIKSON, E. H. (1945), Ego Development and Historical Change. In *The Psychoanalytic Study of the Child, 2*:391-396. New York: International Universities Press.

—— (1950), *Childhood and Society.* New York: W. W. Norton.

FENICHEL, O. (1937), The Scoptophilic Instinct and Identification. *Int. J. Psychoanal., 18*:6-34.

—— (1941), *Problems of Psychoanalytic . Technique.* Albany, N. Y.: Psychoanalytic Quarterly.

—— (1945), *The Psychoanalytic Theory of Neurosis.* New York: W. W. Norton.

FERENCZI, S. (1930), The Principle of Relaxation and Neocatharsis. *Int. J. Psychoanal., 11*:428-443.

—— (1931), Child-Analysis in the Analysis of Adults. *Int. J. Psychoanal., 12*:468-482.

FISHER, C. (1953), Studies on the Nature of Suggestion. Parts I and II. *J. Am. Psychoanal. Assn., 1*:222-255; *1*:406-437.

Fox, H. M. (1951), Teaching Integrated Medicine: Report of a Five-Year Experiment at Peter Bent Brigham Hospital. *J. Med. Educ., 26*:421-429.

—— (1953), Psychiatric Research in a General Hospital. *New England J. Med., 249*:351-354.

FREUD, A. (1946), *The Ego and the Mechanisms of Defense.* New York: International Universities Press.

—— (1952), The Role of Bodily Illness in the Mental Life of Children. In *The Psychoanalytic Study of the Child, 7*:65-91. New York: International Universities Press.

FREUD, S. (1893), *Studies on Hysteria.* New York: Nervous and Mental Disease Monographs, 1936.

—— (1905), Three Essays on the Theory of Sexuality. *Standard Edition, 7*:123-243. London: Hogarth Press, 1953.

—— (1908), Character and Anal Erotism. *Standard Edition, 9*:167-175. London: Hogarth Press, 1959.

—— (1915), Further Recommendations in the Technique of Psycho-Analysis: Observations on Transference-Love. *Collected Papers,* 2:377-391. London: Hogarth Press, 1924.

—— (1922), *Group Psychology and the Analysis of the Ego.* London: International Psychoanalytic Press, pp. 2, 78.

—— (1923), *The Ego and the Id.* London: Hogarth Press, 1927.

—— (1937), Analysis Terminable and Interminable. *Int. J. Psychoanal., 18:*373-405.

—— (1938), Construction in Analysis. *Collected Papers, 5:*358-371. London: Hogarth Press, 1950.

—— (1938a), Splitting of the Ego in the Defensive Process. *Collected Papers, 5:*372-376. London: Hogarth Press, 1950.

FROMM-REICHMANN, F. (1950), *Principles of Intensive Psychotherapy.* Chicago: University of Chicago Press.

GILL, M. (1954), Psychoanalysis and Exploratory Psychotherapy. *J. Am. Psychoanal. Assn., 2:*771-797.

GITELSON, M. (1951), Psychoanalysis and Dynamic Psychiatry. *Arch. Neurol. & Psychiat., 66:*280-288.

GLOVER, E. (1924), 'Active Therapy' and Psychoanalysis. *Int. J. Psychoanal., 5:*269-311.

—— et al. (1937), Symposium on the Theory of the Therapeutic Results of Psychoanalysis. *Int. J. Psychoanal., 18:*125-189.

GREENSHILL, M. H. & KILGORE, S. R. (1950), Principles of Methodology in Teaching Psychiatric Approach to Medical Officers. *Psychosom. Med., 12:*38-48.

GRINKER, R. R. (1947), Teaching Psychiatry to Physicians. *Am. J. Orthopsychiat., 17:*617-621.

GROEN, J. (1956), Post-Graduate Teaching and Its Integration in Medical Practice. *J. Med. Educ., 31:*181-186.

GROTJAHN, M. (1950), The Process of Maturation in Group Psychotherapy and the Group Therapist. *Psychiatry, 13:*63-67.

Group for the Advancement of Psychiatry, Committee on Preventive Psychiatry. Promotion of Mental Health in the Primary and Secondary Schools: An Evaluation of Four Projects. GAP Report No. 18 January, 1951.

HACKETT, T. P. & WEISMAN, A. D. (1960), Psychiatric Management of Operative Syndromes. *Psychosom. Med., 22:*356-372.

HART, B. (1929), *Psychopathology.* Cambridge: Cambridge University Press, Second Edition.

HARTMANN, H. (1951), Technical Implications of Ego Psychology. *Psychoanal. Quart., 20:*31-43.

—— & KRIS, E. (1946), The Genetic Approach in Psychoanalysis. In *The Yearbook of Psychoanalysis, 2:*1-22. New York: International Universities Press.

JOKL, R. H. (1927), The Mobilizing of the Sense of Guilt: A Contribution to the Problem of Active Therapy. *Int. J. Psychoanal., 1*:479-485.

JONES, E. (1913), The Good Complex. In *Essays in Applied Psychoanalysis.* London: International Psychoanalytic Press, 1923, pp. 204-226.

KAHANA, R. J. (1959), Teaching Medical Psychology through Psychiatric Consultation. *This Volume,* pp. 98-107.

KAUFMAN, M. R. (1953), Role of Psychiatrist in General Hospital. *Psychiat. Quart., 27*:34.

KLEIN, M. (1929), Infantile Anxiety Situations Reflected in a Work of Art and in the Creative Impulse. *Int. J. Psychoanal., 10*:436-443.

KLIGERMAN, S. (1952), Program of Teaching Psychodynamic Orientation to Resident Physicians in Medicine. *Psychosom. Med., 14:* 277-283.

KNAPP, P. H. (1960), Acute Bronchial Asthma. II. Psychoanalytic Observations in Fantasy. Emotional Arousal and Partial Discharge. *Psychosom. Med., 22*:88-105.

KNIGHT, R. P. (1952), An Evaluation of Psychotherapeutic Techniques. *Bull. Menninger Clin., 16*:113-124.

KRIS, E. (1950), On Preconscious Mental Processes. *Psychoanal. Quart., 19*:540-560.

—— (1951), Ego Psychology and Interpretation in Psychoanalytic Therapy. *Psychoanal. Quart., 20*:15-29.

—— (1952), *Psychoanalytic Explorations in Art.* New York: International Universities Press.

LEE, S. S. (1958), A Fresh Look at Outpatient Department Problems. *Hospitals, 32*:5.

LEVIN, S. Nursing Faculty Groups. In *An Experiment in Education: A Psychoanalytic Group Approach and Its Use in Nursing* (to be published).

LEVINE, M. (1942), Psychiatry for Internists. *Am. J. Orthopsychiat., 17:* 598-601.

—— (1949), *Psychotherapy in Medical Practice.* New York: Macmillan.

LIDZ, T. et al. (1956), An Outline for a Curriculum for Teaching Psychiatry in Medical Schools. (Prepared by the Committee on Medical Education of the American Psychiatric Association.) *J. Med. Educ., 31*:115-128.

LINDEMANN, E. (1945), Psychiatric Aspects of the Conservative Treatment of Ulcerative Colitis. *Arch. Neurol. & Psychiat., 53*:322.

—— (1946), Psychotherapeutic Opportunities for General Practitioner. *Bull. New England Med. Center, 8*:248-254.

LIPSITT, D. R. (1961), Institutional Dependency: A Rehabilitation Problem. In *Mental Patients in Transition,* eds. M. Greenblatt, D. Levinson, G. Klerman. Springfield, Ill.: C. C Thomas.

—— (1962), Dependency, Depression and Hospitalization: Toward an Understanding of a "Conspiracy." *Psychiat. Quart., 36:*537-554.

LOEWENSTEIN, R. M. (1951), The Problem of Interpretation. *Psychoanal. Quart., 20:*1-14.

—— (1957), A Contribution to the Psychoanalytic Theory of Masochism. *J. Am. Psychoanal. Assn., 5:*197-234.

LOW, B. (1935), The Psychological Compensations of the Analyst. *Int. J. Psychoanal., 16:*1-8.

LUDWIG, A. O. (1954), Rheumatoid Arthritis. In *Recent Developments in Psychosomatic Medicine,* eds. E. D. Wittkower and R. A. Cleghorn. New York: J. B. Lippincott.

MACALPINE, I. (1950), The Development of the Transference. *Psychoanal. Quart., 19:*501-539.

MARGOLIN, R. J. (1953), New Perspectives for Teachers: An Evaluation of Mental Health Institute. *Ment. Hyg., 37:*394-442.

MARGOLIN, S. (1953), Report of Panel on Psychotherapy. *J. Am. Psychoanal. Assn., 1:*550-561.

MENNINGER, W. C. (1953), Psychiatry and Practice of Medicine. *Bull. Menninger Clin., 17:*170-179.

MORENO, J. L. (1940), Mental Catharsis and Psychodrama. *Sociometry, 1:*128.

MURRAY, J. M. (1950), Personal Communication.

MUSHATT, C. (1954), Psychological Aspects of Non-Specific Ulcerative Colitis. In *Recent Developments in Psychosomatic Medicine,* eds. E. D. Wittkower and R. A. Cleghorn. New York: J. B. Lippincott.

—— (1959), Loss of Sensory Perception Determining Choice of Symptoms. In *On the Mysterious Leap from the Mind to the Body,* ed. Felix Deutsch. New York: International Universities Press.

NUNBERG, H. (1928), Problems of Therapy. In *Practice and Theory of Psychoanalysis.* New York: Nervous and Mental Disease Monographs, 1948.

ORMSBY, R. (1948), Interpretation in Casework Therapy. *J. Soc. Casework* (April).

PEDERSON-KRAG, G. (1946), Unconscious Factors in Group Therapy. *Psychoanal. Quart., 15:*180-189.

PINCOFFS, M. C. (1954), Editorial: Certain Trends in Undergraduate Medical Education. *Annals Internal Med., 41:*1250-1253.

PRANGE, A. J., JR., & ABSE, D. W. (1957), Psychic Events Accompanying an Attack of Poliomyelitis. *Brit. J. Med. Psychol., 30:*75-87.

RANK, O. (1948), *Will Therapy.* New York: A. A. Knopf.

RAPAPORT, D. (1951), The Autonomy of the Ego. *Bull. Menninger Clin., 15:*113-123.

REDL, F. (1942), Group Emotion and Leadership. *Psychiatry, 5:*573-596.

—— (1944), Diagnostic Group Work. *Am. J. Orthopsychiat., 14:*53-67.

——— (1944a), *Problems of Clinical Work with Children*. Proceedings of the Second Brief Psychotherapy Council, Institute for Psychoanalysis, Chicago, Ill.

REICH, W. (1933), *Charakteranalyse*. Vienna: Published by the author.

REIDER, N. (1955), Type of Transference to Institutions. In *The Yearbook of Psychoanalysis, 10:*170-176. New York: International Universities Press.

REIK, T. (1941), *Masochism in Modern Man*. New York: Farrar & Rinehart.

RICHMOND, M. E. (1917), *Social Diagnosis*. New York: Russell Sage Foundation.

ROBINSON, V. P. (1930), *A Changing Psychology in Social Case Work*. Chapel Hill: University of North Carolina Press.

ROGERS, C. R. (1942), *Counseling and Psychotherapy*. Boston: Houghton Mifflin.

——— (1951), *Client Centered Therapy*. Boston: Houghton Mifflin.

ROMANO, J. (1950), Basic Orientation and Psychiatric Education of Medical Students. *J. A. M. A., 143:*409-412.

——— & ENGEL, G. L. (1947), Teaching Experiences in General Hospitals. *Am J. Orthopsychiat., 17:*602-604.

ROSENBERG, P. P. & FULLER, M. L. (1955), Human Relations Seminar: A Group Work Experiment in Nursing Education. *Ment. Hyg., 39:* 406-432.

——— ——— (1957), Human Relations Seminar for Nursing Students. *Nursing Outlook, 5:*724-726.

SASLOW, G. (1948), Experiment with Comprehensive Medicine. *Psychosom. Med., 10:*165-175.

SCHMIDEBERG, M. (1935), Reassurance as a Means of Analytic Technique. *Int. J. Psychoanal., 16:*307-324.

——— (1939), The Role of Suggestion in Analytic Therapy. *Psychoanal. Rev., 26:*219-229.

SCHROEDER, T. (1925), The Psycho-Analytic Method of Observation. *Int. J. Psychoanal., 6:*155-170.

SILVERMAN, S. (1956), Teaching Psychoanalytic Psychiatry to Medical Residents. *J. Med. Educ., 31:*436-443.

SLAVSON, S. R. (1947), Differential Dynamics of Activity and Interview Group Therapy. *Am. J. Orthopsychiat., 18:*295-299.

SOLON, J. A., SHEPS, C. G. & LEE, S. S. (1958), Staff Perceptions of Patients' Use of a Hospital Out-Patient Department. *J. Med. Educ., 33:*10.

——— ——— ——— (1960), Patterns of Medical Care: A Hospital's Outpatients. *Am. J. Public Health, 50:*8.

SPERLING, M. (1946), Psychoanalytic Study of Ulcerative Colitis in Children. *Psychoanal. Quart., 15:*302-329.

STEARNS, S. (1953), Some Emotional Aspects of Treatment of Diabetes Mellitus and Role of Physicians. *New England J. Med., 249:*471-476.

STEIGER, W. A., HANSEN, A. V. & RHOADS, J. M. (1956), Experiences in the Teaching of Comprehensive Medicine. *J. Med. Educ., 31:*241-248.

STEKEL, W. (1950), *Technique of Analytic Psychotherapy.* New York: Liveright.

STERBA, R. (1934), The Fate of the Ego in Analytic Therapy. *Int. J. Psychoanal., 15:*117-126.

STERN, A. (1942), On the Counter-Transference in Psychoanalysis. *Psychoanal. Rev., 11:*166-174.

STONE, L. (1951), Psychoanalysis and Brief Psychotherapy. *Psychoanal. Quart., 20:*215-236.

SUTHERLAND, A. M. & ORBACH, C. E. (1953), Psychological Impact of Cancer and Cancer Surgery: II. Repressive Reactions Associated with Surgery for Cancer. *Cancer, 6:*958-962.

THOMAS, G. W. (1943), Group Psychotherapy: A Review of the Recent Literature. *Psychosom. Med., 5:*166-180.

WAELDER, R. (1937), The Problem of the Genesis of Psychical Conflict in Earliest Infancy. *Int J. Psychoanal., 18:*406-473.

—— (1939), Kriterien der Deutung. *Int. Z. Psychoanal., 24:*136-145.

—— (1945), Present Trends in Psychoanalytic Theory and Practice. In *The Yearbook of Psychoanalysis, 1:*84-89. New York: International Universities Press.

WALTERS, T. A. (1961), Experiences in Psychiatric Education of Non-Psychiatrists. *Psychosomatics, 2:*1-8.

WEISS, E. (1953), Psychotherapy in General Practice. *Postgrad. Med., 14:*238-244.

WERMER, H. (1960), Discussion of Anna Freud's Paper on "The Child Guidance Clinic and the Community." In *Recent Developments in Psychoanalytic Child Therapy,* ed. J. Weinreb. New York: International Universities Press, pp. 61-64.

WHITAKER, C. A. (1949), Teaching Practicing Physicians to do Psychotherapy. *South. Med. J., 42:*899-903.

WHITEHORN, J. C., HANAU, S. B. & ROBINSON, R. L. (eds.), Psychiatry and Medical Education: Report of the 1951 Conference held at Cornell University, Ithaca, New York, June 21-27, 1951. Washington, D.C.: American Psychiatric Association, 1952.

WITMER, H. L. (ed.) (1947), *Teaching Psychotherapeutic Medicine. An Experimental Course for General Physicians.* New York: Commonwealth Fund.

WOLF, S. & WOLFF, H. G. (1951), Notes on Symposium: Internist as Psychiatrist. *Annals Internal Med., 34:*212-216.

ZETZEL, E. R. (1953), Treatment of Peptic Ulcer. *New England J. Med.*, *248*:976-982.

ZINBERG, N. E. (1959), Regression and Physical Illness. Paper presented at Harvard Psychiatric Conference.

—— (1963), Some Aspects of Regression. In *Normal Psychology of the Aging Process,* eds. N. Zinberg and I. Kaufman. New York: International Universities Press.

—— & EDINBURGH, G. (1964), *Psychiatric Consultation in an Interdisciplinary Setting.* Smith College Studies in Social Work, pp. 126-139.

——, SHAPIRO, D. & GRUEN, W. (1962), A Group Approach to Nursing Education. *This Volume,* pp. 283-289.

# Index

# Index

*Index by Henrietta Gilden*